Enhanced Recovery After Surgery and Perioperative Medicine

Editors

MICHAEL SCOTT
ANTON KRIGE
MICHAEL P.W. GROCOTT

ANESTHESIOLOGY CLINICS

www.anesthesiology.theclinics.com

Consulting Editor
LEE A. FLEISHER

March 2022 • Volume 40 • Number 1

ELSEVIER

1600 John F. Kennedy Boulevard • Suite 1800 • Philadelphia, Pennsylvania, 19103-2899

http://www.theclinics.com

ANESTHESIOLOGY CLINICS Volume 40, Number 1
March 2022 ISSN 1932-2275, ISBN-13: 978-0-323-76189-5

Editor: Joanna Collett
Developmental Editor: Arlene Campos

Anesthesiology Clinics (ISSN 1932-2275) is published quarterly by Elsevier Inc., 360 Park Avenue South, New York, NY 10010-1710. Months of issue are March, June, September, and December. Periodicals postage paid at New York, NY and at additional mailing offices. Subscription prices are $100.00 per year (US student/resident), $375.00 per year (US individuals), $464.00 per year (Canadian individuals), $986.00 per year (US institutions), $1016.00 per year (Canadian institutions), $100.00 per year (Canadian student/resident), $225.00 per year (foreign student/resident), $498.00 per year (foreign individuals), and $1016.00 per year (foreign institutions). To receive student and resident rate, orders must be accompanied by name of affiliated institution, date of term, and the *signature* of program/residency coordinator on institutions letterhead. Orders will be billed at individual rate until proof of status is received. Foreign air speed delivery is included in all *Clinics'* subscription prices. All prices are subject to change without notice. POSTMASTER: Send address changes to *Anesthesiology Clinics,* Elsevier Health Sciences Division, Subscription Customer Service, 3251 Riverport Lane, Maryland Heights, MO 63043. Customer Service (orders, claims, online, change of address): Elsevier Health Sciences Division, Subscription Customer Service, 3251 Riverport Lane, Maryland Heights, MO 63043. **Tel:1-800-654-2452 (U.S. and Canada); 314-447-8871 (outside U.S. and Canada). Fax: 314-447-8029. E-mail: journalscustomerservice-usa@elsevier.com (for print support); journalsonlinesupport-usa@elsevier.com (for online support).**

Reprints. For copies of 100 or more of articles in this publication, please contact the Commercial Reprints Department, Elsevier Inc., 360 Park Avenue South, New York, NY 10010-1710. Tel.: 212-633-3874; Fax: 212-633-3820; E-mail: reprints@elsevier.com.

Anesthesiology Clinics, is also published in Spanish by McGraw-Hill Inter-americana Editores S. A., P.O. Box 5-237, 06500 Mexico D. F., Mexico.

Anesthesiology Clinics, is covered in *MEDLINE/PubMed (Index Medicus), Current Contents/Clinical Medicine, Excerpta Medica, ISI/BIOMED*, and *Chemical Abstracts*.

Contributors

CONSULTING EDITOR

LEE A. FLEISHER, MD, FACC, FAHA
Professor of Anesthesiology and Critical Care, Professor of Medicine, Perelman School of Medicine, University of Pennsylvania, Philadelphia, Pennsylvania, USA

EDITORS

MICHAEL SCOTT, MBChB, FRCP, FRCA, FFICM
Professor of Anesthesiology and Critical Care Medicine, Hospital of the University of Pennsylvania, Division Chief, Surgical and Neuroscience Critical Care Medicine, Medical Director, PENN E-LERT Telemedicine ICU Program, Senior Fellow, Leonard Davis Institute of Health Economics, University of Pennsylvania, Philadelphia, Pennsylvania, USA; Affiliate Professor in Anesthesiology, Virginia Commonwealth University School of Medicine, Richmond, Virginia, USA; Honorary Senior Lecturer, Surgical Outcomes Research Centre, University College London, London, United Kingdom

ANTON KRIGE, MBChB, DIMC, FRCA, FFICM
Honorary Professor, School of Medicine, University of Central Lancashire, Consultant in Intensive Care Medicine and Anaesthesia, Royal Blackburn Teaching Hospital, Perioperative Medicine Lead, East Lancashire Hospitals NHS Trust, Anaesthesia Lead, National Institute Health Research, Greater Manchester Clinical Research Network, Blackburn, United Kingdom

MICHAEL P.W. GROCOTT, BSc, MBBS, MD, FRCA, FRCP, FFICM
Director Designate, Southampton NIHR Biomedical Research Centre, University Hospital Southampton NHS Foundation Trust/University of Southampton, Head, Anaesthesia, Perioperative and Critical Care Medicine Research Unit, University Hospital Southampton NHS Foundation Trust, Professor, School of Clinical and Experimental Sciences, University of Southampton, Southampton, United Kingdom

AUTHORS

GEETA AGGARWAL, MBBS, MRCP, FRCA
Consultant Anaesthetist, Royal Surrey Hospital NHS Foundation Trust, Guildford, Surrey, United Kingdom

MIKE CHARLESWORTH, MSci, MBChB, PGCert, FRCA, MSc, FFICM
Consultant Anaesthetist, Department of Cardiothoracic Anaesthesia, Critical Care and ECMO, Wythenshawe Hospital, Manchester University NHS Foundation Trust, Manchester, United Kingdom

W. BRENTON FRENCH, MD
Department of Surgery, Virginia Commonwealth University Health System, Richmond, Virginia, USA

CHRISTOPHER N. JONES, MBBS(LOND), FRCA, MD(Res)
Consultant Anaesthetist, Royal Surrey NHS Foundation Trust, Royal Surrey County Hospital, Guildford, Surrey, United Kingdom

LEIGH J.S. KELLIHER, MBBS, BSc, FRCA, MD
Consultant Anaesthetist, Department of Anaesthetics, Royal Surrey County Hospital NHS Foundation Trust, Guildford, Surrey, United Kingdom

ANDREW KLEIN, MBBS, FRCA, FFICM
Consultant Anaesthetist, Department of Cardiothoracic Anaesthesia and Critical Care, Royal Papworth Hospital NHS Foundation Trust, Trumpington, Cambridge, United Kingdom

ANTON KRIGE, MBChB, DIMC, FRCA, FFICM
Honorary Professor, School of Medicine, University of Central Lancashire, Consultant in Intensive Care Medicine and Anaesthesia, Royal Blackburn Teaching Hospital, Perioperative Medicine Lead, East Lancashire Hospitals NHS Trust, Anaesthesia Lead, National Institute Health Research, Greater Manchester Clinical Research Network, Blackburn, United Kingdom

JAVIER D. LASALA, MD
Associate Professor, Department of Anesthesiology and Perioperative Medicine, The University of Texas MD Anderson Cancer Center, Houston, Texas, USA

MATTHEW D. McEVOY, MD
Professor of Anesthesiology and Surgery, Department of Anesthesiology, Vanderbilt University School of Medicine, Vice-Chair of Perioperative Medicine, Program Director, Perioperative Medicine Fellowship, Medical Director, Hi-RiSE Perioperative Optimization Clinic, Director, Perioperative Consult Service, Co-Chair, VUMC ERAS Executive Steering Committee, Vanderbilt University Medical Center, Nashville, Tennessee, USA

GABRIEL E. MENA, MD
Professor, Department of Thoracic and Cardiovascular Surgery, Department of Anesthesiology and Perioperative Medicine, The University of Texas MD Anderson Cancer Center, Houston, Texas, USA

JAISHEL PATEL, MBChB, BSc, FRCA
Clinical Fellow in Oncoanaesthesia, Royal Surrey NHS Foundation Trust, Royal Surrey County Hospital, Guildford, Surrey, United Kingdom

CAROL J. PEDEN, MBChB, MD, FRCA, FFICM, MPH
Adjunct Professor of Clinical Anesthesiology, Keck School of Medicine of USC, University of Southern California, Los Angeles, California, USA; Adjunct Professor of Clinical Anesthesiology, Perelman School of Medicine, University of Pennsylvania, Philadelphia, Pennsylvania, USA; Executive Director for Clinical Quality the Blue Cross Blue Shield Association, Chicago, Illinois, USA

BRITANY L. RAYMOND, MD
Assistant Professor, Department of Anesthesiology, Vanderbilt University School of Medicine, Director of Undergraduate Medical Education, Vanderbilt University Medical Center, Nashville, Tennessee, USA

CHRISTA L. RILEY, MD
Fellow, Surgical Critical Care, Department of Anesthesiology and Critical Care, Penn Medicine, Philadelphia, Pennsylvania, USA; Anesthesiologist and Intensivist, Department of Anesthesiology, Hunter Holmes McGuire VA Medical Center, Richmond, Virginia, USA

MICHAEL SCOTT, MBChB, FRCP, FRCA, FFICM
Professor of Anesthesiology and Critical Care Medicine, Hospital of the University of Pennsylvania, Division Chief, Surgical and Neuroscience Critical Care Medicine, Medical Director, PENN E-LERT Telemedicine ICU Program, Senior Fellow, Leonard Davis Institute of Health Economics, University of Pennsylvania, Philadelphia, Pennsylvania, USA; Affiliate Professor in Anesthesiology, Virginia Commonwealth University School of Medicine, Richmond, Virginia, USA; Honorary Senior Lecturer, Surgical Outcomes Research Centre, University College London, London, United Kingdom

ELLEN M. SOFFIN, MD, PhD
Department of Anesthesiology, Critical Care and Pain Management, Hospital for Special Surgery, New York, New York, USA

PAULA SPENCER, MSHA, PMP, CPHIMS
Virginia Commonwealth University Health System, Chesterfield, Virginia, USA

THOMAS W. WAINWRIGHT, PT
Professor, Orthopaedic Research Institute, Bournemouth University, Bournemouth, Dorset, United Kingdom

ANDRES ZORRILLA-VACA, MD
Department of Anesthesiology, Brigham and Women's Hospital, Boston, Massachusetts, USA

CHRISTA L. RILEY, MD
Fellow, Surgical Critical Care, Department of Anesthesiology and Critical Care Medicine, Philadelphia, Pennsylvania, USA; Anesthesiologist and Intensivist, Department of Anesthesiology, Hunter Holmes McGuire VA Medical Center, Richmond, Virginia, USA

MICHAEL SCOTT, MBChB, FRCP, FRCA, FFICM
Professor of Anesthesiology and Critical Care Medicine, Hospital of the University of Pennsylvania, Division Chief, Surgical and Neuroscience Critical Care Medicine, Medical Director, PENN E-LERT Telemedicine ICU Program, Senior Fellow, Leonard Davis Institute of Health Economics, University of Pennsylvania, Philadelphia, Pennsylvania, USA; Affiliate Professor in Anesthesiology, Virginia Commonwealth University, School of Medicine, Richmond, Virginia, USA; Honorary Senior Lecturer, Surgical Outcomes Research Centre, University College London, London, United Kingdom

ELLEN M. SOFFIN, MD, PhD
Department of Anesthesiology, Critical Care and Pain Management, Hospital for Special Surgery, New York, New York, USA

PAULA SPENCER, MSHA, PMP, CPHIMS
Virginia Commonwealth University Health System, Chesterfield, Virginia, USA

THOMAS W. WAINWRIGHT, PT
Professor, Orthopaedic Research Institute, Bournemouth University, Bournemouth, Dorset, United Kingdom

ANDRES ZORRILLA-VACA, MD
Department of Anesthesiology, Brigham and Women's Hospital, Boston, Massachusetts, USA

Contents

> Enhanced recovery after surgery (ERAS) is a series of evidence-based perioperative care protocols designed to improve outcomes following surgery. The concept was founded on the principle of producing a predictable quality outcome by reducing morbidity and shortening hospital stay. The key objective of ERAS is to incorporate optimized multimodal perioperative care in a variety of different surgical specialties to reduce injury and stress during the perioperative period and promote a return to normal function rapidly.

> The idea that perioperative outcomes may be improved through the implementation of measures that modify the surgical stress response has been around for several decades. Many techniques have been trialled with varying success. In addition, how the response to modification is measured, what constitutes a positive result and how this translates into clinical practice is the subject of debate. Modification of the stress response is the principal tenet behind the enhanced recovery after surgery (ERAS) movement which has seen the development of guidelines for perioperative care across a variety of surgical specialties bringing with them significant improvements in outcomes.

> Opioid-based analgesia in the perioperative period can provide excellent pain control, but this approach exposes the patient to avoidable side effects and possible harm. Optimal analgesia, an approach that targets the fastest functional recovery with adequate pain control while minimizing side effects, can be achieved with opioid minimization. Many different options for nonopioid multimodal analgesia exist and have been shown to be efficacious, with certain modalities being more beneficial for specific

This article provides a broad perspective on the salient perioperative issues encountered when caring for patients undergoing pancreatic surgery in the setting of pancreatic cancer. It describes the epidemiology of pancreatic cancer, the indications for and evolution of pancreatic resection surgery, the challenges faced perioperatively including patient selection, optimization, anesthetic considerations, postoperative analgesia, fluid management, and nutrition and discusses some of the common complications and their management. It finishes by outlining the future directions for research and development required to continue improving outcomes for these patients.

The Enhanced Recovery After Surgery Society published guidelines for bariatric surgery reviewing the evidence and providing specific care recommendations. These guidelines emphasize preoperative nutrition, multimodal analgesia, postoperative nausea and vomiting prophylaxis, anesthetic technique, nutrition, and mobilization. Several studies have since evaluated these pathways, showing them to be safe and effective at decreasing hospital length of stay and postoperative nausea and vomiting. This article emphasizes anesthetic management in the perioperative period and outlines future directions, including the application of Enhanced Recovery After Surgery principles in patients with extreme obesity, diabetes, and metabolic disease and standardization of the pathways to decrease heterogeneity.

The aims of "Fast track" cardiac anesthesia including shortening time to tracheal extubation and to hospital discharge in selected patients. The evidence is weak and recommendations are mostly based on observational, nonrandomized data and expert opinion. The majority of outcomes studied include: time to tracheal extubation, hospital/ICU length of stay, procedure-related financial costs, and the type/amount of opioids used in the peri-operative period. There should be a shift in focus to generating higher quality evidence supporting the use of enhanced recovery protocols in cardiac surgical patients and finding ways to tailor enhanced recovery principles to all cardiac surgical patients. Research should focus on the quality of care for individual patients and the delivery of health care to the public.

Gynecologic surgery encompasses over a quarter of inpatient surgical procedures for US women, and current projections estimate an increase of the US female population by nearly 50% in 2050. Over the last decade, US hospitals have embraced enhanced recovery pathways in many specialties. They have increasingly been used in multiple institutions worldwide, becoming the standard of care for patient optimization. According to the last updated enhanced recovery after surgery (ERAS) guideline published in 2019, there are several new considerations behind each practice in ERAS protocols. This article discusses the most updated evidence regarding ERAS programs for gynecologic surgery.

This article focuses on the anesthetic considerations for major cancer urology surgeries such as cystectomies, nephrectomies, and radical prostatectomies. It aims to explore the anesthetic considerations for both open and minimally invasive techniques.

Emergency laparotomy is a high-risk surgical procedure with mortality and morbidity up to 10 times higher than for a similar procedure performed electively. An enhanced recovery approach has been shown to improve outcomes. A focus on rapid correction of underlying deranged acute physiology and proactive management of conditions associated with aging such as frailty and delirium are key. Patients are at high risk of complications and prevention and avoidance of failure to rescue are essential to improve outcomes. Other enhanced recovery components such as opioid-sparing analgesia and early postoperative mobilization are beneficial.

ANESTHESIOLOGY CLINICS

SERIES OF RELATED INTEREST

Critical Care Clinics

THE CLINICS ARE AVAILABLE ONLINE!
Access your subscription at:
www.theclinics.com

SERIES OF RELATED INTEREST

Critical Care Clinics

Foreword

Enhanced Recovery After Surgery and Perioperative Care: A Continually Evolving Approach to Surgical Care

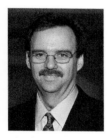

Lee A. Fleisher, MD, FACC, FAHA
Consulting Editor

Since Henrik Kehlet first described Enhanced Recovery After Surgery (ERAS), the approach to modern surgical and anesthetic techniques has continued to evolve. While the approach started with abdominal procedures, it has now been applied to most surgical procedures, including emergency procedures. In this issue of *Anesthesiology Clinics*, an outstanding group of authors has reviewed the most recent evidence and approaches to many common procedures.

In order to commission an issue on ERAS, it was easy to find 3 leaders in the field who can teach us the latest information: Michael Scott, Anton Krige, and Michael Grocott. Michael James Scott, MBChB, FRCP, FRCA, FFICM is Professor and Division Chief in Critical Care Medicine in the Department of Anesthesiology at the Perelman School of Medicine at the University of Pennsylvania. He was National Clinical Advisor in the UK National Health System (NHS). He is currently President of ERAS USA and has coauthored key guidelines. Anton Krige, MBChB, DIMC, FRCA, FFICM is a specialist in Anaesthesia and Intensive Care Medicine and has been practicing as a NHS hospital consultant since 2005 at the East Lancashire Hospitals NHS Trust. He is a member of the Institute for Functional Medicine. Michael Grocott, BSc, MBBS, MD, FRCA, FRCP, FFICM is the Professor of Anaesthesia and Critical Care Medicine at the University of Southampton and a UK National Institute of Health Research (NIHR) Senior Investigator. He is UK NIHR National Specialty Lead for anesthesia, perioperative medicine, and pain and Chair of the Board of the UK National Institute of Academic Anaesthesia. Mike is an elected vice-president of the Royal

Anesthesiology Clin 40 (2022) xiii–xiv
https://doi.org/10.1016/j.anclin.2021.11.014
1932-2275/22/© 2021 Published by Elsevier Inc.

anesthesiology.theclinics.com

College of Anaesthetists and vice-chair of the UK Centre for Perioperative Care. Together, they have edited an important issue that is relevant to all clinicians.

Lee A. Fleisher, MD, FACC, FAHA
Perelman School of Medicine
University of Pennsylvania
3400 Spruce Street, Dulles 680
Philadelphia, PA 19104, USA

E-mail address:
Lee.Fleisher@pennmedicine.upenn.edu

Preface

Enhanced Recovery After Surgery and Perioperative Medicine Driving Value-Based Surgical Care

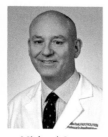

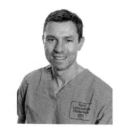

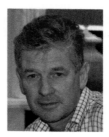

Michael Scott, MBChB, FRCP, FRCA, FFICM

Anton Krige, MBChB, DIMC, FRCA, FFICM

Michael P.W. Grocott, BSc, MBBS, MD, FRCA, FRCP, FFICM

Editors

Surgical volumes continue to increase around the world, particularly in major surgery. Treatments for both benign conditions and cancer have improved, and patient expectation has increased, driving surgical volumes.

While surgical technique is key for good outcomes, patient factors and perioperative pathways play an important role. Over the last 20 years, the development of enhanced recovery after surgery (ERAS) and the increasing recognition that what we do to patients around surgery affects them just as much as the surgery itself have led to the development of a new specialty, Perioperative Medicine (POM). Good perioperative care pathways can't make poor surgery good but can make good surgery optimal.

But all is not well. The increase in patients' comorbid conditions and increasing age and frailty mean few patients receiving surgery have optimal health and good reserve. Inconsistent perioperative care remains one of the key drivers of poor surgical outcomes, and its adoption remains a barrier to optimizing surgical outcomes around the world.

In the drive for value-based care in the United States, ERAS and POM have been vehicles to win hearts and minds of providers and politicians. Organization of health systems is key as well as the challenge to finance the stakeholders in a fair and transparent fashion from central governments.

The COVID-19 pandemic has created a backlog of major surgery at a time when services are still restricted and beds that otherwise would be used for surgery are being

Anesthesiology Clin 40 (2022) xv–xvi
https://doi.org/10.1016/j.anclin.2021.11.013
1932-2275/22/© 2021 Published by Elsevier Inc.

used for emergent admissions. This has refocused health systems on how to get the most surgery done out of a system with limited beds, and so, ERAS and POM are even more important than ever.

This issue of *Anesthesiology Clinics* is a follow-up from the 2015 issue "Anesthetic Care for Abdominal Surgery" with the aim of updating key articles and complementing it. All articles are written by experts in their field, who have personal experience in surgical pathway creation, implementation, and optimization. An example of using ERAS as a core structure to remap a US health system's delivery of surgery and perioperative care is included. There is an update of managing the stress response as well as fluids and hemodynamics. Finally, there is a series of individual articles addressing some of the more recent advances in pathways in major surgical specialties, such as cardiac surgery, gynecologic surgery, oncologic surgery, and liver surgery. The recognition of the increasing morbidity and costs in emergency general surgery has led to a massive increase in the literature in the last 5 years, which is summarized succinctly by the authors.

Michael Scott, MBChB, FRCP, FRCA, FFICM
Surgical and Neuroscience Critical Care Medicine
PENN E-LERT Telemedicine ICU Program
University of Pennsylvania
3400 Spruce Street
Philadelphia, PA 19104, USA

Anton Krige, MBChB, DIMC, FRCA, FFICM
Anaesthesia and Critical Care
Royal Blackburn Teaching Hospital
Haslingden Road, Blackburn BB2 3HH, UK

Michael P.W. Grocott, BSc, MBBS, MD, FRCA, FRCP, FFICM
NIHR Southampton Biomedical Research Centre
University Hospital Southampton/University of Southampton
Tremona Road, Southampton, SO16 6YD, UK

E-mail addresses:
michael.scott@pennmedicine.upenn.edu (M. Scott)
Anton.Krige@elht.nhs.uk (A. Krige)
mike.grocott@soton.ac.uk (M.P.W. Grocott)

Implementing Enhanced Recovery After Surgery Across a United States Health System

Paula Spencer, MSHA, PMP, CPHIMS[a],
Michael Scott, MBChB, FRCP, FRCA, FFICM[b],*

KEYWORDS

- Enhanced recovery after surgery • Perioperative medicine • Value-based health care
- Governance structure

KEY POINTS

- Enhanced Recovery After Surgery can serve as a framework for implementing adoption of best practice across the whole perioperative pathway in all surgical specialties.
- Implementation requires reorganizing the health system model with executive support, governance restructuring and a transformation team.
- Change management using LEAN principles can help drive and map change.
- Engagement of all bedside providers is key to build the multidisciplinary team.
- We used a vertical and horizontal implementation model to accelerate implementation across all surgical specialties in the health system.

BRIEF HISTORY AND OVERVIEW

Enhanced recovery after surgery (ERAS) is a series of evidence-based perioperative care protocols designed to improve outcomes following surgery. The concept was founded on the principle of producing a predictable quality outcome by reducing morbidity and shortening hospital stay. The key objective of ERAS is to incorporate optimized multimodal perioperative care in a variety of different surgical specialties to reduce injury and stress during the perioperative period and promote a return to normal function rapidly.

In 2017, the percent of gross domestic product attributed to health care goods and services was at 17.9%. With an average annual spend growth estimated at 5.5%,

[a] Virginia Commonwealth University Health System, 7826 Hampton Green Drive, Chesterfield, VA 23832, USA; [b] Hospital of the University of Pennsylvania, Department of Anesthesiology, PENN E-LERT Telemedicine ICU Program, Leonard Davis Institute of Health Economics, University of Pennsylvania, 3400 Spruce Street, Philadelphia, PA 19104, USA
* Corresponding author.
E-mail address: Michael.Scott@Pennmedicine.Upenn.edu

Anesthesiology Clin 40 (2022) 1–21
https://doi.org/10.1016/j.anclin.2021.11.011
1932-2275/22/© 2022 Elsevier Inc. All rights reserved.

health care spending could reach as much as 19.4% by the year 2027. For Medicare specifically, an average annual spend growth of 7.4% is anticipated during the same period.[1,2]

Factors contributing to these numbers include increases in prices, utilization, and intensity of services. Operating room (OR) utilization continues to increase to meet the increased demand for elective surgical services even as the aging population is leading to an increase in 2 of the major common emergency surgical procedures: fractured neck of femur and emergency laparotomy. In short, the US economy has been unable to bend the cost curve despite continual efforts.[2]

Government and private payers alike are moving from volume to value to control costs and place increased emphasis on better outcomes. Making ERAS principles the standard of care is one way to move providers in that direction. These value-based payment models mean hospitals and surgery centers must find a way to deliver care via reliable processes that afford better predictability of desirable outcomes, thus resulting in better cost control. With ERAS, these savings are realized through less need for intensive care, reduced utilization of pharmaceuticals and parenteral nutrition, reduced complication rates, and shorter hospital length of stay with fewer (or unchanged) readmission rates.[3,4]

Increasingly, there is pressure for hospital systems to reduce their focus on costs and expand efforts to improve quality. Medicare payments are shifting away from volume toward value (quality outcomes). Although other payers may lag behind Medicare in adopting value-based care, there is little reason to expect the fee-for-service model will last for much longer.[5] Leaders at Virginia Commonwealth University Health System (VCU Health) understood that across surgical specialties and regardless of superior surgical technique, perioperative and anesthesia care, patients can experience extended length of hospital stay, postoperative complications, and slow return of organ function. In addition, surgical care had a high degree of variability in processes across all care areas: surgical clinics, ORs, and acute care units, that was responsible for wide cost variance, placing the organization at risk with future payment models.

Strategies that can achieve the aims of excellent clinical care, fewer complications and reduced costs, are core to the value system of health care provider organizations.

Comprehensive implementation of an ERAS program that follows the surgical patient's journey can help achieve these aims in the surgical population (**Fig. 1**).

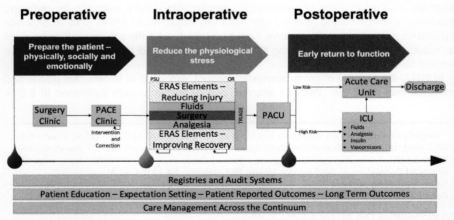

Fig. 1. ERAS implementation follows the surgical patient's journey. ICU, intensive care unit; PACU, post anesthesia care unit; PSU, presurgery unit.

In the fall of 2016, VCU Health had implemented their first ERAS pathway: Colorectal Surgery Enhanced Recovery Protocol. Reductions in length of stay, cost per case, and complications were immediately realized. In February 2017, hospital leadership sponsored the launch of a system-wide ERAS endeavor, introducing the program at surgical grand rounds, and initiating projects with 4 more specialties to design a common pathway centered on the patient.

Although the authors were starting to see improvements in these specialty areas, the authors were also discovering key areas where implementation was suboptimal and where practices were not sustained. The authors conducted a series of lessons learned discussions, a retrospective analysis of their successes and failures, and an assessment of their progress toward the goal of system-wide implementation. Based on their findings, the authors proposed a new approach to transform care more rapidly across all surgical services, engaging key resources in each vertical care phase to design standard work with the intent of delivering ERAS care principles to all elective surgery patients.

The authors' new vertical implementation strategy launched in early 2018 and was running toward completion by summer of 2021.

In this article, the authors describe how they used ERAS pathways across the full range of surgical specialties to establish a new perioperative process for all surgical patients. It aligned with VCU Health goals to improve quality and patient satisfaction and to control costs with consideration of the increasing shift toward alternative payment models, such as bundled payment models.

ORGANIZING AROUND THE HEALTH SYSTEM MODEL
Executive Buy-In

The work to transform surgical patient care successfully requires consistent, active, and engaged sponsorship on the part of executives across the health system. The level of buy-in required for success increases when looking across all surgical specialties, as almost all health system leaders will now have a stake. Before committing to this work, organizations should spend the time to educate and engage senior leaders in physician practice, nursing, administration, and allied health professions across the entire care.

Executives need to understand the following:
- Why ERAS is important
- The risk of not implementing
- How ERAS aligns with the vision and direction of the organization
- How to articulate these concepts through consistent, structured communications across the organization from front-line team members to the board of directors

The program's executive sponsor and clinical leads set goals and expectations for the program. They will need to emphasize the importance of developing efficient, standardized processes that integrate the clinical principles of ERAS to ensure high-quality, consistent patient experiences.

A Governance Structure for Change

ERAS governance at VCU Health started with forming a focused ERAS steering committee consisting of key leaders in surgery, anesthesia, nursing, allied health, quality and safety, and operations. The steering committee, co-chaired by the quality and safety officer and the vice president (VP) of perioperative services, is supported by a combination of ERAS program champion teams and reinforced by the operational structure for clinical governance.

Together, these oversight teams signify the unified, committed sponsorship of ERAS that is necessary for sustained success (**Fig. 2**).

Two key clinical groups lead the foundational work to establish the system-wide program. The ERAS Nursing Committee and ERAS Provider Champions Team members include committed champions representing anesthesia, surgery, nursing, pharmacy, and allied health professionals. They are influential leaders among their peers and well respected in their field. These individuals, who exhibit strong listening and collaboration skills, may be in the early stages of their careers and, therefore, years of experience should not be the primary deciding factor when selecting champions. These influencers are a key ingredient to ERAS implementation success and must be actively supported by the program sponsor, the executive steering committee, and operations.

The Perioperative Executive Committee (PEC) is the main governing body for surgery operations. The chief operations officer, department chairs from anesthesia and each surgery department, and the VP of perioperative services comprise the membership of the committee. This committee is responsible for the following:

- Approving policies
- Supporting operational guidelines
- Holding team members accountable to deliver a standard patient experience that incorporates evidence-based best practices

They have ultimate approval over any major clinical process decisions.

The Quality, Safety, and Regulatory (QSR) subcommittee of PEC is established to monitor and improve patient and staff safety, quality, regulations, and compliance. Membership includes a physician from each surgical department and anesthesia, and representatives from OR nursing, quality coordinator, educator, OR supply chain, information systems, and scheduling. The committee is responsible for the following:

- Identifying key performance indicators
- Reviewing regulatory issues
- Ensuring compliance with requirements

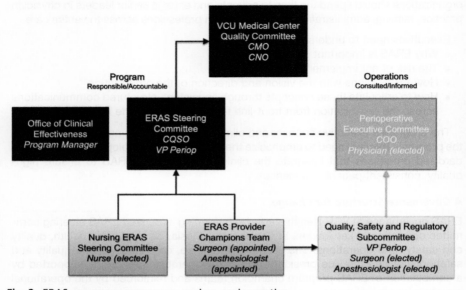

Fig. 2. ERAS program governance. periop, perioperative.

- Promoting standardization of patient experience
- Monitoring data

The Enhanced Recovery After Surgery Transformation Team

Once appropriate oversight and clinical governance are established, more detailed program planning can ensue, starting with building the team that will carry out the work of the improvement projects. Because ERAS is a team sport and requires the engagement of everyone from patients and families to doctors, nurses, allied health professionals, registrars, food services staff, administrators, and others, it is critically important that an interdisciplinary team be enlisted to design the change. Clinical sponsors and champions for each surgical pathway project and vertical care-phase task force include the department chair, surgical champion, nurse director, nurse champion, and unit dyad leaders, where applicable.

The key roles for the team and the associated responsibilities for each are outlined in the program documentation and made available for all team members to reference (**Table 1**). A clear understanding of these roles and responsibilities will provide the right starting point for a successful transformation.

Change Management

Despite general agreement with the clinical principles of ERAS, the authors have encountered pockets of resistance in the form of both active resisters, those who voice opposition, and passive resisters, those who fail to change by not engaging in the design or participating in the implementation of protocols.[6] It is important to understand the emotional and personal factors that contribute to resistance and prepare accordingly. A key strategy to overcome resistance is to ensure a variety of providers and clinicians are provided with the opportunity to participate in designing the change.

A formalized change management process is imperative to sustainable transformation. Direct supervisors are best at addressing how ERAS impacts the individual and the team, the effect on daily work, and how individuals will benefit. Key messages here focus on the "why" of the change and include how a well-implemented ERAS program benefits everyone involved (**Fig. 3**).

Communications should use standard formats and channels at regular intervals to best engage team members in the change. Examples include the following:

- Weekly e-mails with a printable page
- Grand rounds presentations
- Cascading message kits

The target audience, front-line staff, consists of individuals who have devoted a large portion of their lives to the care of other human beings. Hence, the purpose is to improve the care for patients in a measurably better way (patient-centered, clinically relevant outcomes) and to get better at taking care of patients.

ROLE OF THE OPERATING ROOM TEAM

By recognizing that ERAS is a value stream for the patient, from the time the patient decides to have surgery through the return to baseline function and full recovery, the team can work together to provide the best possible care.

- The OR team: surgeons, anesthesia providers, nursing, technicians, and others, must work together to achieve a sustained change of practice for the intraoperative period, stressing the importance of communication and focusing on treating the whole patient.

Table 1
Key roles and responsibilities for an enhanced recovery after surgery transformation team

Role	Description	Responsibilities
Program sponsor	Primary decision maker for the program; serves as champion for program and project management processes	• Ensure alignment with organizational strategy • Secure support of key stakeholders across the organization
Executive steering committee	Support the program and resolve conflict	• Participates in regularly scheduled steering committee meetings • Contributes to project decisions that impact the organization at a greater level • Ensures appropriate interdisciplinary representation within the clinical project team • Reinforces project expectations with team members • Approves expenses to support successful implementation
Clinical champion	Lead their clinician teams, provide for 2-way feedback of information and issues Each specialty area should have a surgery, anesthesia, and nursing champion	• Identifies gaps in performance: redesign as needed, involving all affected stakeholders • Identifies barriers to implementations • Updates best practices and associated processes • Drives best practice identification and operational redesign • Has front-line accountability for design and implementation • Assists in the development of metrics to demonstrate compliance with best practice examples • Charters and populates project teams • Receives requests from colleagues • Provides timely feedback to support project progress • Proactively engages members of other clinical disciplines to facilitate the completion of tasks
Program manager	Coordinates across multiple concurrent projects running over a long period of time	• Manages program level decisions and issues • Coordinates interdependencies across projects • Leads stakeholder analysis • Secures IT resources for the projects via the IT management team

(continued on next page)

Table 1 (continued)		
Role	Description	Responsibilities
Project manager/ process engineer	Dedicated manager for each project within the program to ensure timely, quality delivery	• Manages project schedule, scope, and communications • Facilitates meetings • Records and maintains meeting agendas, minutes, and key decisions • Manages project risks and issues
Clinical informaticist	Clinicians trained in EMR design and focused on electronic workflows are essential to the successful integration of the EMR with redesigned workflows	• Documents current and future process flows and data flow diagrams • Elicits user requirements for EMR solutions • Recommends best available technical solutions to meet customer requirements while adhering to established guidelines for system design in conjunction with EMR analysts • Partners with EMR analysts to develop technical specifications • Conducts EMR demonstrations for clinical users • Obtains requestor acceptance of production build
Project team	Led by specialty champions, composed of clinical and administrative front-line workers representing all roles that participate in the patient care process	• Participates actively in the workflow redesign • Provides front-line input for key decisions • Tests changes and provides iterative feedback • Engages colleagues in the change • Seeks input from subject matter experts in clinical care, regulatory and compliance, operations, and finance

- Good processes are the foundation on which to build a successful ERAS program in which the team knows what to do and when to do it, has access to the resources needed, and knows what to expect of others.
- When members of the OR team engage with the patient throughout all 6 phases of the value stream, the patient care is coordinated and personalized, resulting in the best possible outcomes.
- Nursing, surgeon, and anesthesiologist responsibilities are clearly delineated by role (**Table 2**). Pharmacists and anesthesia technicians ensure the right drugs and equipment are available at the right time to the correct OR team.

Vertical and Horizontal Implementation Model

At VCU Health, the authors started their ERAS transformation with a single pathway for colorectal surgery, a common approach used by most health care provider organizations. The authors then built on that success and, following a horizontal specialty-

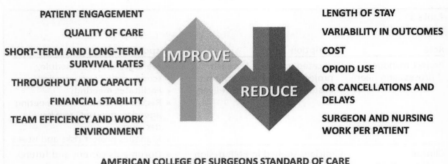

PATIENT ENGAGEMENT

QUALITY OF CARE

SHORT-TERM AND LONG-TERM SURVIVAL RATES

THROUGHPUT AND CAPACITY

FINANCIAL STABILITY

TEAM EFFICIENCY AND WORK ENVIRONMENT

IMPROVE

REDUCE

LENGTH OF STAY

VARIABILITY IN OUTCOMES

COST

OPIOID USE

OR CANCELLATIONS AND DELAYS

SURGEON AND NURSING WORK PER PATIENT

AMERICAN COLLEGE OF SURGEONS STANDARD OF CARE
OPPORTUNITY FOR VCU HEALTH TO BE A U.S. LEADER
MARKET DEMAND FOR VALUE-DRIVEN CARE

Fig. 3. Why is ERAS important to VCU health?

based approach, expanded to 4 more surgery types. As the authors worked on these separate projects, they began to recognize inefficiencies in their approach. Slight variations were being introduced at the specialty level with no clinical significance leading to difficulty designing and delivering the expected care in venues that serve patients across multiple specialties. These variations increased opportunity for error, an effect that was opposite of the goal.

Another unintended consequence was the developing perception of an ERAS patient versus a "non-ERAS" patient. This concerned the authors because they understood the 22 key elements of care for ERAS to be commonly applicable across all patients, therefore, making the ERAS/non-ERAS labeling of patients an opportunity for important care elements that may change a patient's surgical outcome to be missed.

Knowing that the core ERAS elements are common to all surgery types, the authors concluded that ERAS can be most successful when core processes are efficient and reliable. By building a foundation of common ERAS elements at every point of interaction with the patient and developing standard guidelines for analgesia and fluids for each surgery type, they can accelerate the deployment of surgical specialty pathways and build up their reliability for delivering the highest quality care. The authors grouped the elements by care phase and added a series of task forces to address these vertical cross-sections.

These new vertically aligned teams were given responsibility to

- Address design and implementation of ERAS key elements applicable to all surgery types
- Optimize workflows and documentation that support consistent delivery of best-practice care using LEAN principles
- Produce a framework for all specialty pathways
- Optimize and fortify the system foundation on which to build

The revised methodology, the blending of vertical and horizontal approaches, addresses fundamental change by implementing ERAS principles across surgical specialties as standard work, introducing variation by specialty only where clinically indicated (**Fig. 4**).

The authors took the following steps to stand up their new approach:

- Defined the scope to include all adult (18 years and older) patients undergoing inpatient elective procedures that require general anesthesia

Table 2
Operating room team roles in enhanced recovery after surgery care delivery

Role/Care Phase	Surgeon	Anesthesia	Nursing
The decision for surgery until day of surgery	• Define the acuity of surgery • Participate in preoperative optimization of patient's comorbid conditions	• Direct and staff preoperative clinic for assessment and optimization • Coordinate the medical optimization needed for the patient's planned operation	Provide guidance for the patient and family to maximize the patient's ability to be well prepared and medically optimized for surgery Educate patients about pain management and early recovery expectations
Day of surgery	• Minimize the surgical stress response and control the surgical factors affecting the perioperative course • Choose appropriate antibiotics and preoperative medications • Use minimally invasive approaches where applicable • Use separate closure trays in appropriate cases	• Perform nerve blocks to decrease opioid consumption • Ensure administration of key perioperative medications (antibiotics, deep vein thrombosis prophylaxis, preoperative nonopioid analgesics) in addition to the anesthetic plan • For cases with moderate or significant fluid shifts, use a flow-based fluid approach to decrease the possibility of overresuscitation or underresuscitation intraoperatively	• Verify appropriate carbohydrate loading and hydration • Administer appropriate premedications to minimize opioid use for pain management • Actively warm patients to maintain normothermia in the OR • Reinforce education and expectations • Ensure equipment and supplies are appropriate for the procedure being done and applicable infection prevention protocols are followed (surgery team manager)
During acute care period	Encourage mobilization, normalization of bodily functions, and removal of drains		Continue to aid the patient through deescalation of care with a focus on early return to baseline function

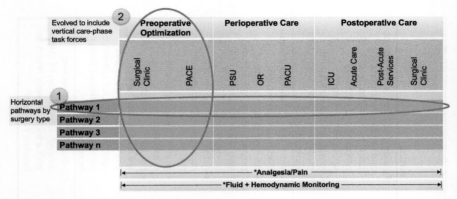

Fig. 4. Vertical and horizontal implemental model.

- Developed a single patient-centered pathway that spans the period from decision for surgery through 90 days after surgery and encompasses all surgical specialties
- Convened vertical care-phase aligned interprofessional teams with internal consulting resources to develop a systematic framework using LEAN thinking
- Integrated project oversight with perioperative operations governance
- Formalized organizational change management strategy
- Focused on a sustainable infrastructure built around staff and other capabilities, through resource optimization, training and development, analytics, and information technology tools

Designing the Change

To achieve system-wide implementation, the authors needed to systematize the delivery of clinical best practice across surgical departments, changing the way they executed the care delivery process. This begins with shifting how they approach change from reactive to fundamental.

Reactive change: Limits an organization to a focus on keeping day-to-day operations running at the current level of performance; constantly putting out fires or applying Band-Aids using tactics such as routine problem solving or reaction to a special circumstance

Fundamental change: Focuses on determining or redefining the essential structure, resulting in a new system of performance

---

Reactive change can be put into place quickly, producing immediate impact; however, disadvantages are as follows:

- Does not result in improvement
- Only restores the previous level of function
- Often involves a tradeoff or compromise in the form of increased cost, such as additional work or new resources
- Rarely considers the full care continuum
- Has the potential for creating unforeseen problems in other upstream or downstream processes[7]

Fundamental change is needed for improvement and should be used when

- The needed improvement extends beyond addressing special circumstances
- An opportunity exists to positively impact more than one aspect of the system
- A lasting impact is desired

System design or redesign is often used to address multifactorial problems that require a systems approach to reach a reliable resolution and involves a change to what work is done or how it is done.[7] The teams are guided by process improvement professionals through a series of activities to support them in successfully designing the new process.

Current state process mapping
To identify and eliminate waste in processes, the first step is to map the current state workflows with the project team, focusing on what actually happens, as opposed to what is supposed to happen. Mapping the current state is necessary to establish a shared understanding of the surgical continuum of care. Team awareness of the baseline process is instrumental in identifying gaps and successfully moving toward the ideal future state. Having the visual of a process map allows the team to better identify challenges and opportunities for improvement.

Voice of the customer
According to the Institute for Healthcare Improvement, "compared to other industries, healthcare has been slow to identify who the customer really is. Because of the complexity of the healthcare system, internal customers—physicians, hospitals, insurers, government, payers—have often driven processes. It is critically important that value be defined by the primary customer: the patient."[8]

Voice of the Customer (VOC) is a method for gathering and analyzing customers' needs when designing or improving a process. Common tools used include surveys, interviews, and panel discussions. Customers' responses are then analyzed to identify the "critical customer requirements" a process must achieve. Taking the time to internalize customers' needs, wants, and expectations helps to design a process that serves them better while preventing waste and addressing quality and safety issues.

To compile VOC input for the ERAS implementation, VCU Health contacted members of the Patient and Family Advisory Council and other patients. This information was shared with project team members to help set the stage for identifying value-add process steps.

Voice of the business
Although the primary customer is the patient, health care must also comply with regulations from a multitude of governing bodies and payers. To ensure this perspective is not lost, the authors also examined the Voice of the Business (VOB). VOB is a method for understanding how a process aligns with the organization's wider needs by doing the following:

- Understanding organizational priorities, such as strategy, financial stewardship, operational plans, major investments, marketing initiatives, employee satisfaction, and key performance indicators
- Identifying key regulatory and compliance issues associated with the process
- Considering the needs of suppliers and other stakeholders

In preparation for ERAS implementation, the project team identified internal guidelines and expectations, regulatory requirements, and interdependencies across all care venues.

Value-add/non-value-add analysis
Value-add/non-value-add analysis adds an extra layer to process mapping by considering how well the process meets its requirements. This analysis helps us understand some important things about the process:

- The inputs and resources required to complete various steps in this process
- How long the process takes to complete
- What data are collected during the process, and what additional data are needed
- Which parts of the process add value, and which do not
- Which process steps are causing delays, waste, quality problems, compliance issues, or frustrations for the customer

With VOC and VOB in mind, the project team assessed the current state to identify customer value-add, business value-add, and non-value-add process steps.

Impact/effort analysis and prioritization

From the mapping and value-add/non-value-add assessment, a list of improvement opportunities was identified. The team then conducted an impact/effort analysis and prioritized the improvement opportunities based on analysis results.

Prioritization is critical during this time to ensure the most impactful opportunities are addressed and to reduce the bias individual team members may have toward improving portions of the process. As a result of the prioritization process, the team was able to identify items that were low-effort implementations, such as adjustments to patient education, versus those that would take considerable resources and efforts, such as a complete process redesign of a particular phase of care, and plan accordingly to maximize benefit.

Future state process mapping

Often processes are created within silos, which may result in suboptimal handoff at transition of care. Here, the team focused on a systems view of the patient's journey along the surgical continuum to develop more flexible processes, allowing for more patient choice and convenience. Redesigned processes and tools ensure that information gathered along the way is shared at the appropriate time in the process. For example, information collected from the patient during preanesthesia assessment is shared with the day-of-surgery staff. Most importantly, the future state incorporated the new ERAS principles into the process, ensuring that the standards of care would be hardwired into the care pathway.

Virginia Commonwealth University Health Quality Standards for Enhanced Recovery After Surgery

The ERAS Society has developed evidence-based pathways for multiple surgical procedures. Within each pathway, there are recommendations for preoperative, intraoperative, and postoperative elements of an ERAS pathway. VCU Health uses these pathways, coupled with evidence within specific domains, to develop system-wide quality standards for addressing ERAS elements across surgical procedures.

Each VCU Health Quality Standard represents a fundamental change in clinical practice needed to address ERAS care elements and provides a tool for securing approval and managing expectations regarding consistent care methods rooted in current scientific evidence.[9] These standards are designed for all team members involved in the care continuum. They provide guidance, serve as a reference point when questions arise, and reflect executive support through a strong governance process.

The VCU Health Quality Standards template outlines key information regarding the associated clinical care topic. This predetermined format ensures that the governance groups that maintain oversight of these standards receive consistent information on how each standard is developed, while also providing staff with the necessary information to manage patient care to the standard.

How it is done:
- A surgeon-led interprofessional team is convened.
- They use clinical evidence design and document a standard.
- The material is socialized among stakeholders, allowing an opportunity for feedback and refinement.
- The surgery lead brings the document to the QSR for acceptance and implementation guidance.
- The document is sent to PEC for formalization.
- The standard is published to the intranet and disseminated.
- The electronic health record and other system tools are updated to further reinforce the change in practice.

Formal exceptions to the quality standards can be brought before the QSR for approval provided there is evidence to support the exception and the request is based on patient factors, not individual clinician preferences.

Enhanced Recovery After Surgery by Care-Phase

To reinforce the importance of the ERAS principles to every phase of patient care, the vertical task force teams identified the top 5 care points for each and posted them in clinical areas for easy reference. Intraoperative care points are specified for each role (**Table 3**).

The preoperative assessment communication and education clinic

Moving the discovery of the patient's clinical needs earlier in the process allows for more reliable scheduling, efficient optimization, and improved patient satisfaction. At VCU Health, the preoperative assessment communication and education (PACE) clinic serves as the medical clearinghouse for complex patients who have elected for a scheduled surgery.

The clinic is staffed by advanced practice providers under the supervision of an anesthesiologist. Patients are referred to the clinic based on a combination of the surgical procedure complexity and the patient's comorbidity status. A preoptimization algorithm serves as guidance for diagnostics, laboratory testing, and other preoperative preparations. Patients at high risk for complications are seen in clinic, and a physical examination and assessment are performed to develop a preoptimization plan, which may include additional specialty consults and/or treatments to improve the patient's medical status before surgery. The PACE team communicates this plan to the surgeon so that the patient's progress can be monitored.

Intraoperative pathways

Each specialty service works with anesthesia to develop an intraoperative pathway for their common procedures. This pathway serves as a "playbook" to help achieve and sustain success in ERAS by aligning anesthesia, surgeon, nursing, pharmacy, and equipment (**Fig. 5**).

Perioperative and postoperative analgesia

Optimal analgesia is achieved when both the type of surgery and the patient's individual presentation are accounted for.

To restore function and reduce stress response, it is especially important to do the following:
- Set patient expectations for pain management
- Use multimodal approach with planned deescalation
- Minimize opioids

Table 3
Intraoperative care points by role

Preoperative Nursing

Give premedications	Multimodal pain (acetaminophen, gabapentin, nonsteroidal anti-inflammatory drugs) Deep vein thrombosis prophylaxis (heparin, enoxaparin)
Keep patient warm	Use warming device Transport with warmed blankets to OR
Place saline locked intravenous line	Avoid unnecessary fluid infusions If no carbohydrate drink/preload: may infuse up to 500 mL
Education patient about pain management	Scheduled pain medication to reduce pain Nonnarcotic pain relief methods Goal: Manage pain in order to enable early mobilization
Clip hair	Reduces risk of surgical site infection Avoid hair clipping in OR

Anesthesiologist

Consider analgesia technique	Reduce opioid need perioperatively: neuroaxial block, thoracic epidural analgesia/TAP or truncal blocks Consider adjuncts: Ketamine, Precedex, lidocaine
Continue goal-directed fluid therapy	Maintain euvolemia but avoid fluid excess using hemodynamic monitors if necessary Optimize the cardiac output and hemoglobin Maintain MAP with vasopressors if needed
Allow rapid awakening/prevent postoperative nausea and vomiting (PONV)	Avoid sedative premedication if possible Use short-acting anesthetic agents PONV prophylaxis: use 2 different class of drugs Avoid PONV triggers where possible
Keep patient warm	Warming device Fluid warming
Monitor neuromuscular block	Monitor both neuromuscular block and reversal

Recovery room (post anesthesia care unit [PACU]) nursing

Continue goal-directed fluid therapy	Fluid bolus as charted, up to 500 mLs targeted on blood pressure and urine output Maintenance fluids at 1 mL/1 kg per hour
Education patient about pain management	Scheduled pain medication to control pain Minimize opiates: Prioritize nonnarcotic pain relief methods Goal: Manage pain in order to enable early mobilization
Prepare patient to be out of bed	Patient should be sitting upright with head of bed at least 30° as tolerated
Start digestive process early	Offer clear liquids in the PACU Provide protein drinks as soon as tolerated Maintain glucose control
Keep patient warm	Use warming device Use warmed blankets for patient comfort

Abbreviations: MAP, mean arterial pressure; TAP, trans abdominis plane.

Intraoperative Pathway for Elective Adult – [X] Surgery
NOTE: **PATIENT** *related factors* **WILL** *lead to change from Pathway.*
This change is an **ESSENTIAL** *part of medical judgment.*

Element	Pathway	[Approach A] E.g. [XX]	[Approach B] E.g. [XX]
SA-Anes Macro			
Blood Utilization	Intraop Plan (if adequate starting Hgb)		
Frailty & Geriatric Patients	Preoperative		
	Day of Surgery		
Analgesia (use judgment in elderly, or in severe Heart, Liver, Renal disease)	Preoperative		
	Intraoperative		
PONV Prophylaxis	Risk Factors (Sum: 0–4)		
	Approach (per Risk Factor)		
	Note		
Antibiotic	Preferred		
	B-lactam Allergy		
Intraop Fluid & Hemodynamic Therapy (use judgment in severe heart & renal disease)	Fluid Plan		
	Maintenance Plan (via Alaris pump)		
	Warning Signs & Vasoactive Infusion		
Normothermia	Intraoperative		
DVT Prophylaxis	Intraoperative		
Other Notes			
Equipment			
Position, Rx, or Neuromonitoring			

Anesthesia Champion: [Name]   Surgical Champion: [Name]
STM Lead: [Name]   Last Updated: [Date]

Fig. 5. Intraoperative pathway playbook. DVT, deep vein thrombosis; gtt, ; Hbg, hemoglobin; Rx, prescription; SA, ; SN-6, .

- Choose oral over intravenous medication routes
- Use intravenous medications for breakthrough pain where oral medications are ineffective
- Reduce all drug doses according to age and glomerular filtration rate

A rescue plan should always be available. This will do the following:

- Ensure patient safety so complications are not missed
- Address the type of pain with an appropriate modality of analgesia
- Avoid the default of strong opioids, which can then delay patient's recovery, particularly when this occurrence is at night

When an opioid-sparing analgesia approach is in place, take-home opioids should not exceed 7 days in duration. Exceptions may be approved by the attending surgeon if extenuating circumstances exist.

Fluids and hemodynamics

Proper management of fluids and hemodynamics is a key determinant in all-cause outcomes.

Fluid administration ranges are set according to specialty and procedure and provided in the intraoperative pathways.

Best practices when managing fluid administration include the following:

- Working in milliliters per kilogram, ideal body weight
- Using hemodynamic monitoring for American Society of Anesthesiologists (ASA) 3, ASA 4, high-risk surgery
- Knowing what types of monitors are best and when
- Using balanced crystalloid solutions
- Escalating monitoring for bleeding greater than 10 mL/kg, systemic inflammatory response, fluid shifts, hemodynamic instability
- Zoning," 5 to 10 mL/kg at start, 2 to 4 mL/kg per hour plus blood loss, optimize at end

These practices will help to avoid hypovolemia and hypervolemia and reduce the likelihood of acute kidney injury.

Postoperative recovery

Engaged, empowered patients are key to changing outcomes. Setting goals with patients that they can work toward independently and providing tools they can use to track their progress will encourage patients to actively participate in their recovery and be better prepared to continue a rapid return to baseline function after discharge.

Patient engagement tools used in the nursing units at VCU Health include the following:

- Admission (comfort) kits
- Aromatherapy
- Gum
- Patient diaries (**Fig. 6**)
- Unit mobility game boards (**Fig. 7**)
- Step tracking apps or devices
- In-room patient communication boards
- Protein drinks
- Progressive care sleep precautions

Electronic Medical Record and Order Sets

The result of combining a process design with ERAS principles is creating standardized care pathways that reduce waste and increase value to the patient. Developing the right preoptimization plan for a patient is rooted in a holistic understanding of the patient's baseline function through a targeted set of studies and assessments. Electronic medical record (EMR) functionality can be used to suggest the most appropriate pathways based on documented results/characteristics and then flex the order set to the most appropriate tests, medications, and dosing. To maximize this type of functionality, EMR documentation flows must mirror the flow of clinical care and use structured templates to capture data in a way that can be processed in coded algorithms. The algorithms guide the provider to develop a care plan that reflects the most current evidence, allowing the provider to place their focus on addressing any nonroutine needs of the patient.

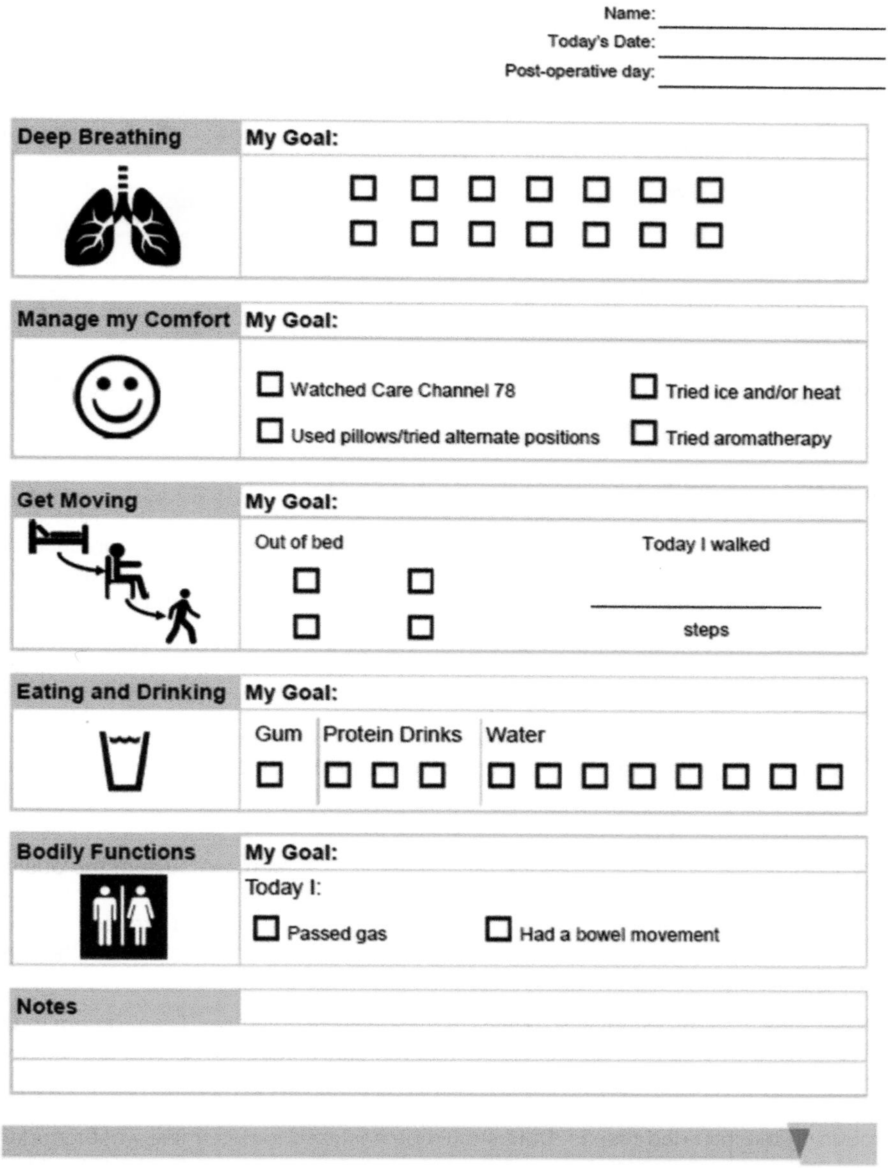

Name: _____
Today's Date: _____
Post-operative day: _____

Deep Breathing	My Goal:
	☐ ☐ ☐ ☐ ☐ ☐ ☐ ☐ ☐ ☐ ☐ ☐ ☐ ☐

Manage my Comfort	My Goal:
☺	☐ Watched Care Channel 78 ☐ Tried ice and/or heat ☐ Used pillows/tried alternate positions ☐ Tried aromatherapy

Get Moving	My Goal:
	Out of bed Today I walked ☐ ☐ ☐ ☐ _____ steps

Eating and Drinking	My Goal:
	Gum Protein Drinks Water ☐ ☐ ☐ ☐ ☐ ☐ ☐ ☐ ☐ ☐ ☐ ☐

Bodily Functions	My Goal:
	Today I: ☐ Passed gas ☐ Had a bowel movement

Notes	

Fig. 6. Postoperative patient diary.

An Example of Patient Optimization Compliance Tracking

- Patient misses an appointment for intravenous iron.
- The designated nurse on the surgeon's team sees the missed appointment on the optimization tracking dashboard.
- The nurse contacts the patient to understand why the appointment was missed, educate the patient about the importance of treatment, and take corrective action.

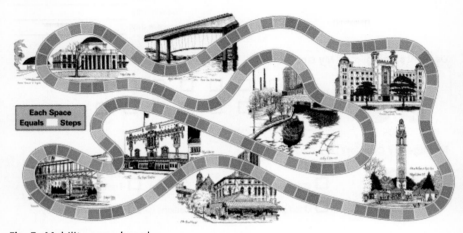

Each Space
Equals ___ Steps

Fig. 7. Mobility game board.

Custom views and tracking tools can improve compliance of good practice by serving as an aid for the care team to follow the patient throughout the surgical care journey and intervene as needed to keep the patient on course for the best possible outcome.

Results

What quality indicators to use: measuring standards

Although the interdisciplinary team, feedback opportunities, and approval from executives are important to the initial adoption of a quality standard, the ongoing utilization by front-line staff can be measured through both process and outcome measures by the following:

- Identifying the outcome you want to measure as a representative of the quality standard
- Determining data points you will use as markers of the desired process
- Ensuring the EMR is designed in a way to collect these data points within the clinical workflow

It is critical to approach these data from a learning perspective. The program must be supported by a suite of data analytics that not only measures compliance with the process but also looks at surgical outcomes and the correlation between the two. The purpose of the data is to compare processes to outcomes to ensure the standards are producing the intended results. Data should be analyzed to determine whether additional resources are needed to support the change or whether the standard should be refined to achieve the desired patient outcomes.

Using data visualization tools to build data sets

Large complex data sets can be produced from the EMR; however, selecting appropriate visualization tools for the presentation of data is important to conveying the right messages and supporting additional analysis. The correct data visualizations will first provide insight into individual performance compared with the group for the desired outcome and then allow drill-down capability for an individual to see performance on the associated process measures providing a feedback loop for reinforcing desired practice. The authors used dashboards and run charts as a basis to demonstrate sustained improvement (**Fig. 8**).

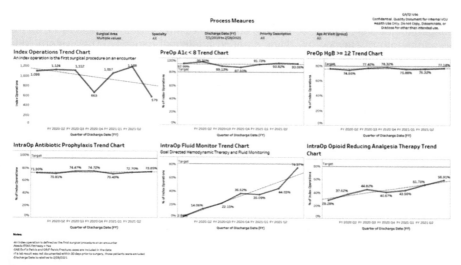

Fig. 8. ERAS process measures.

Continuing to inspire stakeholders and reinforce their value

High accountability and resiliency are characteristics needed to move large projects through change even if the change is one that is readily accepted or "is the right thing to do." The best way to engage medical professionals in change is using meaningful data.

Measures of comparison must be used as "vital signs" to help health care leaders understand recent performance and where improvement is needed. In addition, the data must be valid and as transparent as possible to ensure the team or teams have confidence in the protocols.

By aligning these system goals with the professional ethics of providers, the authors shift the focus from improving comparative measures toward improving patient outcomes, something that medical professionals can get behind.

SUMMARY

A major component of successful organizational change is ensuring that the people have a clear understanding of the benefits of the change they are being asked to make. ERAS has a compelling platform for change in that it provides benefits for all involved.

For patients, ERAS encourages active engagement in the care process leading to improved short-term and long-term clinical outcomes and improved satisfaction. Methods for multimodal opioid-sparing analgesia included in ERAS pathways reduce the probability of patients developing opioid dependence, a key area of concern in today's patients.

Surgeons benefit from increased OR capacity and timely availability, predictable case booking, and avoidance of cancellations and delays caused by unprepared patients.

An ERAS program engages the entire care team across the continuum of care. Decreased nursing and attending work per patient leads to improved efficiency and, subsequently, a more positive work environment. Provider organizations benefit at the highest levels by improving throughput, increasing capacity, reducing costs to create financial stability for value-based payment models, and improving publicly reported measures, which make them more market competitive.

For VCU Health, implementing ERAS across surgical specialties has fundamentally changed the delivery of care across the entire perioperative pathway and reduced the average length of stay by 0.5 days, creating additional capacity. The system-wide approach also affords the opportunity to be a US leader in pathway development for areas such as emergency general surgery and positions the organization to be highly competitive in both local and national markets.

CLINICS CARE POINTS

- Enhanced recovery after surgery can be used as a framework for perioperative surgical care to improve quality, reduce variation, and improve patient satisfaction while increasing value in health care.
- Executive leadership support is key to implementing an enhanced recovery after surgery program.
- A dedicated support team comprising a director, medical director, and quality improvement and data analysts is necessary to tackle the enormity of health system transformation.
- Surgical and anesthesia champions are needed with dedicated time.
- Advanced practice providers and nurses need to be involved in pathway organization.
- Vertical and horizontal implementation of enhanced recovery after surgery elements accelerated the standardization of perioperative pathways across the health system.
- Using the electronic medical record can help drive real-time compliance of enhanced recovery after surgery elements and produce audits but requires a lot of new resources in current electronic medical record versions.
- Data assessing the compliance of enhanced recovery after surgery elements and complications, length of stay, can improve the process and guide ongoing quality improvement projects.

DISCLOSURE

P. Spencer: none. M. Scott: speaker, expenses for travel: Baxter, Edwards Advisory Board: Edwards, Trevena, Merck, Baxter, Deltex.

REFERENCES

1. National Health Expenditure Projections 2018-2027 Forecast Summary. Available at: https://www.cms.gov/Research-Statistics-Data-and-Systems/Statistics-Trends-and-Reports/NationalHealthExpendData/Downloads/ForecastSummary.pdf. Accessed November 14, 2021.
2. Meyer H. Healthcare spending will hit 19.4% of GDP in the next decade, CMS projects. Mod Healthc 2019.
3. Joliat GR, Ljungqvist O, Wasylak T, et al. Beyond surgery: clinical and economic impact of enhanced recovery after surgery programs. BMC Health Serv Res 2018;18:1008.
4. Sanchez J, Barach P, Johnson JK, et al, editors. Surgical patient care: improving safety, quality, and value. 1st edition. New York: Springer International Publishing; 2017.
5. Available at: https://hcp-lan.org/2018-apm-measurement/#1466615406342d34e0 eeb-f073. Accessed November 14, 2021.
6. Eryılmaz M, Eryılmaz F. (2015). Active and passive resistance to organizational change: a case of entrepreneurship minor program in a public university. 10.4018/978-1-4666-8487-4.ch003.

7. Langley GJ, Moen R, Nolan KM, et al. The improvement guide: a practical approach to improving organizational performance. 2nd edition. San Francisco (CA): Jossey-Bass; 2009. p. P109–37.
8. Going Lean in Health Care. IHI innovation series white paper. Cambridge (MA): Institute for Healthcare Improvement; 2005. Available at: www.IHI.org.
9. Woolf SH, Grol R, Hutchison A, et al. Clinical guidelines: potential benefits, limitations, and harms of clinical guidelines. Br Med J 1999;318(7182):527–30.

Modifying the Stress Response – Perioperative Considerations and Controversies

Leigh J.S. Kelliher, MBBS, BSc, FRCA, MD[a],*,
Michael Scott, MBChB, FRCP, FRCA, FFICM[b,c,d]

KEYWORDS

- Stress response to surgery • Metabolic response to surgery
- Modification of the stress response • Enhanced recovery after surgery • Anesthesia
- Perioperative care

KEY POINTS

- The 'surgical stress response' describes the complex and interdependent physiological processes that occur following trauma/tissue injury.
- There are a variety of perioperative interventions that may alter these processes and therefore modify the stress response.
- Definitive clinical evidence for the benefit of any single stress-modifying perioperative intervention is lacking.
- Combining perioperative interventions to form comprehensive care pathways, e.g. ERAS pathways, has produced improvements in clinical outcomes.

The idea that perioperative outcomes may be improved through the implementation of measures that modify the surgical stress response has been around for several decades, generating a great deal of research.[1,2] The term "stress response" describes the characteristic wide-ranging physiologic changes that occur following a surgical insult/trauma. These are complex, interdependent, and often incompletely understood molecular processes and consequently, there is a multitude of ways in which modification may be attempted and many different techniques trialled.[2] In addition, how the response to modification is measured, what constitutes a positive result and how this translates into clinical practice has and continues to be the subject of debate. Toward the end of the 1990s interest grew in combining individual interventions and adopting a global approach to perioperative care aimed at producing "stress-free anesthesia and

---

[a] Department of Anaesthetics, Royal Surrey County Hospital NHS Foundation Trust, Egerton Road, Guildford, Surrey GU2 7AS, UK; [b] Hospital of the University of Pennsylvania, 3400 Spruce Street, Philadelphia, PA 19104, USA; [c] Leonard Davis Institute of Health Economics, University of Pennsylvania, Philadelphia, PA, USA; [d] Surgical Outcomes Research Centre, University College London, London, UK
* Corresponding author.
E-mail address: lkelliher@nhs.net

Anesthesiology Clin 40 (2022) 23–33
https://doi.org/10.1016/j.anclin.2021.11.012
1932-2275/22/© 2021 Elsevier Inc. All rights reserved.

anesthesiology.theclinics.com

surgery to improve postoperative recovery and reduce morbidity.[3] This is the principal tenet behind the enhanced recovery after surgery (ERAS) movement which has seen the development of guidelines for perioperative care across a variety of surgical specialties[4] bringing with them significant improvements in outcomes, including reductions in length of hospital stay and postoperative morbidity.[5,6] While the benefits seen with the implementation of ERAS pathways are likely the result of multiple factors, included among these is how they modify the stress response. Another key aspect of recovery after surgery is the restoration of normal metabolism. ERAS pathways promote a patient that is eating, sleeping, and mobilizing as soon as possible after surgery by not just reducing stress but improving the metabolic response to this stress response. An overview of the complex relationship between surgical injury, the SIRS response and the metabolic response, and how perioperative interventions can impact these are illustrated in **Fig. 1**. This metabolic response is generally characterized as a state of insulin resistance causing transient hyperglycemia. However, patients can present for surgery with a disrupted metabolic state before stress is incurred. This is commonly seen in patients who have protein malnutrition or who have cancer. Cancer drives a catabolic state which is hard to reverse without controlling cancer.

There is a lot of literature written on the stress response so this chapter is focused on interventions to reduce this. The impact of some common elements of ERAS pathways on surgical stress as well as that of more novel/controversial techniques is summarized here.

NUTRITION

The physiologic response to surgery includes several characteristic metabolic changes that ultimately result in increased breakdown of glycogen and skeletal muscle to mobilize glucose stores and the creation of a generally insulin-resistant, catabolic state.[7] The

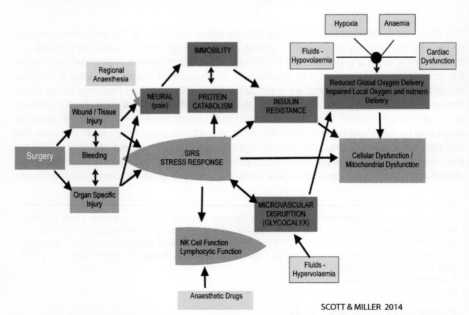

SCOTT & MILLER 2014

Fig. 1. Overview of the surgical stress response and perioperative interventions that may impact it. NK, natural killer; SIRS, systemic inflammatory response syndrome.

negative effect of this may be compounded by prolonged perioperative starvation times and the presence of preexisting malnutrition (eg, in patients with cancer) which, left unchecked, increases the risk of postoperative complications and poor outcomes.[8–10] Minimization of starvation times, administration of a preoperative carbohydrate "loading," early return to enteral feeding postoperatively and adequate perioperative nutritional support/supplementation have all been shown to mitigate the metabolic changes, reduce postoperative insulin-resistance, and catabolism[11,12] and consequently reduce the incidence of complications such as poor wound healing, infection and decreased mobility, and promote functional recovery.[13,14] These measures, alongside assessment of patients' nutritional status and recognition of those at highest risk, are constitutive to enhanced recovery pathways across all surgical specialties and the European Society for Clinical Nutrition and Metabolism (ESPEN) has produced comprehensive guidelines for the management of perioperative nutrition.[15]

THERMOREGULATION

Hypothermia is common under anesthesia and is the result of a combination of physical exposure and a loss of the body's ability to thermoregulate.[16] Evidence from a variety of settings including critical care, military research, postcardiac arrest, and during cardiopulmonary bypass has demonstrated that hypothermia is a trigger for stress, primarily through the release of catecholamines and activation of the hypothalamic–pituitary–adrenocortical axis.[17] The elevation in circulating catecholamines, cortisol, and other factors such as thyroid hormone has a variety of downstream sequelae including metabolic disturbance, immunosuppression, and the release of inflammatory mediators. The magnitude of this phenomenon is proportional to the degree of hypothermia, but even mild hypothermia can elicit a response which may, in turn, further compound the stress response seen because of the surgical insult.[18,19] The clinical consequences of intraoperative hypothermia include changes in drug metabolism, coagulopathy, increased transfusion requirements, shivering, and delayed recovery as well as an increase in infective and cardiac complications.[19–21] A proactive approach to maintaining normothermia perioperatively can modify the degree of stress which is induced thus mitigating the clinical risks and a variety of consensus guidelines exist aimed at achieving this end.[22]

HEMODYNAMICS AND OXYGEN DELIVERY

Successful hemodynamic management exists in equilibrium with surgical stress. The greater the stress response, the more salt and water retention, inflammation, and capillary permeability occur which in turn may result in a situation whereby both intravascular hypovolemia and tissue edema exist simultaneously. The ultimate consequence of this is reduced oxygen delivery to end-organ tissues and an increase in oxidative stress (OS) at a cellular level setting in motion a downward spiral of events that manifest clinically as an increase in the incidence of postoperative complications and mortality.[23] Fluid management becomes extremely challenging and involves negotiating a fine margin between too little and too much fluid, both of which will further contribute to ongoing stress and complications.[23,24] Getting fluid management correct from the outset—avoiding hypotension, fluid overload, electrolyte disturbance, and optimizing oxygen delivery to the tissues—is essential for preventing excessive stress and inflammation.[24] Finding the best way to achieve this has been the subject of a vast amount of research but to date, no one regimen has been shown to be superior. Most consensus guidelines of perioperative care for major surgical procedures advocate a tailored approach with the judicious use of balanced crystalloid fluids and vasopressors, guided by invasive blood pressure measurement and some form of cardiac output monitoring.[4,24,25] Maintenance of oxygen delivery with an adequate cardiac output and oxygen-carrying capacity is also important in high-risk surgeries. Maintaining hemoglobin above that which can cause organ dysfunction (usually 7–9 g/dL), while avoiding overzealous blood transfusion is key using a restrictive blood transfusion policy. Preoperative optimization of hemoglobin by screening and identifying causes of anemia and correcting them with intravenous iron therapy is becoming increasingly common in major surgery.

SURGICAL APPROACH

The degree of tissue trauma inflicted at the time of surgery is a major determinant of the magnitude of the stress response and there is a significant body of evidence demonstrating a reduction in various aspects of the stress response with laparoscopic surgery when compared with the equivalent open technique. A randomized controlled trial comparing markers of the stress response in laparoscopic versus open cholecystectomy demonstrated postoperative catecholamine, cortisol, IL-6, glucose, and CRP levels were all significantly higher following open surgery[26] and several other studies in cholecystectomy patients have demonstrated better preservation of immune function (cytokine levels, T-cell ratios, and function) with the laparoscopic approach.[27] A study comparing markers of the stress response following open, laparoscopic, and robotic colorectal surgery found them to be higher in the open surgery group, but comparable between laparoscopic and robotic surgery[28] and another in patients undergoing major urologic surgery demonstrated lower IL-6, IL-10, and granulocytic elastase with laparoscopic surgery.[29] Similar evidence exists for multiple other surgical procedures.[30] It should be noted that not all evidence supports this effect with several studies finding no difference in certain aspects of the stress response between equivalent laparoscopic and open procedures and a few suggesting that the response may even be greater following laparoscopy. A systematic review of the effect of laparoscopic surgery on the OS response (the balance of prooxidants and antioxidants) found that many studies were of low quality with a great heterogeneity between them in terms of design, method, measured OS markers, duration of investigation, and types of operations investigated. Results between studies were discordant necessitating further robust work be conducted before firm conclusions may be reached.[31]

In terms of clinical outcomes, laparoscopic surgery has been associated with reduced postoperative pain, fewer wound infections, shorter length of hospital stay, and faster return to normal activities for a variety of surgeries,[32–35] although several systematic reviews have found the evidence for many of the procedures to be of low quality. A systematic review of Cochrane systematic reviews identified 36 such studies evaluating laparoscopic versus open surgery. The authors concluded that overall evidence supports an advantage with laparoscopic surgery.[35]

The mechanisms behind the benefits of laparoscopic surgery are doubtless multiple and while a reduction in the stress response may be contributory the evidence to date does not demonstrate a causative link. In any event, the move toward more minimally invasive surgical procedures (laparoscopic, lap-assisted, robotic, endoscopic, single port, natural orifice) has been inexorable and has been accompanied by a general improvement in perioperative outcomes over the last decades.

ANESTHETIC FACTORS
Total Intravenous Anesthesia Versus Volatile Anesthesia

The idea that the stress response (and hence clinical outcomes) may be differentially affected using either volatile anesthesia or propofol-based total intravenous anesthesia

(TIVA) is controversial. Evidence, principally from the laboratory, has highlighted various biological mechanisms that lend plausibility to this theory.[36] One such is that volatile anesthetic agents have been shown to promote the expression of hypoxia-inducible factors (HIF).[37] These are transcription factors, released in response to hypoxia, that promote angiogenesis and glycolysis and form the basis of the ischemic preconditioning phenomenon seen with volatile anesthesia.[38] HIFs have also been implicated in the promotion of tumor growth and metastases leading to speculation that they may play a role in early tumor recurrence following cancer surgery. By contrast, laboratory evidence suggests that propofol does not elicit a HIF response and may even inhibit it.[39] Despite this clinical evidence of a beneficial effect with TIVA is mixed and of low quality with several recent systematic reviews commenting that prospective randomized controlled trials are required before any conclusions may be drawn.[40–42]

Regional Anesthesia

By far the most studied the regional anesthetic technique in terms of the stress response to major surgery is thoracic epidural (TEA). Several studies have demonstrated how TEA ameliorates the catecholamine and cortisol response to surgery, reducing postoperative catabolism;[43,44] however, evidence also suggests that it has little/no effect on the inflammatory cytokine response.[45] Clinical benefits of TEA include excellent pain relief—it is recommended in guidelines for a variety of open upper abdominal and thoracic surgeries[4,46,47]—and reduced incidence of cardiac, pulmonary, and thromboembolic complications[48–50] although it should be noted that several studies have failed to show these effects. The high failure rate, potential complications of insertion, and complexities of successful management of TEA, alongside the reduced analgesic requirements associated with minimally invasive surgery, has seen a variety of alternatives emerge including wound catheters, abdominal field blocks, and single-shot intrathecal opioids. While reportedly effective, robust evidence directly comparing these techniques with TEA is lacking.

Opioids

Despite the drive to adopt opioid-sparing strategies for perioperative analgesia to accelerate postoperative recovery, worldwide, opioid drugs remain ubiquitous for the management of severe pain. They exert their analgesic effect principally via agonism of the μ-opioid receptor, both peripherally and centrally. Opioids have been shown to modulate the stress response both directly and indirectly. By reducing nociceptive transmission in the sensory pathways of the spinal cord they may, in turn, reduce the central activation of the sympathetic nervous system, reducing catecholamine release, and moderating the cardiovascular response to surgical stimulation.[51] In addition, opioid receptors have been identified within the sympathetic nervous system itself and therefore may exert some of their action by directly reducing sympathetic activity.[52] High-dose fentanyl has been shown to prevent the increase in circulating catecholamines and completely suppress the circulatory response in patients undergoing cholecystectomy[53] and cardiac surgery.[54] As well as blunting the sympathetic response to surgery, opioids may act on the hypothalamic–pituitary–adrenocortical axis to reduce the release of both ACTH and cortisol[55,56] although evidence for this is mixed, and the clinical consequences are unclear. Finally, opioids have been implicated in causing postoperative immunosuppression either because of their effect on cortisol levels or via a direct action on cellular components of the immune system.[57] Evidence for this is effect is conflicting and mostly limited to in vitro animal studies. What is certain is that opioid analgesics are associated with several side effects that negatively impact recovery after surgery, namely respiratory depression, sedation, constipation, nausea, and vomiting and it is also true that poorly controlled pain is both a trigger and perpetuating factor in surgical stress. As a result, most current guidelines for fast-track recovery pathways advocate adopting an effective, opioid-sparing, multimodal analgesic strategy, tailored to the requirements of the surgical procedure, the institution, and the individual.[4]

Steroids

Cortisol is perhaps the principal "stress" hormone, playing a key role in the surgical stress response. It, therefore, follows that the perioperative use of exogenous corticosteroids will modify the innate stress response. In addition to reducing inflammation, corticosteroid therapy produces a wide range of effects throughout the body including alterations in carbohydrate, lipid, and protein metabolism and changes in water and electrolyte balance. The use of corticosteroids has a multisystemic impact, from cardiovascular, musculoskeletal, and gastrointestinal to endocrine and immune systems.[57] Consequently, they are indicated for a vast array of conditions spanning the whole of clinical medicine, including perioperative care, whereby low-dose steroid (typically dexamethasone between 0.05 mg/kg and 0.1 mg/kg) is used widely for its antiemetic, antiinflammatory and analgesic effect and has been shown to improve the quality of recovery for a variety of surgeries.[58–60] Concerns have been raised over the safety of perioperative steroid administration with the suggestion that it may lead to an increased incidence of wound infection, dehiscence or even an early recurrence of cancer because of the immunosuppression and hyperglycemia it induces. However, the evidence to date seems to show that these concerns are unfounded with several meta-analyses failing to demonstrate these effects.[61,62] Research into this issue continues and the results are awaited.[63] More recently there has been a resurgence of interest in the use of high-dose (>0.1 mg/kg) perioperative steroids for improving parameters of recovery. A systematic review identified 11 RCTs examining the use of high-dose dexamethasone in hip and knee arthroplasty with the meta-analysis showing a reduction in postoperative nausea and vomiting and pain and a faster recovery with high-dose steroids. There was no difference in complications between groups.[64] Further work to elucidate both the optimal dose of steroid in this setting and the effect of this intervention on subpopulations at higher risk of postoperative pain is underway with 3 further RCTs due to report their results soon.[65] The perioperative use of high-dose methylprednisolone (15–30 mg/kg) has also been evaluated in a variety of surgeries. In hepatic resection, it has been shown to reduce markers of the stress response (IL-6, IL-8, CRP) (although the clinical implications of this were unclear)[66,67] and a metanalysis of 28 studies (including 25 RCTs) in mandibular surgery found that use of high-dose methylprednisolone was associated with less postoperative pain, swelling and trismus.[68] Finally, a systematic review of the use of high dose methylprednisolone in 51 studies in cardiac and noncardiac surgery found no significant difference in adverse effect between groups, but also no significant difference in postoperative pain or hospital stay—although pulmonary complications were reduced in trauma patients given methylprednisolone.[69] Currently, the evidence is insufficient to recommend the routine use of high-dose steroids in perioperative care, but this may change as more data emerges.

ß-Blockers

Perioperative ß-blockade blunts sympathetic activity and thereby diminishes the neuroendocrine response to surgery. It has been postulated that by using them for this indication it may be possible to reduce the physiologic stress of surgery and thereby reduce complications and improve outcomes. Despite the biological plausibility of this idea, clinical research examining this question has yielded conflicting results with some studies demonstrating harm from this intervention—an increased incidence of postoperative hypotension, stroke, and mortality.[70] A recent meta-analysis of 83 RCTs (14,967 patients) found the evidence for all-cause mortality with perioperative ß-blockade was uncertain and that further, large, placebo-controlled trials were required.[71]

A variety of other agents aimed at modifying surgical stress and improving postoperative outcomes have been investigated, including α2-agonists (clonidine, dexmedetomidine)[72] and melatonin;[73] however, to date there is no high-quality evidence supporting their use in this setting.

SUMMARY

The interplay between pathologic processes, surgery, and its physiologic sequelae and clinical outcomes is complex and incompletely understood. Research in this area is challenging, particularly in the face of constantly evolving practice, new technologies, and pharmaceutical agents and changing patient demographics. Finding definitive evidence for specific perioperative interventions is often difficult with studies yielding a variety of conflicting results. Fast track surgical programs, such as ERAS, aim to optimize patients' recovery from surgery by reducing its physiologic impact—"stress-free surgery and anesthesia"—by using multiple perioperative interventions. While definitive evidence to support any one of these interventions alone may be lacking, perhaps the improvement in clinical outcomes (reduced length of hospital stay, reduced morbidity) seen as the advent of fast-track pathways demonstrates that in combination they are effective in achieving their aim.

CLINICS CARE POINTS

- For patients undergoing major surgery, a perioperative care pathway comprising multimodal interventions with the overall aim of minimising the stress of anaesthesia and surgery is recommended.

- A pragmatic approach to perioperative care is to consider the benefits and risks of individual perioperative interventions in the context of local skills and resources to produce a pathway tailored to the patients and institution in question.

- Optimising nutritional status is important and often overlooked, particularly where surgery is time critical (e.g. cancer surgery).

REFERENCES

1. Kehlet H. The stress response to surgery: release mechanisms and the modifying effect of pain relief. Acta Chir Scand Suppl 1989;550:22–8.
2. Novak-Jankovič V, Paver-Eržen V. How can anesthetists modify stress response during perioperative period?. In: Gullo A, editor. Anaesthesia, pain, Intensive care and emergency medicine — a.P.I.C.E. Milano: Springer; 2002. https://doi.org/10.1007/978-88-470-2099-3_89.
3. Kehlet H. The surgical stress response: should it be prevented? Can J Surg 1991; 34(6):565–7.
4. Available at: https://erassociety.org/guidelines/list-of-guidelines/. Accessed October 14, 2021.
5. Jones C, Kelliher L, Dickinson M, et al. Randomized clinical trial on enhanced recovery versus standard care following open liver resection. Br J Surg 2013; 100(8):1015–24. https://doi.org/10.1002/bjs.9165.

6. Rawlinson A, Kang P, Evans J, et al. A systematic review of enhanced recovery protocols in colorectal surgery. Ann R Coll Surg Engl 2011;93(8):583–8.

7. Cuthbertson DP. Observations on the disturbance of metabolism produced by injury to the limbs. Q J Med 1932;1:233–46.

8. Gillis C, Carli F. Promoting perioperative metabolic and nutritional care. Anesthesiology 2015;123:1455–72.

9. Alazawi W, Pirmadid N, Lahiri R, et al. Inflammatory and immune responses to surgery and their clinical impact. Ann Surg 2016;64:73–80.

10. Aahlin EK, Tranø G, Johns N, et al. Risk factors, complications and survival after upper abdominal surgery: a prospective cohort study. BMC Surg 2015;15:83.

11. Soop M, Nygren J, Thorell A, et al. Preoperative oral carbohydrate treatment attenuates endogenous glucose release 3 days after surgery. Clin Nutr 2004;23:733–41.

12. Breuer JP, von Dossow V, von Heymann C, et al. Preoperative oral carbohydrate administration to ASA III-IV patients undergoing elective cardiac surgery. Anesth Analg 2006;103:1099–108.

13. Andersen HK, Lewis SJ, Thomas S. Early enteral nutrition within 24h of colorectal surgery versus later commencement of feeding for postoperative complications. Cochrane Database Syst Rev 2006;(4):CD004080.

14. Osland E, Yunus RM, Khan S, et al. Early versus traditional post- operative feeding in patients undergoing resectional gastrointestinal sur- gery: a meta-analysis. J Parenter Enteral Nutr 2011;35:473–87.

15. Weimann A, Braga M, Carli F, et al. ESPEN guideline: clinical nutrition in surgery. Clin Nutr 2017;36(3):623–50. https://doi.org/10.1016/j.clnu.2017.02.013.

16. Sessler DI. Mild perioperative hypothermia. N Engl J Med 1997;336(24):1730–7. https://doi.org/10.1056/NEJM199706123362407.

17. Goldstein DS. Adrenal responses to stress. Cell Mol Neurobiol 2010;30(8):1433–40. https://doi.org/10.1007/s10571-010-9606-9.

18. Pozos RS, Danzl DF. In: Medical aspects of harsh environments, vol. 1. U.S. Army. Office of the surgeon general. Borden Institute; 2002. p. pp351–82.

19. Sessler DI. Perioperative thermoregulation and heat balance. Lancet 2016;387(10038):2655–64. https://doi.org/10.1016/S0140-6736(15)00981-2.

20. Kurz A, Sessler DI, Lenhardt R. Perioperative normothermia to reduce the incidence of surgical-wound infection and shorten hospitalization. Study of Wound Infection and Temperature Group. N Engl J Med 1996;334:1209–15. https://doi.org/10.1056/NEJM199605093341901.

21. Frank SM, Fleisher LA, Breslow MJ, et al. Perioperative maintenance of normothermia reduces the incidence of morbid cardiac events. A randomized clinical trial. JAMA 1997;277:1127–34. https://doi.org/10.1001/jama.277.14.1127.

22. Available at: https://www.nice.org.uk/guidance/cg65/chapter/Context. Accessed October 14, 2021.

23. Miller TE, Myles PS. Perioperative fluid therapy for major surgery. Anesthesiology 2019;130:825–32.

24. Holte K, Sharrock NE, Kehlet H. Pathophysiology and clinical implications of perioperative fluid excess. Br J Anaesth 2002;89(4):622–32.

25. Thiele RH, Raghunathan K, Brudney CS, et al. Perioperative Quality Initiative (POQI) I Workgroup. American Society for Enhanced Recovery (ASER) and Perioperative Quality Initiative (POQI) joint consensus statement on perioperative fluid management within an enhanced recovery pathway for colorectal surgery. Perioper Med (Lond) 2016;5:24. https://doi.org/10.1186/s13741-016-0049-9. Erratum in: Perioper Med (Lond). 2018 Apr 10;7:5. PMID: 27660701; PMCID: PMC5027098.

26. Karayiannakis AJ, Makri GG, Mantzioka A, et al. Systemic stress response after laparoscopic or open cholecystectomy: a randomized trial. Br J Surg 1997; 84(4):467–71.
27. Gupta A, Watson DI. Effect of laparoscopy on immune function. Br J Surg 2001; 88(10):1296–306. https://doi.org/10.1046/j.0007-1323.2001.01860.x.
28. Shibata J, Ishihara S, Tada N, et al. Surgical stress response after colorectal resection: a comparison of robotic, laparoscopic, and open surgery. Tech Coloproctol 2015;19(5):275–80. https://doi.org/10.1007/s10151-014-1263-4.
29. Miyake H, Kawabata G, Gotoh A, et al. Comparison of surgical stress between laparoscopy and open surgery in the field of urology by measurement of humoral mediators. Int J Urol 2002;9:329–33.
30. Buunen M, Gholghesaei M, Veldkamp R, et al. Stress response to laparoscopic surgery: a review. Surg Endosc 2004;18(7):1022–8. https://doi.org/10.1007/s00464-003-9169-7.
31. Yiannakopoulou EC, Nikiteas N, Perrea D, et al. Effect of laparoscopic surgery on oxidative stress response: systematic review. Surg Laparosc Endosc Percutaneous Tech 2013;23(2):101–8. https://doi.org/10.1097/sle.0b013e3182827b33.
32. Jaschinski T, Mosch CG, Eikermann M, et al. Laparoscopic versus open surgery for suspected appendicitis. Cochrane Database Syst Rev 2018;(11):CD001546. https://doi.org/10.1002/14651858.CD001546.pub4.
33. Piessen G, Lefèvre JH, Cabau M, et al, AFC and the FREGAT working group. Laparoscopic versus open surgery for gastric gastrointestinal stromal tumors: what is the impact on postoperative outcome and oncologic results? Ann Surg 2015;262(5):831–9. https://doi.org/10.1097/SLA.0000000000001488 [discussion 829–40].
34. Jien, He MD, Xiaohua, et al. Laparoscopic versus open surgery in the treatment of hepatic hemangioma. Medicine 2021;100(8):e24155. https://doi.org/10.1097/MD.0000000000024155.
35. Carr BM, Lyon JA, Romeiser J, et al. Laparoscopic versus open surgery: a systematic review evaluating Cochrane systematic reviews. Surg Endosc 2019; 33(6):1693–709. https://doi.org/10.1007/s00464-018-6532-2.
36. Evans MT, Wigmore T, Kelliher LJS. The impact of anaesthetic technique upon outcome in oncological surgery. BJA Educ 2019;19(1):14–20. https://doi.org/10.1016/j.bjae.2018.09.008.
37. Benzonana LL, Perry NJ, Watts HR, et al. Isoflurane, a commonly used volatile anesthetic, enhances renal cancer growth and malignant potential via the hypoxia-inducible factor cellular signaling pathway in vitro. Anesthesiology 2013;119(3):593–605. https://doi.org/10.1097/ALN.0b013e31829e47fd.
38. Cai Z, Luo W, Zhan H, et al. Hypoxia-inducible factor 1 is required for remote ischemic preconditioning of the heart. Proc Natl Acad Sci U S A 2013;110(43): 17462–7. https://doi.org/10.1073/pnas.1317158110.
39. Behmenburg F, van Caster P, Bunte S, et al. Impact of anesthetic regimen on remote ischemic preconditioning in the rat heart in vivo. Anesth Analg 2018; 126(4):1377–80. https://doi.org/10.1213/ANE.0000000000002563.
40. Soltanizadeh S, Degett TH, Gögenur I. Outcomes of cancer surgery after inhalational and intravenous anesthesia: a systematic review. J Clin Anesth 2017;42: 19–25. https://doi.org/10.1016/j.jclinane.2017.08.001.
41. Yap A, Lopez-Olivo MA, Dubowitz J, et al, Global Onco-Anesthesia Research Collaboration Group. Anesthetic technique and cancer outcomes: a meta-analysis of total intravenous versus volatile anesthesia. Can J Anaesth 2019;

66(5):546–61. https://doi.org/10.1007/s12630-019-01330-x. Erratum in: Can J Anaesth. 2019 Aug;66(8):1007-1008. PMID: 30834506.

42. Chang CY, Wu MY, Chien YJ, et al. Anesthesia and long-term oncological outcomes: a systematic review and meta-analysis. Anesth Analg 2021;132(3): 623–34. https://doi.org/10.1213/ANE.0000000000005237.

43. Holte K, Kehlet H. Epidural anaesthesia and analgesia - effects on surgical stress responses and implications for postoperative nutrition. Clin Nutr 2002;21(3): 199–206. https://doi.org/10.1054/clnu.2001.0514.

44. Kouraklis G, Glinavou A, Raftopoulos L, et al. Epidural analgesia attenuates the systemic stress response to upper abdominal surgery: a randomized trial. Int Surg 2000;85(4):353–7.

45. Norman JG, Fink GW. The effects of epidural anesthesia on the neuroendocrine response to major surgical stress: a randomized prospective trial. Am Surg 1997; 63(1):75–80.

46. Joshi GP, Bonnet F, Shah R, et al. A systematic review of randomized trials evaluating regional techniques for postthoracotomy analgesia. Anesth Analg 2008; 107(3):1026–40. https://doi.org/10.1213/01.ane.0000333274.63501.ff.

47. Manion SC, Brennan TJ, Bruno R. Thoracic epidural analgesia and acute pain management. Anesthesiology 2011;115:181–8.

48. Beattie WS, Badner NH, Choi P. Epidural analgesia reduces postoperative myocardial infarction: a meta-analysis. Anesth Analg 2001;93(4):853–8.

49. Guay J. The benefits of adding epidural analgesia to general anesthesia: a meta-analysis. J Anesth 2006;20:335–40.

50. Pöpping DM, Elia N, Marret E, et al. Protective effects of epidural analgesia on pulmonary complications after abdominal and thoracic surgery: a meta-analysis. Arch Surg 2008;143(10):990–9. https://doi.org/10.1001/archsurg.143.10.990.

51. Schlereth T, Birklein F. The sympathetic nervous system and pain. Neuromol Med 2008;10:141–7.

52. Hung CF, Chang WL, Liang HC, et al. Identification of opioid receptors in the sympathetic and parasympathetic nerves of guinea-pig atria. Fundam Clin Pharmacol 2000;14(4):387–94. https://doi.org/10.1111/j.1472-8206.2000.tb00420.x.

53. Klingstedt C, Giesecke K, Hamberger B, et al. High- and low-dose fentanyl anaesthesia: circulatory and plasma catecholamine responses during cholecystectomy. Br J Anaesth 1987;59(2):184–8. https://doi.org/10.1093/bja/59.2.184.

54. Naguib AN, Tobias JD, Hall MW, et al. The role of different anesthetic techniques in altering the stress response during cardiac surgery in children: a prospective, double-blinded, and randomized study. Pediatr Crit Care Med 2013;14(5): 481–90. https://doi.org/10.1097/PCC.0b013e31828a742c.

55. Watanabe K, Kashiwagi K, Kamiyama T, et al. High-dose remifentanil suppresses stress response associated with pneumoperitoneum during laparoscopic colectomy. J Anesth 2014;28(3):334–40. https://doi.org/10.1007/s00540-013-1738-x.

56. Haroutounian S. Postoperative opioids, endocrine changes, and immunosuppression. Pain Rep 2018;3(2):e640. https://doi.org/10.1097/PR9.0000000000000640.

57. McKay LI, Cidlowski JA. Physiologic and pharmacologic effects of corticosteroids. In: Kufe DW, Pollock RE, Weichselbaum RR, et al, editors. Holland-frei cancer medicine. 6th edition. Hamilton, ON: BC Decker; 2003. Available at: https://www.ncbi.nlm.nih.gov/books/NBK13780/.

58. Mihara T, Ishii T, Ka K, et al. Effects of Steroids on Quality of Recovery and Adverse Events after General Anesthesia: Meta-Analysis and Trial Sequential Analysis of Randomized Clinical Trials. PLoS One 2016;11(9):e0162961.

59. Zhuo Y, Yu R, Wu C, et al. The role of perioperative intravenous low-dose dexamethasone in rapid recovery after total knee arthroplasty: a meta-analysis. J Int Med Res 2021. https://doi.org/10.1177/0300060521998220.

60. Murphy GS, Szokol JW, Greenberg SB, et al. Preoperative dexamethasone enhances quality of recovery after laparoscopic cholecystectomy: effect on in-hospital and postdischarge recovery outcomes. Anesthesiology 2011;114:882–90.

61. Toner AJ, Ganeshanathan V, Chan MT, et al. Safety of perioperative glucocorticoids in elective noncardiac surgery: a systematic review and meta-analysis. Anesthesiology 2017;126:234–48.

62. Waldron NH, Jones CA, Gan TJ, et al. Impact of perioperative dexamethasone on postoperative analgesia and side-effects: systematic review and meta-analysis. Br J Anaesth 2013;110(2):191–200. https://doi.org/10.1093/bja/aes431.

63. Corcoran TB, Myles PS, Forbes AB, et al, on behalf of the Australian and New Zealand College of Anaesthetists Clinical Trials Network (ANZCA), and the Australian Society for Infectious Diseases (ASID) Clinical Research Network. The perioperative administration of dexamethasone and infection (PADDI) trial protocol: rationale and design of a pragmatic multicentre non-inferiority study. BMJ Open 2019;9:e030402. https://doi.org/10.1136/bmjopen-2019-030402.

64. Yue C, Wei R, Liu Y. Perioperative systemic steroid for rapid recovery in total knee and hip arthroplasty: a systematic review and meta-analysis of randomized trials. J Orthop Surg Res 2017;12(1):100. https://doi.org/10.1186/s13018-017-0601-4.

65. Nielsen NI, Kehlet H, Gromov K, et al. Preoperative high-dose Steroids in total knee and hip arthroplasty - protocols for three randomized controlled trials. Acta Anaesthesiol Scand 2020;64(9):1350–6. https://doi.org/10.1111/aas.13656.

66. Schmidt SC, Hamann S, Langrehr JM, et al. Preoperative high-dose steroid administration attenuates the surgical stress response following liver resection: results of a prospective randomized study. J Hepatobiliary Pancreat Surg 2007; 14(5):484–92. https://doi.org/10.1007/s00534-006-1200-7.

67. Yamashita Y, Shimada M, Hamatsu T, et al. Effects of preoperative steroid administration on surgical stress in hepatic resection: prospective randomized trial. Arch Surg 2001;136(3):328–33. https://doi.org/10.1001/archsurg.136.3.328.

68. Nagori SA, Jose A, Roy ID, et al. Does methylprednisolone improve postoperative outcomes after mandibular third molar surgery? A systematic review and meta-analysis. Int J Oral Maxillofac Surg 2019;48(6):787–800. https://doi.org/10.1016/j.ijom.2018.09.005.

69. Sauerland S, Nagelschmidt M, Mallmann P, et al. Risks and benefits of preoperative high dose methylprednisolone in surgical patients. Drug Saf 2000;23:449–61.

70. POISE Study Group, Devereaux PJ, Yang H, Yusuf S, et al. Effects of extended-release metoprolol succinate in patients undergoing non-cardiac surgery (POISE trial): a randomised controlled trial. Lancet 2008;371(9627):1839–47. https://doi.org/10.1016/S0140-6736(08)60601-7.

71. Blessberger H, Lewis SR, Pritchard MW, et al. Perioperative beta-blockers for preventing surgery-related mortality and morbidity in adults undergoing non-cardiac surgery. Cochrane Database Syst Rev 2019;9(9):CD013438. https://doi.org/10.1002/14651858.CD013438.

72. Devereaux PJ, Sessler DI, Leslie K, et al. Clonidine in patients undergoing noncardiac surgery. N Engl J Med 2014;370(16):1504–13.

73. Andersen LPH, Werner MU, Rosenberg J, et al. A systematic review of perioperative melatonin. Anaesthesia 2014;69:1163–71.

Opioid-Sparing Perioperative Analgesia Within Enhanced Recovery Programs

Matthew D. McEvoy, MD[a,b,]*, Britany L. Raymond, MD[a,b],
Anton Krige, MBChB, DIMC, FRCA, FFICM[c]

KEYWORDS

- Opioid • Nonopioid • Opioid-sparing • Multimodal • Analgesia • Recovery
- Side effects • Intravenous

KEY POINTS

- Opioid-based analgesia can provide excellent pain control but exposes the patient to avoidable side effects and complications.
- Optimal analgesia is an approach that targets the fastest functional recovery with adequate pain control while minimizing side effects.
- Opioid-sparing analgesia appears to be of benefit in the perioperative period.
- Many different options for nonopioid multimodal analgesia exist and have been shown to be efficacious, with certain modalities being more beneficial for specific surgeries.

INTRODUCTION

Perioperative pain management plays a central role in functional recovery after surgery and can be related to overall patient satisfaction with the surgical and anesthesia experience.[1,2] Although opioids are extremely effective to treat pain, they do so at the expense of adverse side effects that can interfere with functional recovery.[3] In addition, acute exposure to opioids in the perioperative period can also lead to the long-term risk of developing persistent postoperative opioid use (PPOU).[1,4] Recognition of these drawbacks has prompted providers to shift away from opioid-only based regimens and has encouraged the exploration of alternative analgesic strategies.

[a] Department of Anesthesiology, Vanderbilt University School of Medicine, 1301 Medical Center Drive, TVC 4619, Nashville, TN 37221, USA; [b] Perioperative Medicine Fellowship, Hi-RiSE Perioperative Optimization Clinic, Perioperative Consult Service, VUMC ERAS Executive Steering Committee, Vanderbilt University Medical Center, 1301 Medical Center Drive, TVC 4648, Nashville, TN 37232, USA; [c] Department of Anaesthesia and Critical Care, Royal Blackburn Teaching Hospital, Haslingden Road, Blackburn BB2 3HH, UK
* Corresponding author. 1301 Medical Center Drive, TVC 4648, Nashville, TN 37232.
E-mail address: matthew.d.mcevoy@vumc.org

Anesthesiology Clin 40 (2022) 35–58
https://doi.org/10.1016/j.anclin.2021.11.001
1932-2275/22/© 2022 Elsevier Inc. All rights reserved.
anesthesiology.theclinics.com

Abbreviations	
ERP	Enhanced Recovery Program
NOMA	non-opioid multimodal analgesia
PPOU	persistent postoperative opioid use
CWIC	continuous wound infiltration catheters
TEA	thoracic epidural analgesia
RCT	randomized controlled trial

The concept of an Enhanced Recovery Program (ERP) is a multicomponent approach aimed at reducing the stress of surgery experienced by the patient and improving the metabolic response, thereby speeding the return of functional recovery.[5] One of the central principles of ERP is the application of nonopioid multimodal analgesic (NOMA) interventions to reduce the reliance on opioid-based medications.[5] ERPs provide a framework to decrease the amount of perioperative opioids used while still targeting excellent pain control. Compared with traditional care, ERPs have been shown to successfully reduce perioperative opioid use and complications while still providing adequate analgesia.[6] This is particularly important in the opioid epidemic era, as clinicians are looking for guidance on the management of acute postoperative pain and the appropriate use of opioids.

Recent consensus statements have discussed potential strategies to address acute postoperative pain management with focus on preventing PPOU, and the feasibility and relative merits, if any, of opioid-free anesthesia and analgesia for ERPs.[4,6–8] Specifically, the reports noted that opioid-free, or at least opioid-minimizing, ERP care pathways are feasible and able to be used in routine practice. Opioid reduction has been associated with reduced postoperative ileus and length of stay.[9,10] In light of recent, conflicting reports of the effect of some multimodal agents, such as gabapentinoids, on postoperative complications,[11,12] and the recent report that opioid-free analgesia may be associated with harm,[13] it is important to consider the evidence behind a practical approach to appropriate opioid minimization in the perioperative period.

Within any ERP, the goal should be to deliver "optimal" or "effective" analgesia, which has been defined as a "technique that optimizes patient comfort and facilitates functional recovery with the fewest medication side effects," regardless of the particular analgesics used (**Fig. 1**).[7] It has been noted that this may not correspond with the lowest pain score possible, which is important to discuss with patients during the preoperative education phase. As such, a practical goal is that the pain is "tolerable," which is best defined as not keeping the patient from sleeping, not waking the patient from sleep, and not inhibiting them from participating in their recovery (eg, drinking, eating, ambulating). In short, the goal is to reduce pain interference in the recovery process while also preventing side effects from the analgesics used. Thus, the approach to treating pain should be multifaceted, including a combination of techniques such as neural blockade, intravenous (IV), and oral multimodal analgesia. The overall combination of analgesic components is not as important as targeting the goal of optimal/effective analgesia.

However, opioids have been the backbone for treating perioperative pain and are still used extensively, if not exclusively, in most surgical specialties. In light of the fact that opioids are excellent analgesics, many perioperative physicians may ask why there is such a focus on opioid minimization or elimination from perioperative care. In short, *minimizing opioid analgesia for patients reduces the adverse effects of opioid use.* The short-term side effects of opioids, including nausea, vomiting, ileus,

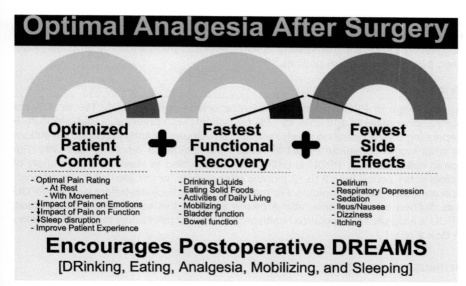

Fig. 1. Optimal analgesia. This figure illustrates the core components of providing optimal analgesia. Pain after surgery can have profound effects on patient recovery. However, the complete elimination of pain may also have untoward effects, as listed in the figure. Optimal analgesia after surgery is an approach to pain control that facilitates a positive patient experience through optimized patient comfort that facilitates functional recovery while minimizing adverse drug events. (Reproduced with permission from POQI, www. thepoqi.org.)

urinary retention, and somnolence can cause patient distress and delay enteral intake, mobilization, and hospital discharge in the surgical patient.[14] In addition, postoperative delirium (itself a risk factor for the development of dementia and longer-term cognitive dysfunction) in the elderly patient is a frequent complication that delays discharge and can be caused both by uncontrolled pain and its treatment with opioids.[15–17] Finally, traditional use of an opioid-based pain management regimen is likely to be associated with developing tolerance and hyperalgesia.[14] In contrast, non–opioid-based approaches may reduce the incidence of developing chronic postsurgical pain, and could potentially decrease the recurrence of and increase survival for certain cancers based on tumor biology, although there is conflicting data concerning the latter.[18,19] These advantages have led to the adoption of a multifaceted approach using various analgesic components to greatly reduce the need to give any opioids during the perioperative period. For all the reasons detailed earlier, opioid-sparing pathways should be considered a best practice.[20]

PERSISTENT POSTOPERATIVE OPIOID USE
Epidemiology

In light of the opioid epidemic in the United States and many other countries, anesthesiologists and surgeons are uniquely positioned to play a significant role in reducing opioid use for surgical patients, for whom opioids continue to be first-line analgesic agents while nonopioid medications are inconsistently prescribed.[1,2] Crucially, several studies suggest that surgery is associated with an increased risk of long-term opioid use, a phenomenon known as PPOU.[3,4] As such, efforts to reduce the risk of PPOU can have a direct effect on opioid use at the population level. In addition, decreasing the risk of PPOU could also have indirect benefits on population-level opioid use by reducing the incidence of diversion and overdose, particularly in the light of studies suggesting a substantial amount of opioid overprescription and large amounts of unused pills among surgical patients.[5,6,7]

Incidence

A wide range of PPOU rates have been reported—approximately 1% to 20% for opioid-naïve patients and 35% to 77% for patients with previous opioid exposure—depending on the definition used. Kent and colleagues recently proposed definitions of what would constitute PPOU to reduce this incidence reporting variability. For opioid-naïve patients, PPOU is defined as having filled at least a 60-day supply of opioid in the period from 3 to 12 months after surgery, which allows for normal postoperative weaning from opioids. For patients who used opioids before surgery, PPOU was defined as an increase above baseline during this same period. Regardless, PPOU is a significant population health problem. Major risk factors for PPOU are listed in **Box 1**.

DEFINING ERP STRATEGIES

A key component of developing an analgesic strategy for an ERP is to be clear on the goal and the overall approach. As such, definitions for terms such as opioid-based, opioid-sparing, and opioid-free analgesia are important when applied operationally to patient care. Traditional perioperative pain management was *opioid-based*, meaning that the primary medications used for analgesia were opioids, and nonopioid therapies were seldomly used in a scheduled or structured fashion. In contrast, the current trend in perioperative care includes a massive reduction in the use of opioid-based patient-controlled analgesia (PCA) regimens.[21] *Opioid-free* analgesia is an approach to pain management that strictly avoids the use of opioids, which is sometimes confused as a goal rather than a strategy. There have been reported successes with this approach, and early evidence suggested that not only can this strategy be used in routine practice, but pain scores and patient satisfaction may be better.[6] Nonetheless, total abstinence from opioid use does not ensure an uncomplicated postoperative course, as nonopioid analgesics can also be associated with side effects that inhibit surgical recovery. Finally, *opioid-sparing* strategies promote structured and

---

Box 1
Risk factors for persistent postoperative opioid use

Preoperative opioid use

History of psychiatric disorder

History of substance use disorder

Presence of preoperative pain conditions

History of smoking

Type of surgery
  Total knee arthroplasty
  Thoracotomy—open or video-assisted
  Breast surgery
  Spine surgery
  Craniotomy

scheduled use of NOMAs, including regional and neuraxial analgesia, to achieve the goal of optimal analgesia. However, the judicious use of opioids is not viewed as a failure, and if opioids are required, there are clear guidelines for doing so.[20,22]

APPROACH TO AN OPIOID-SPARING ERP

A practical approach to implementing an opioid-sparing strategy is to adhere to the principle that nonopioid agents are used first, used in a scheduled manner, and discontinued last (**Fig. 2**). Conversely, opioids are used last, used only as needed, and discontinued first. To deliver optimal analgesia using such a strategy, a well-structured and planned multimodal approach should be constructed that covers the entire perioperative care arc, from the preoperative period into the postdischarge recovery phase (**Fig. 3**).[7,8] It should be noted that the literature is replete with a wide variety of successful opioid-sparing analgesic combinations across many types of surgery.[21,23–25] From the published literature to date, it would appear that reducing opioid use is beneficial in the perioperative period, and high compliance with opioid-sparing ERP care pathways is strongly associated with an overall reduction in opioid consumption and improved patient outcomes. In the following discussion, we present an overview of the most recent data on a wide variety of nonopioid analgesic options, including information about the benefits of use and areas of controversy. In the accompanying tables, we will present a summary of which components have been associated with opioid reduction for specific types of surgery.

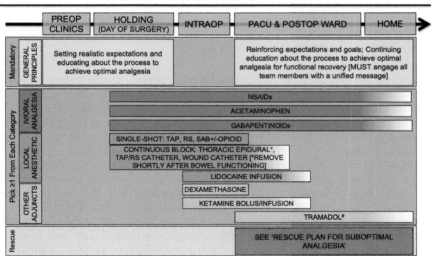

TREATMENT ALGORITHM FOR ACHIEVING OPTIMAL ANALGESIA AFTER COLORECTAL SURGERY

Fig. 2. Multimodal plan within ERAS. This figure illustrates suggested components of a multimodal approach to pain management in an ERP for colorectal surgery. Of note, the plan should be comprehensive, encompassing all phases of perioperative care from preoperative to postdischarge. However, current evidence is insufficient to determine how many components should be selected to maximize pain control, reduce opioid burden, and avoid the side effects of all analgesics used. See **Table 1** for specific dosing recommendations for different analgesic components. ERP, Enhanced Recovery Pathway. (Reproduced with permission from POQI, www.thepoqi.org.)

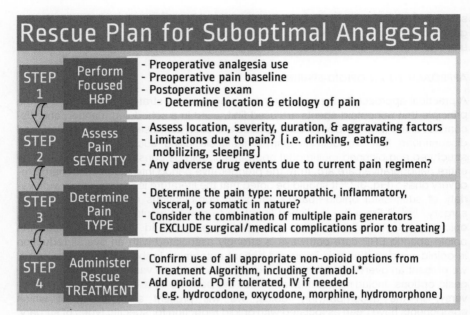

Fig. 3. Structured rescue plan. This figure illustrates a structured approach as a rescue plan for a patient experiencing suboptimal pain control. Except in extreme cases, this step-by-step process should lead to appropriate management that continues the principles being used with the goal of delivering optimal analgesia. See **Table 1** for specific dosing recommendations for different analgesic components.

MULTIMODAL ANALGESIA
Primary Options—Regional Anesthesia/Analgesia

Neuraxial analgesia
Thoracic epidural analgesia. Compared with parenteral opioid-based analgesia, thoracic epidural analgesia (TEA) has been shown to be associated with superior postoperative pain control,[26,27] reduced pulmonary morbidity,[28] and earlier return of bowel function for open abdominal surgery.[29,30] However, in the era of minimally invasive surgery, the overall benefit of TEA for patients undergoing laparoscopic colorectal procedures is uncertain.[31,32] From a practical perspective, using TEA as a routine care component of ERPs for open abdominal surgery is of benefit.[33] In addition, TEA may be particularly beneficial for specific populations, such as those with significant pulmonary disease or a history of chronic pain.[34] To ensure that TEA does not prolong the length of stay, it is prudent to have a plan to wean the infusion and remove the catheter within 2 to 4 days after surgery, depending on the typical recovery timeline (eg, colorectal surgery [CRS] vs Whipple) while supplementing with oral, nonopioid multimodal agents as soon as possible in the postoperative period. Whether TEA can be supplanted by other regional techniques, such as rectus sheath catheters (RSCs), is being investigated.[35] This is important to note as recent meta-analyses have reported TEA failure rates as high as 30% in some centers and that ~20% of patients experience postoperative hypotension, a complication increasingly known to be associated with acute kidney and myocardial injury.[36–39]

Intrathecal opioids. Two meta-analyses of randomized controlled trials (RCTs) have reported that the use of a single-shot of intrathecal hydrophilic opioid (eg, morphine, hydromorphone, and diamorphine) is associated with significantly lower pain scores and reduced opioid requirements.[40,41] These benefits are likely more pronounced in patients undergoing abdominal surgery as opposed to other types of surgery. Interestingly, these meta-analyses included studies covering large dose ranges (100–4000 µg). Current research and practice trends suggest that lower doses are more commonly used (eg, <300 µg) because of dose-dependent side effects and respiratory depression.[42] Of note, this finding was replicated in the most recent meta-analysis on intrathecal opioids, but only with intrathecal morphine doses of greater than 500 µg[41] From a practical perspective, some centers use a spinal dose of bupivacaine as a carrier for the opioid and to cover the stimulation and pain from the incision in the immediate perioperative period; there is often a resulting sympathetic block that can require management of hypotension intraoperatively; however, this is typically not severe. There is a practical benefit of hybrid techniques where intrathecal opiates are used to provide visceral analgesia and then truncal blocks without or with continuous infusion catheters are used for somatic pain. This is becoming a more common approach in the United Kingdom for nonseptic emergency laparotomy or rescue of laparoscopic colorectal cases converted to open and is gaining traction in North America as well.

Truncal and chest wall plane blocks
Advances in ultrasound technology have led to an exponential rise in the incorporation of truncal and chest wall blocks for routine analgesia of abdominal and thoracic surgery (**Table 1**).[43] Meta-analyses indicate that truncal blocks for abdominal surgical procedures are associated with superior analgesia and decreased postoperative opioid consumption compared with opioid analgesia alone.[44–48] Some of these blocks are technically simple to perform and have minimal side effects and complications (eg, rectus sheath and erector spinae), while some are quite challenging (eg, quadratus lumborum). Some studies have boasted equivocal analgesic efficacy compared with neuraxial analgesia, although data are mixed.[49–51] Although wound infiltration offers similar short-term analgesia, these plane blocks provide superior long-term analgesia in the setting of a multimodal analgesic regimen.[52,53] The placement of these blocks preoperatively, rather than postoperatively, may offer some benefit in terms of early analgesia and opioid consumption.[54] However, the full impact of preoperative versus postoperative placement on longer-term outcomes remains unknown.

Concerning the choice of local anesthetic, ropivacaine, bupivacaine, and liposomal bupivacaine have all been used in ERPs with good results, although liposomal formulations have recently been challenged.[55–58] In short, the latest evidence would suggest

Table 1		
Examples of chest wall and truncal blocks		
Chest Wall		Paravertebral
		PECs (PECtoralis and serratus plane blocks)
		Erector spinae plane (ESP)
		Transversus thoracis plane
Truncal/ Abdominal Wall		Paravertebral
		Q Quadratus lumborum blocks (QL)
		Transversus abdominus plane (TAP) blocks/catheter
		Rectus sheath block/catheters (RSC)
		Wound infiltration and continuous wound infusion catheters (CWIC)

that there is no difference when using any of these local anesthetic formulations. However, it should be noted that additives, such as dexamethasone, epinephrine, and opioids, are effective at prolonging the duration of regional blocks.[59]

Continuous wound infiltration catheters

Continuous wound infiltration catheters (CWICs) offer sustained postoperative analgesia through wound infiltration analgesia using specially designed wound soaker catheters.[60] RSCs seem to be superior to them for midline in at least 1 RCT but they have the advantage of simplicity for 2 reasons. First, the surgeon can place them into the length of the wound in the preperitoneal space before closing. Second, CWICs can be used in any wound orientation, unlike RSC, which are for midline incisions only. A practical example of this is used as a rescue technique in laparoscopic hepatobiliary surgery that gets converted to an open approach. At the start of the case, one might use intrathecal opiate and IV lidocaine as primary analgesia; then, once converted to open the surgeon could place CWIC in the incisions that are often subcostal or in a "hockey stick" shape and the lidocaine infusion could be discontinued.

Tables 2 and 3 delineate details for how these regional anesthesia techniques can be applied for various operations.

Nonopioid Adjuvants

Lidocaine

IV lidocaine infusions are effective to reduce systemic inflammation and are indicated as part of a multimodal analgesic approach for visceral surgery when other local anesthetic approaches such as regional analgesia are not possible. In open and laparoscopic abdominal surgery, IV lidocaine infusions have been shown to result in a significant reduction in postoperative pain intensity at rest, with cough, and movement, as well as opioid consumption for up to 48 hours postoperatively.[61–64] From a functional recovery perspective, IV lidocaine infusions are associated with earlier return of bowel function and shorter length of stay.[61–64] Lidocaine infusions should be used with caution in patients with any cardiovascular instability and concomitant use of alpha agonists or certain beta-blockers (eg, sotalol), and in patients with allergies to other amide local anesthetics. Side effects are more pronounced in patients with liver dysfunction, pulmonary diseases when the predominant problem is carbon dioxide retention, and congestive heart failure. Lidocaine is typically administered as a bolus (100–150 mg or 1.5–2.0 mg/kg) followed by an infusion of 1 to 2 mg/kg/h through the end of surgery. The most recent meta-analyses suggest that continued perioperative administration of IV lidocaine is associated with a decrease in postoperative pain and opioid consumption and possibly faster return of bowel function and decreased length of hospital stay.[65–67] Of note, the ALLEGRO study, which is nearing the end of recruitment in the United Kingdom, is a large multicenter NIHR funded study of lidocaine versus placebo in CRS with primary end-point reduction in ileus/speed return of bowel function. The results of the trial have the potential to standardize the use of lidocaine as prophylaxis for ileus in CRS, which remains the greatest factor in the prolonged length of stay (https://srmrc.nihr.ac.uk/trials/allegro-2/).

N-methyl-ᴅ-aspartate antagonists

Ketamine. Perioperative inhibition of N-methyl-ᴅ-aspartate (NMDA) receptors with clinically available NMDA antagonists such as ketamine may be associated with improved perioperative pain and decreased opioid use.[68–71] Ketamine has also been shown to be of particular benefit in patients on chronic opioids, but this has not been specifically tested in chronic pain patients undergoing CRS.[72] Perioperative

Table 2
Suggested use of local anesthetics in blocks and intravenous by type of elective surgery

	IT LA ± opioid ± LA in joint	TEA	RSC	CWIC (catheter infusion in surgical donor site)	IV Lidocaine gtt	Hybrid – Intrathecal opiate + RSC	Hybrid – Intrathecal opiate + CWIC
Oesophagectomy		X					
Major colorectal—laparo/open transverse	X				X		
Major colorectal—open midline		X	X			X	X
Major liver resection—laparoscopic	X				X		
Major liver resection—open		X					X
Whipple (pancreatectomy)—laparo	X				X		
Whipple (pancreatectomy)—open		X					X
Radical cystectomy—laparo with Pfannestiel	X				X		
Radical cystectomy—open midline		X				X	X
Major open vascular		X					
Major gynae—laparo/open transverse	X				X		
Major gynae—open midline		X				X	X
Hip/Knee replacement	X						
Radical neck dissection with free flap				X			
Radical neck dissection w/o free flap					X		

Abbreviations: FI, fascia iliaca; gtt, infusion; IT, intrathecal; LA, local anesthetic; SIFI, suprainguinal fascia iliaca.

Table 3
Suggested use of local anesthetics in blocks and intravenous by type of emergency surgery

	Spinal (LA+Opioid)	TEA	RSC	CWIC	IV Lidocaine gtt	Hybrid–Intrathecal Opiate + RSC	Hybrid – Intrathecal Opiate + CWIC	Peripheral Nerve Block Infusion – Surgically Placed	Facscia Iliaca Block (FI or SIFI)
Emergency midline laparotomy	X	X	X	X	X	X			
Neck of femur	X								X
Vascular surgery amputations	X	X						X	

ketamine, including boluses as well as intraoperative and postoperative low-dose infusions for up to 48 hours, has been shown to result in significant reductions in pain, opioid consumption, and postoperative nausea and vomiting (PONV) with no significant side effect profile.[73–75] The intraoperative boluses ranged from 0.15 to 1 mg/kg and perioperative infusions ranged from 1 to 5 µg/kg/min, with a postoperative infusion rate of 2.5 mcg/kg/min.

Magnesium. Systemic infusions of perioperative magnesium may reduce postoperative pain and opioid consumption.[76–78] The optimal dosing is uncertain, as some studies include both a bolus followed by an infusion, whereas others only use an infusion without a loading bolus. Typical boluses are 30 to 50 mg/kg and the infusion rates range from 4 to 15 mg/kg/h. None of the studies in a systematic review reported clinical toxicity related to toxic serum levels of magnesium.[76]

Memantine. Although traditionally used in the treatment of Alzheimer dementia, memantine has recently emerged as a nonopioid analgesic alternative.[79] It is a long-acting NMDA antagonist with a half-life between 60 and 80 hours.[80] It also has a lower side effect profile and is generally better tolerated than ketamine.[81] Memantine preferentially binds to pathologically active channels, suggesting promise in areas of opioid-induced hyperalgesia and central sensitization.[82,83] Although most data support its use for chronic neuropathic pain[84–86] and fibromyalgia,[87,88] it is gaining popularity in the perioperative setting. The limited evidence available is promising, showing reductions in pain intensity and analgesic consumption.[89,90] It can also be used as an oral agent to help transition patients from ketamine infusions.[82]

Steroids
Glucocorticoid steroids may have analgesic benefits possibly related to anti-inflammatory properties and should be considered as part of a multimodal perioperative pain regimen. Several meta-analyses examined perioperative dexamethasone and indicated that patients who received dexamethasone (4–10 mg or >0.1 mg/kg) had lower pain scores, used less opioids, and required less rescue analgesia.[91–93] Glucocorticoids are also powerful antiemetics, thus providing an additional value to ERPs.[94] The concern for significant hyperglycemia (>180 mg/dL) has not been confirmed, even in bariatric patients receiving these doses of dexamethasone.[95] Meta-analysis review revealed glucocorticoid administration only slightly increases average peak glucose concentrations by 20 mg/dL, which is unlikely to have a significant clinical impact.[96] In addition, this same analysis addressed the theoretic concerns of immunosuppression and determined the concerns for wound infection were unfounded.

Acetaminophen (paracetamol)
Acetaminophen (paracetamol), when administered as part of a multimodal regimen, is associated with a significant reduction in pain and opioid usage, which may result in a decrease in some opioid-related side effects.[97–103] One meta-analysis concerning studies using a single dose of IV acetaminophen (paracetamol, typically 1g) given before surgery was associated with significantly lower early pain at rest and movement, postoperative opioid consumption, and PONV versus placebo.[98] A separate meta-analysis concerning studies using 1g or 15 mg/kg of IV acetaminophen (paracetamol) given 10 to 30 minutes before induction/incision (vs the same dose given 10–30 min before the end of surgery/before skin closure) was associated with a reduction in 24-h opioid consumption and a lower incidence of postoperative vomiting in the preventive acetaminophen (paracetamol) group.[97] Some studies including

pharmacokinetic outcomes reported higher postoperative plasma concentrations and larger proportions of patients achieving target plasma concentrations after IV dosing compared with oral dosing.[104] However, for patients who can take oral medications preoperatively, there does not appear to be evidence of a clear benefit of the IV formulation if the oral dose is given 30 to 60 minutes to surgery.[104] As such, decision-making should take into account both convenience and cost.[104]

Nonsteroidal anti-inflammatory drugs

Nonsteroidal anti-inflammatory drugs (NSAIDs), whether nonselective or selective cyclooxygenase-2 inhibitors (COX-2), when administered as part of a multimodal regimen, are associated with a reduction in pain and opioid usage, which may result in a decrease in some opioid-related side effects.[105–110] A systematic review noted that preoperative COX-2 inhibitors significantly reduced postoperative pain, analgesic consumption, antiemetic use, and improved patient satisfaction compared with preoperative placebo.[107] In the studies examining celecoxib, the doses used were 200 or 400 mg PO, and for parecoxib, they were 40 mg PO.[111]

The use of COX-2 inhibitors has minimal effect on coagulation, even at supratherapeutic doses.[112] However, it is uncertain whether the perioperative use of NSAIDs carries additional risk of harm. Although it is unlikely that NSAIDs increase the risk of renal injury in euvolemic patients who do not have contraindications to receiving these medications,[113] caution should be undertaken in patients who are hypotensive or thought to be hypovolemic. In addition, there is a concern for the potential for an association with increased anastomotic leak, but the literature surrounding this question is inconclusive and some studies show no risk of harm specifically in an ERP for CRS.[114,115] As such, insufficient evidence is available to recommend against routine use of NSAIDs, especially COX-2 inhibitors, as these medications are effective in treating pain and reducing opioid use in the perioperative period.[116,117]

Gabapentinoids

Several meta-analyses including studies concerning intra-abdominal surgery suggest that gabapentinoids (gabapentin and pregabalin) when given as a single dose preoperatively are associated with a decrease in postoperative pain and opioid consumption at 24 hours.[118–124] For gabapentin, a preoperative dose of 300 to 1200 mg is associated with lower pain scores (both at rest and with movement) and reduced opioid consumption.[120,122,123] It should be noted that one small RCT found that a single preoperative dose of gabapentin 600 mg PO did not significantly reduce opioid consumption or pain scores on postoperative day 1 or 2 for patients presenting for colectomy.[125] However, opioid consumption and pain scores were lower at all time points in the gabapentin group compared with placebo, but there were only 36 patients per group and it was underpowered to detect any difference. As noted by the authors, continuing doses in the postoperative period may confer added benefit given the pharmacokinetics of gabapentin. This corresponds with the dosing regimens reported in successful ERPs for CRS where gabapentin is used as one component to reduce opioid consumption in the perioperative period.[21,25] However, the exact contribution of gabapentin to these positive outcomes is unknown. For pregabalin, a recent meta-analysis indicated that pain scores at rest were reduced with all doses of pregabalin (mostly 75–300 mg) but pain scores with movement were only reduced with the 300 mg dose. There were no significant differences in side effects between the 3 dose levels of pregabalin. The opioid-sparing effect of pregabalin appeared to be limited to doses 100 mg to 300 mg but not ≤75 mg at 2h after surgery.[121] Although most of the studies in the meta-analysis involve abdominal hysterectomy and cholecystectomy, none were in

CRS patients. A more recent meta-analysis found no difference between gabapentinoids and placebo in terms of pain scores.[126] However, the authors did note approximately a 30% reduction in opioid consumption with the use of gabapentinoids, as well as a significant reduction in PONV, while also noting an increase in postoperative dizziness. Overall, the evidence would suggest that gabapentinoids may be of benefit for reducing opioid consumption in the perioperative period, but use can come with an increase in some side effects, which is likely most pronounced in the elderly. From a practical perspective, the institutions at which the authors work use a structured plan for gabapentinoid use and assessment of side effects. These plans recommend standard dosing for adult patients that can be reduced based on renal function and age or possibly increased if the patient takes a larger dose at home on a regular basis.

Alpha-2 adrenergic agonists

A Cochrane review of dexmedetomidine infusions for pain found reduced opioid consumption, but no significant difference in pain scores compared with placebo, and there was more hypotension in the dexmedetomidine group.[127] Dexmedetomidine has been added both perineurally to nerve blocks and intravenously to prolong nerve block.[128,129] However, the extended duration provided by the IV administration of dexmedetomidine is shorter than that provided by perineural administration. A recent extensive review of perioperative alpha agonists comparing dexmedetomidine and clonidine found similar reductions in opioid consumption and weak antiemetic effects, but as expected, both drugs had adverse effects on hemodynamics.[130] In summary, perioperative administration of dexmedetomidine or clonidine can reduce morphine consumption up to 24h and to a similar extent as acetaminophen (paracetamol), but not as much as other NSAIDs. These alpha agonists have other side effects such as sedation and hypotension that have to be considered.[131] Typical dose ranges are 1 to 5 mcg/kg orally, IV or perineurally for clonidine and 0.5 mcg/kg IV bolus followed by an infusion of 0.2 to 0.7 mcg/kg/h or 0.5mcg/kg perineurally for dexmedetomidine.

Special Opioids

Tramadol

Overall, there is limited evidence for the use of tramadol in CRS. However, one study compared postoperative pain control with an opioid IV-PCA to IV tramadol and found that the patients in the non-PCA (tramadol) group needed less rescue analgesia, and none required escalation of analgesic therapy to IV-PCA.[132] In addition, another study included scheduled tramadol as part of an ERP.[133] Although this was only one component of the ERP, overall pain scores and other outcomes were improved. If tramadol is to be used, one study would suggest caution with its use in patients undergoing major abdominal surgery who are more than 75 years, American Society of Anesthesiologists (ASA) 3 or 4, or have impaired mobility or frailty, as use in this setting was associated with delirium.[134] Based on the evidence that exists in CRS, we recommend considering tramadol as an analgesic adjunct.

Methadone

Methadone has a complex pharmacologic profile. It exerts agonist activity at the μ, kappa, and delta-opioid receptors, and functions as an antagonist at NMDA receptors. It has a rapid onset with variable metabolism.[135] The prolonged duration of action of methadone has been used to significantly reduce postoperative opioid consumption.[136–139] A meta-analysis of 10 RCTs demonstrated that methadone results in better patient satisfaction, lower pain scores, and reduced opioid consumption compared with alternative opioid regimens.[140,141] In addition, 2 recent RCTs demonstrated significant reductions in postoperative opioid use and pain in the first few days after surgery and out to 1 year.[141] In short, methadone may be the opioid that helps greatly limit the use of other opioids. The exact role and possible benefit of methadone within ERPs remain to be elucidated.[142]

Practical Implementation

At this point, it is important to consider the practical application of the preceding data for someone implementing an ERP. At a high level, **Fig. 2** illustrates a summary view of perioperative planning and the components to be considered. **Tables 2 and 3** detail how these components can be best used according to the type of surgery and whether it is elective or emergent. **Table 4** displays the recommended dose ranges

Table 4
Recommended dosing strategies by phase of care for nonopioid multimodal analgesics

Analgesic Component	Phase of Care		
	Preoperative	Intraoperative	Postoperative
Oral Medications			
Celecoxib	200-400 mg	n/a	200-400mg q12
Clonidine	0.1-0.3 mg	n/a	0.1-0.3 mg q12h
Gabapentin	300-1200 mg	n/a	300-1200 mg q8h
Ketorolac	20 mg	n/a	10 mg q4-6h
Memantine	5-10 mg	n/a	5-10 mg q12
Paracetamol/ Acetaminophen	1000 mg	n/a	1000 mg q8
Pregabalin	75-300 mg	n/a	75-300 mg q12
Tramadol	50-100 mg	n/a	50-100 mg q4-6h
Intravenous Medications			
Clonidine	n/a	1-5 mcg/kg	n/a
Dexamethasone	n/a	4-10 mg or >0.1mg/kg	n/a
Dexmedetomidine	n/a	0.5 mcg/kg bolus followed by an infusion of 0.2-0.7 mcg/kg/h	0.2-0.7 mcg/kg/h infusion
Ketamine	n/a	0.15-1 mg/kg bolus followed by infusion 1-5 micrograms/kg/min	2-2.5 mcg/kg/min infusion
Ketorolac	15-30 mg		15-30 mg q6h
Lidocaine	n/a	1.5–2.0 mg/kg bolus followed by infusion 2 mg/kg/h	1-2 mg/min infusion
Magnesium	n/a	30-50 mg/kg bolus followed by infusion 4-15 mg/kg/h	4-15 mg/kg/h infusion
Methadone[a]	5-20 mg		n/a
Paracetamol/ Acetaminophen	1000 mg		1000 mg q8h
Parecoxib	40 mg		20-40 mg q12h
Tramadol	50-100 mg		50-100 mg q4-6h

for each analgesic component and any specific contraindications (relative or absolute) that have been reported in routine practice. Finally, any ERP should have a structured plan for rescue analgesia when the typical pathway is not sufficient to meet the needs of the patient.[8] **Fig. 3** provides an example of what a rescue plan should entail, although individual implementations of this may vary by program.

FUTURE DIRECTIONS

Much of the push toward opioid minimization has come through enhanced recovery after surgery (ERAS). However, as some have pointed out, even though many publications and guidelines note that opioid minimization is associated with improved outcomes, many ERAS protocols contain unproven elements in regards to analgesia.[33] As such, future research should include a more thorough investigation of the current components used to reduce opioids and opioid-related adverse events in the perioperative period. Major ongoing RCTs include trials investigating the efficacy of lidocaine and ketamine.[a] As there is debate in the literature as to the benefit (or lack thereof), additional research should also include prospective trials concerning gabapentinoids, NSAIDs, muscle relaxants, and other commonly used nonopioid analgesic components. Finally, as opioid-free anesthesia and analgesia may work for some patients, research on the role of methadone as an opioid-sparing opioid within ERPs is warranted.[142]

SUMMARY

Traditional opioid-based analgesia in the perioperative period can provide excellent pain control, but this approach exposes the patient to avoidable side effects and possible harm. Optimal analgesia within an ERP, an approach that targets the fastest functional recovery with adequate pain control while minimizing side effects, can be achieved with opioid minimization. Many different options for nonopioid multimodal analgesia exist and have been shown to be efficacious, with certain modalities being more beneficial for specific surgeries. However, much research remains to be done to better define the optimal approach for opioid minimization to maximize patient outcomes.

CLINICS CARE POINTS

- Opioid-based analgesia can provide excellent pain control, yet exposes the patient to avoidable side effects and complications
- Optimal analgesia is an approach that targets the fastest functional recovery with adequate pain control while minimizing side effects
- Opioid-sparing analgesia appears to be of benefit in the perioperative period
- Many different options for nonopioid multimodal analgesia exist and have been shown to be efficacious, with certain modalities being more beneficial for specific surgeries

---

[a] IMPAKT (https://clinicaltrials.gov/ct2/show/NCT04625283?term=raymond+and+ketamine&draw=2&rank=1); ROCKET (https://medicine.unimelb.edu.au/research-groups/critical-care-research/critcare/about-us/the-rocket-study); and Lidocaine (https://clinicaltrials.gov/ct2/show/NCT04176419?term=lidocaine+AND+intraoperative&recrs=a&cntry=US&draw=2&rank=6).

DISCLOSURE

Dr M.D. McEvoy receives consultant fees for work on the Takeda Pharmaceuticals Scientific Advisory Board; Drs B.L. Raymond and A. Krige have nothing to disclose.

Neuraxial and Regional Blocks	Intrathecal	Epidural	Perineural
Clonidine	15-75 mcg	1-2 mcg/kg	150-300 mcg
Dexmedetomidine	5 mcg	1 mcg/kg	50–60 mcg
Dexamethasone	4-8 mg	4-10 mg	4 mg
Epinephrine	100-200 mcg	1-5 mcg/mL	100-300 mcg

[a] Studies performed with methadone versus other opioids have typically used doses of 10-20 mg IV, but some have gone as high as (0.3mg/kg); use of lower doses of opioids may be needed if other adjuncts are used but lower doses of methadone are also noted to have pharmacokinetics/dynamics similar to hydromorphone rather than what is achieved with higher doses of methadone and longer half-lives.

REFERENCES

1. Wu CL, Naqibuddin M, Rowlingson AJ, et al. The effect of pain on health-related quality of life in the immediate postoperative period. Anesth Analg 2003;97: 1078–85, table of contents.
2. Dihle A, Helseth S, Paul SM, et al. The exploration of the establishment of cut-points to categorize the severity of acute postoperative pain. Clin J Pain 2006;22:617–24.
3. Benyamin R, Trescot AM, Datta S, et al. Opioid complications and side effects. Pain Physician 2008;11:S105–20.
4. Kent ML, Hurley RW, Oderda GM, et al. American Society for Enhanced Recovery and Perioperative Quality Initiative-4 Joint Consensus Statement on Persistent Postoperative Opioid Use: Definition, Incidence, Risk Factors, and Health Care System Initiatives. Anesth Analg 2019;129:543–52.
5. Kehlet H, Wilmore DW. Evidence-based surgical care and the evolution of fast-track surgery. Ann Surg 2008;248:189–98.
6. Wu CL, King AB, Geiger TM, et al. Fourth Perioperative Quality Initiative W: American Society for Enhanced Recovery and Perioperative Quality Initiative Joint Consensus Statement on Perioperative Opioid Minimization in Opioid-Naive Patients. Anesth Analg 2019;129:567–77.
7. McEvoy MD, Scott MJ, Gordon DB, et al. Perioperative Quality Initiative IW: American Society for Enhanced Recovery (ASER) and Perioperative Quality Initiative (POQI) joint consensus statement on optimal analgesia within an enhanced recovery pathway for colorectal surgery: part 1-from the preoperative period to PACU. Perioper Med (Lond) 2017;6:8.
8. Scott MJ, McEvoy MD, Gordon DB, et al. Perioperative Quality Initiative IW: American Society for Enhanced Recovery (ASER) and Perioperative Quality Initiative (POQI) Joint Consensus Statement on Optimal Analgesia within an Enhanced Recovery Pathway for Colorectal Surgery: Part 2-From PACU to the Transition Home. Perioper Med (Lond) 2017;6:7.
9. Keller DS, Zhang J, Chand M. Opioid-free colorectal surgery: a method to improve patient & financial outcomes in surgery. Surg Endosc 2019;33:1959–66.

10. Alhashemi M, Fiore JF Jr, Safa N, et al. Incidence and predictors of prolonged postoperative ileus after colorectal surgery in the context of an enhanced recovery pathway. Surg Endosc 2019;33:2313–22.

11. Quail J, Spence D, Hannon M. Perioperative Gabapentin Improves Patient-Centered Outcomes After Inguinal Hernia Repair. Mil Med 2017;182:e2052–5.

12. Cozowicz C, Bekeris J, Poeran J, et al. Multimodal Pain Management and Postoperative Outcomes in Lumbar Spine Fusion Surgery: A Population-based Cohort Study. Spine (Phila Pa 1976) 2020;45:580–9.

13. Beloeil H, Garot M, Lebuffe G, et al. Balanced Opioid-free Anesthesia with Dexmedetomidine versus Balanced Anesthesia with Remifentanil for Major or Intermediate Noncardiac Surgery. Anesthesiology 2021;134:541–51.

14. Wanderer JP, Nathan N. Opioids and Adverse Effects: More Than Just Opium Dreams. Anesth Analg 2016;123:805.

15. Oresanya LB, Lyons WL, Finlayson E. Preoperative assessment of the older patient: a narrative review. JAMA 2014;311:2110–20.

16. Bilotta F, Lauretta MP, Borozdina A, et al. Postoperative delirium: risk factors, diagnosis and perioperative care. Minerva Anestesiol 2013;79:1066–76.

17. Leung JM, Sands LP, Lim E, et al. Does preoperative risk for delirium moderate the effects of postoperative pain and opiate use on postoperative delirium? Am J Geriatr Psychiatry 2013;21:946–56.

18. Hayhurst CJ, Durieux ME. Differential Opioid Tolerance and Opioid-induced Hyperalgesia: A Clinical Reality. Anesthesiology 2016;124:483–8.

19. Maher DP, White PF. Proposed mechanisms for association between opioid usage and cancer recurrence after surgery. J Clin Anesth 2016;28:36–40.

20. Shanthanna H, Ladha KS, Kehlet H, et al. Perioperative Opioid Administration. Anesthesiology 2021;134:645–59.

21. McEvoy MD, Wanderer JP, King AB, et al. A perioperative consult service results in reduction in cost and length of stay for colorectal surgical patients: evidence from a healthcare redesign project. Perioper Med (Lond) 2016;5:3.

22. Koepke EJ, Manning EL, Miller TE, et al. The rising tide of opioid use and abuse: the role of the anesthesiologist. Perioper Med (Lond) 2018;7:16.

23. Thiele RH, Rea KM, Turrentine FE, et al. Standardization of care: impact of an enhanced recovery protocol on length of stay, complications, and direct costs after colorectal surgery. J Am Coll Surg 2015;220:430–43.

24. Miller TE, Thacker JK, White WD, et al. Enhanced Recovery Study G: Reduced length of hospital stay in colorectal surgery after implementation of an enhanced recovery protocol. Anesth Analg 2014;118:1052–61.

25. Larson DW, Lovely JK, Cima RR, et al. Outcomes after implementation of a multimodal standard care pathway for laparoscopic colorectal surgery. Br J Surg 2014;101:1023–30.

26. Werawatganon T, Charuluxanun S. Patient controlled intravenous opioid analgesia versus continuous epidural analgesia for pain after intra-abdominal surgery. Cochrane Database Syst Rev 2005;CD004088.

27. Block BM, Liu SS, Rowlingson AJ, et al. Efficacy of postoperative epidural analgesia: a meta-analysis. JAMA 2003;290:2455–63.

28. Popping DM, Elia N, Van Aken HK, et al. Impact of epidural analgesia on mortality and morbidity after surgery: systematic review and meta-analysis of randomized controlled trials. Ann Surg 2014;259:1056–67.

29. Marret E, Remy C, Bonnet F. Postoperative Pain Forum G: Meta-analysis of epidural analgesia versus parenteral opioid analgesia after colorectal surgery. Br J Surg 2007;94:665–73.

30. Hughes MJ, Ventham NT, McNally S, et al. Analgesia after open abdominal surgery in the setting of enhanced recovery surgery: a systematic review and meta-analysis. JAMA Surg 2014;149:1224–30.

31. Liu H, Hu X, Duan X, et al. Thoracic epidural analgesia (TEA) vs. patient controlled analgesia (PCA) in laparoscopic colectomy: a meta-analysis. Hepato-gastroenterology 2014;61:1213–9.

32. Khan SA, Khokhar HA, Nasr AR, et al. Effect of epidural analgesia on bowel function in laparoscopic colorectal surgery: a systematic review and meta-analysis. Surg Endosc 2013;27:2581–91.

33. Memtsoudis SG, Poeran J, Kehlet H. Enhanced Recovery After Surgery in the United States: From Evidence-Based Practice to Uncertain Science? JAMA 2019;321:1049–50.

34. Prabhu AS, Krpata DM, Perez A, et al. Is It Time to Reconsider Postoperative Epidural Analgesia in Patients Undergoing Elective Ventral Hernia Repair?: An AHSQC Analysis. Ann Surg 2018;267:971–6.

35. Wilkinson KM, Krige A, Brearley SG, et al. Thoracic Epidural analgesia versus Rectus Sheath Catheters for open midline incisions in major abdominal surgery within an enhanced recovery programme (TERSC): study protocol for a randomised controlled trial. Trials 2014;15:400.

36. Hamid HKS, Marc-Hernandez A, Saber AA. Transversus abdominis plane block versus thoracic epidural analgesia in colorectal surgery: a systematic review and meta-analysis. Langenbecks Arch Surg 2021;406:273–82.

37. McEvoy MD, Gupta R, Koepke EJ, et al. Physiology g, Preoperative blood pressure g, Intraoperative blood pressure g, Postoperative blood pressure g: Perioperative Quality Initiative consensus statement on postoperative blood pressure, risk and outcomes for elective surgery. Br J Anaesth 2019;122: 575–86.

38. Sessler DI, Bloomstone JA, Aronson S, et al. Physiology g, Preoperative blood pressure g, Intraoperative blood pressure g, Postoperative blood pressure g: Perioperative Quality Initiative consensus statement on intraoperative blood pressure, risk and outcomes for elective surgery. Br J Anaesth 2019;122: 563–74.

39. Sessler DI, Meyhoff CS, Zimmerman NM, et al. Period-dependent Associations between Hypotension during and for Four Days after Noncardiac Surgery and a Composite of Myocardial Infarction and Death: A Substudy of the POISE-2 Trial. Anesthesiology 2018;128:317–27.

40. Meylan N, Elia N, Lysakowski C, et al. Benefit and risk of intrathecal morphine without local anaesthetic in patients undergoing major surgery: meta-analysis of randomized trials. Br J Anaesth 2009;102:156–67.

41. Koning MV, Klimek M, Rijs K, et al. Intrathecal hydrophilic opioids for abdominal surgery: a meta-analysis, meta-regression, and trial sequential analysis. Br J Anaesth 2020;125:358–72.

42. Gehling M, Tryba M. Risks and side-effects of intrathecal morphine combined with spinal anaesthesia: a meta-analysis. Anaesthesia 2009;64:643–51.

43. Koh WU, Lee JH. Ultrasound-guided truncal blocks for perioperative analgesia. Anesth Pain Med 2018;13:128–42.

44. Baeriswyl M, Kirkham KR, Kern C, et al. The Analgesic Efficacy of Ultrasound-Guided Transversus Abdominis Plane Block in Adult Patients: A Meta-Analysis. Anesth Analg 2015;121:1640–54.

45. Zhao X, Tong Y, Ren H, et al. Transversus abdominis plane block for postoperative analgesia after laparoscopic surgery: a systematic review and meta-analysis. Int J Clin Exp Med 2014;7:2966–75.
46. Johns N, O'Neill S, Ventham NT, et al. Clinical effectiveness of transversus abdominis plane (TAP) block in abdominal surgery: a systematic review and meta-analysis. Colorectal Dis 2012;14:e635–42.
47. Siddiqui MR, Sajid MS, Uncles DR, et al. A meta-analysis on the clinical effectiveness of transversus abdominis plane block. J Clin Anesth 2011;23:7–14.
48. Charlton S, Cyna AM, Middleton P, et al. Perioperative transversus abdominis plane (TAP) blocks for analgesia after abdominal surgery. Cochrane Database Syst Rev 2010;CD007705.
49. Yeung JH, Gates S, Naidu BV, et al. Paravertebral block versus thoracic epidural for patients undergoing thoracotomy. Cochrane Database Syst Rev 2016;2: CD009121.
50. Niraj G, Kelkar A, Hart E, et al. Comparison of analgesic efficacy of four-quadrant transversus abdominis plane (TAP) block and continuous posterior TAP analgesia with epidural analgesia in patients undergoing laparoscopic colorectal surgery: an open-label, randomised, non-inferiority trial. Anaesthesia 2014;69:348–55.
51. Niraj G, Kelkar A, Jeyapalan I, et al. Comparison of analgesic efficacy of subcostal transversus abdominis plane blocks with epidural analgesia following upper abdominal surgery. Anaesthesia 2011;66:465–71.
52. Yu N, Long X, Lujan-Hernandez JR, et al. Transversus abdominis-plane block versus local anesthetic wound infiltration in lower abdominal surgery: a systematic review and meta-analysis of randomized controlled trials. BMC Anesthesiol 2014;14:121.
53. Guo Q, Li R, Wang L, et al. Transversus abdominis plane block versus local anaesthetic wound infiltration for postoperative analgesia: A systematic review and meta-analysis. Int J Clin Exp Med 2015;8:17343–52.
54. De Oliveira GS Jr, Castro-Alves LJ, Nader A, et al. Transversus abdominis plane block to ameliorate postoperative pain outcomes after laparoscopic surgery: a meta-analysis of randomized controlled trials. Anesth Analg 2014;118:454–63.
55. Hamada T, Tsuchiya M, Mizutani K, et al. Levobupivacaine - dextran mixture for transversus abdominis plane block and rectus sheath block in patients undergoing laparoscopic colectomy: a randomised controlled trial. Anaesthesia 2016;71:411–6.
56. Cohen SM. Extended pain relief trial utilizing infiltration of Exparel((R)), a long-acting multivesicular liposome formulation of bupivacaine: a Phase IV health economic trial in adult patients undergoing open colectomy. J Pain Res 2012; 5:567–72.
57. Ilfeld BM, Eisenach JC, Gabriel RA. Clinical Effectiveness of Liposomal Bupivacaine Administered by Infiltration or Peripheral Nerve Block to Treat Postoperative Pain. Anesthesiology 2021;134:283–344.
58. Hussain N, Brull R, Sheehy B, et al. Perineural Liposomal Bupivacaine Is Not Superior to Nonliposomal Bupivacaine for Peripheral Nerve Block Analgesia. Anesthesiology 2021;134:147–64.
59. Akkaya A, Yildiz I, Tekelioglu UY, et al. Dexamethasone added to levobupivacaine in ultrasound-guided tranversus abdominis plain block increased the duration of postoperative analgesia after caesarean section: a randomized, double blind, controlled trial. Eur Rev Med Pharmacol Sci 2014;18:717–22.

60. Hughes MJ, Harrison EM, Peel NJ, et al. Randomized clinical trial of perioperative nerve block and continuous local anaesthetic infiltration via wound catheter versus epidural analgesia in open liver resection (LIVER 2 trial). Br J Surg 2015; 102:1619–28.

61. Khan JS, Yousuf M, Victor JC, et al. An estimation for an appropriate end time for an intraoperative intravenous lidocaine infusion in bowel surgery: a comparative meta-analysis. J Clin Anesth 2016;28:95–104.

62. Vigneault L, Turgeon AF, Cote D, et al. Perioperative intravenous lidocaine infusion for postoperative pain control: a meta-analysis of randomized controlled trials. Can J Anaesth 2011;58:22–37.

63. McCarthy GC, Megalla SA, Habib AS. Impact of intravenous lidocaine infusion on postoperative analgesia and recovery from surgery: a systematic review of randomized controlled trials. Drugs 2010;70:1149–63.

64. Marret E, Rolin M, Beaussier M, et al. Meta-analysis of intravenous lidocaine and postoperative recovery after abdominal surgery. Br J Surg 2008;95:1331–8.

65. Bi Y, Ye Y, Ma J, et al. Effect of perioperative intravenous lidocaine for patients undergoing spine surgery: A meta-analysis and systematic review. Medicine (Baltimore) 2020;99:e23332.

66. Huang X, Sun Y, Lin D, et al. Effect of perioperative intravenous lidocaine on the incidence of short-term cognitive function after noncardiac surgery: A meta-analysis based on randomized controlled trials. Brain Behav 2020;10:e01875.

67. Cooke C, Kennedy ED, Foo I, et al. Meta-analysis of the effect of perioperative intravenous lidocaine on return of gastrointestinal function after colorectal surgery. Tech Coloproctol 2019;23:15–24.

68. Wang L, Johnston B, Kaushal A, et al. Ketamine added to morphine or hydromorphone patient-controlled analgesia for acute postoperative pain in adults: a systematic review and meta-analysis of randomized trials. Can J Anaesth 2016;63:311–25.

69. Ding X, Jin S, Niu X, et al. Morphine with adjuvant ketamine versus higher dose of morphine alone for acute pain: a meta-analysis. Int J Clin Exp Med 2014;7: 2504–10.

70. Dahmani S, Michelet D, Abback PS, et al. Ketamine for perioperative pain management in children: a meta-analysis of published studies. Paediatr Anaesth 2011;21:636–52.

71. Bell RF, Dahl JB, Moore RA, et al. Perioperative ketamine for acute postoperative pain. Cochrane Database Syst Rev 2006;CD004603.

72. Loftus RW, Yeager MP, Clark JA, et al. Intraoperative ketamine reduces perioperative opiate consumption in opiate-dependent patients with chronic back pain undergoing back surgery. Anesthesiology 2010;113:639–46.

73. Zakine J, Samarcq D, Lorne E, et al. Postoperative ketamine administration decreases morphine consumption in major abdominal surgery: a prospective, randomized, double-blind, controlled study. Anesth Analg 2008;106:1856–61.

74. Laskowski K, Stirling A, McKay WP, et al. A systematic review of intravenous ketamine for postoperative analgesia. Can J Anaesth 2011;58:911–23.

75. Sami Mebazaa M, Mestiri T, Kaabi B, et al. Clinical benefits related to the combination of ketamine with morphine for patient controlled analgesia after major abdominal surgery. Tunis Med 2008;86:435–40.

76. De Oliveira GS Jr, Castro-Alves LJ, Khan JH, et al. Perioperative systemic magnesium to minimize postoperative pain: a meta-analysis of randomized controlled trials. Anesthesiology 2013;119:178–90.

77. Guo BL, Lin Y, Hu W, et al. Effects of Systemic Magnesium on Post-operative Analgesia: Is the Current Evidence Strong Enough? Pain Physician 2015;18: 405–18.
78. Murphy JD, Paskaradevan J, Eisler LL, et al. Analgesic efficacy of continuous intravenous magnesium infusion as an adjuvant to morphine for postoperative analgesia: a systematic review and meta-analysis. Middle East J Anaesthesiol 2013;22:11–20.
79. Suzuki M. Role of N-methyl-D-aspartate receptor antagonists in postoperative pain management. Curr Opin Anaesthesiol 2009;22:618–22.
80. Ferris SH. Evaluation of memantine for the treatment of Alzheimer's disease. Expert Opin Pharmacother 2003;4:2305–13.
81. Kavirajan H. Memantine: a comprehensive review of safety and efficacy. Expert Opin Drug Saf 2009;8:89–109.
82. Grande LA, O'Donnell BR, Fitzgibbon DR, et al. Ultra-low dose ketamine and memantine treatment for pain in an opioid-tolerant oncology patient. Anesth Analg 2008;107:1380–3.
83. Lipton SA. Paradigm shift in NMDA receptor antagonist drug development: molecular mechanism of uncompetitive inhibition by memantine in the treatment of Alzheimer's disease and other neurologic disorders. J Alzheimers Dis 2004;6: S61–74.
84. Buvanendran A, Kroin JS. Early use of memantine for neuropathic pain. Anesth Analg 2008;107:1093–4.
85. Rogers M, Rasheed A, Moradimehr A, et al. Memantine (Namenda) for neuropathic pain. Am J Hosp Palliat Care 2009;26:57–9.
86. Pickering G, Morel V, Joly D, et al. Prevention of post-mastectomy neuropathic pain with memantine: study protocol for a randomized controlled trial. Trials 2014;15:331.
87. Olivan-Blazquez B, Herrera-Mercadal P, Puebla-Guedea M, et al. Efficacy of memantine in the treatment of fibromyalgia: A double-blind, randomised, controlled trial with 6-month follow-up. Pain 2014;155:2517–25.
88. Olivan-Blazquez B, Puebla M, Masluk B, et al. Evaluation of the efficacy of memantine in the treatment of fibromyalgia: study protocol for a doubled-blind randomized controlled trial with six-month follow-up. Trials 2013;14:3.
89. Morel V, Joly D, Villatte C, et al. Memantine before Mastectomy Prevents Post-Surgery Pain: A Randomized, Blinded Clinical Trial in Surgical Patients. PLoS One 2016;11:e0152741.
90. Rahimzadeh P, Imani F, Nikoubakht N, et al. A Comparative Study on the Efficacy of Oral Memantine and Placebo for Acute Postoperative Pain in Patients Undergoing Dacryocystorhinostomy (DCR). Anesth Pain Med 2017;7:e45297.
91. Waldron NH, Jones CA, Gan TJ, et al. Impact of perioperative dexamethasone on postoperative analgesia and side-effects: systematic review and meta-analysis. Br J Anaesth 2013;110:191–200.
92. Allen TK, Jones CA, Habib AS. Dexamethasone for the prophylaxis of postoperative nausea and vomiting associated with neuraxial morphine administration: a systematic review and meta-analysis. Anesth Analg 2012;114:813–22.
93. De Oliveira GS Jr, Almeida MD, Benzon HT, et al. Perioperative single dose systemic dexamethasone for postoperative pain: a meta-analysis of randomized controlled trials. Anesthesiology 2011;115:575–88.
94. Collaborators DT, West Midlands Research C. Dexamethasone versus standard treatment for postoperative nausea and vomiting in gastrointestinal surgery: randomised controlled trial (DREAMS Trial). BMJ 2017;357:j1455.

95. Hans P, Vanthuyne A, Dewandre PY, et al. Blood glucose concentration profile after 10 mg dexamethasone in non-diabetic and type 2 diabetic patients undergoing abdominal surgery. Br J Anaesth 2006;97:164–70.

96. Toner AJ, Ganeshanathan V, Chan MT, et al. Safety of Perioperative Glucocorticoids in Elective Noncardiac Surgery: A Systematic Review and Meta-analysis. Anesthesiology 2017;126:234–48.

97. Doleman B, Read D, Lund JN, et al. Preventive Acetaminophen Reduces Postoperative Opioid Consumption, Vomiting, and Pain Scores After Surgery: Systematic Review and Meta-Analysis. Reg Anesth Pain Med 2015;40:706–12.

98. De Oliveira GS Jr, Castro-Alves LJ, McCarthy RJ. Single-dose systemic acetaminophen to prevent postoperative pain: a meta-analysis of randomized controlled trials. Clin J Pain 2015;31:86–93.

99. Wong I, St John-Green C, Walker SM. Opioid-sparing effects of perioperative paracetamol and nonsteroidal anti-inflammatory drugs (NSAIDs) in children. Paediatr Anaesth 2013;23:475–95.

100. Apfel CC, Turan A, Souza K, et al. Intravenous acetaminophen reduces postoperative nausea and vomiting: a systematic review and meta-analysis. Pain 2013; 154:677–89.

101. McNicol ED, Tzortzopoulou A, Cepeda MS, et al. Single-dose intravenous paracetamol or propacetamol for prevention or treatment of postoperative pain: a systematic review and meta-analysis. Br J Anaesth 2011;106:764–75.

102. Toms L, McQuay HJ, Derry S, et al. Single dose oral paracetamol (acetaminophen) for postoperative pain in adults. Cochrane Database Syst Rev 2008;CD004602.

103. Remy C, Marret E, Bonnet F. Effects of acetaminophen on morphine side-effects and consumption after major surgery: meta-analysis of randomized controlled trials. Br J Anaesth 2005;94:505–13.

104. Jibril F, Sharaby S, Mohamed A, et al. Intravenous versus Oral Acetaminophen for Pain: Systematic Review of Current Evidence to Support Clinical Decision-Making. Can J Hosp Pharm 2015;68:238–47.

105. De Oliveira GS Jr, Agarwal D, Benzon HT. Perioperative single dose ketorolac to prevent postoperative pain: a meta-analysis of randomized trials. Anesth Analg 2012;114:424–33.

106. Marret E, Kurdi O, Zufferey P, et al. Effects of nonsteroidal antiinflammatory drugs on patient-controlled analgesia morphine side effects: meta-analysis of randomized controlled trials. Anesthesiology 2005;102:1249–60.

107. Straube S, Derry S, McQuay HJ, et al. Effect of preoperative Cox-II-selective NSAIDs (coxibs) on postoperative outcomes: a systematic review of randomized studies. Acta Anaesthesiol Scand 2005;49:601–13.

108. Maund E, McDaid C, Rice S, et al. Paracetamol and selective and non-selective non-steroidal anti-inflammatory drugs for the reduction in morphine-related side-effects after major surgery: a systematic review. Br J Anaesth 2011;106:292–7.

109. Michelet D, Andreu-Gallien J, Bensalah T, et al. A meta-analysis of the use of nonsteroidal antiinflammatory drugs for pediatric postoperative pain. Anesth Analg 2012;114:393–406.

110. Elia N, Lysakowski C, Tramer MR. Does multimodal analgesia with acetaminophen, nonsteroidal antiinflammatory drugs, or selective cyclooxygenase-2 inhibitors and patient-controlled analgesia morphine offer advantages over morphine alone? Meta-analyses of randomized trials. Anesthesiology 2005;103:1296–304.

111. Pandazi A, Kapota E, Matsota P, et al. Preincisional versus postincisional administration of parecoxib in colorectal surgery: effect on postoperative pain control

and cytokine response. A randomized clinical trial. World J Surg 2010;34: 2463–9.

112. Leese PT, Hubbard RC, Karim A, et al. Effects of celecoxib, a novel cyclooxygenase-2 inhibitor, on platelet function in healthy adults: a randomized, controlled trial. J Clin Pharmacol 2000;40:124–32.

113. Myles PS, Power I. Does ketorolac cause postoperative renal failure: how do we assess the evidence? Br J Anaesth 1998;80:420–1.

114. Jamjittrong S, Matsuda A, Matsumoto S, et al. Postoperative non-steroidal anti-inflammatory drugs and anastomotic leakage after gastrointestinal anastomoses: Systematic review and meta-analysis. Ann Gastroenterol Surg 2020;4: 64–75.

115. Hawkins AT, McEvoy MD, Wanderer JP, et al. Ketorolac Use and Anastomotic Leak in Elective Colorectal Surgery: A Detailed Analysis. Dis Colon Rectum 2018;61:1426–34.

116. Chou CI, Shih CJ, Chen YT, et al. Adverse Effects of Oral Nonselective and cyclooxygenase-2-Selective NSAIDs on Hospitalization for Acute Kidney Injury: A Nested Case-Control Cohort Study. Medicine (Baltimore) 2016;95:e2645.

117. Bhangu A, Singh P, Fitzgerald JE, et al. Postoperative nonsteroidal anti-inflammatory drugs and risk of anastomotic leak: meta-analysis of clinical and experimental studies. World J Surg 2014;38:2247–57.

118. Engelman E, Cateloy F. Efficacy and safety of perioperative pregabalin for postoperative pain: a meta-analysis of randomized-controlled trials. Acta Anaesthesiol Scand 2011;55:927–43.

119. Eipe N, Penning J, Yazdi F, et al. Perioperative use of pregabalin for acute pain-a systematic review and meta-analysis. Pain 2015;156:1284–300.

120. Hurley RW, Cohen SP, Williams KA, et al. The analgesic effects of perioperative gabapentin on postoperative pain: a meta-analysis. Reg Anesth Pain Med 2006; 31:237–47.

121. Mishriky BM, Waldron NH, Habib AS. Impact of pregabalin on acute and persistent postoperative pain: a systematic review and meta-analysis. Br J Anaesth 2015;114:10–31.

122. Peng PW, Wijeysundera DN, Li CC. Use of gabapentin for perioperative pain control – a meta-analysis. Pain Res Manag 2007;12:85–92.

123. Seib RK, Paul JE. Preoperative gabapentin for postoperative analgesia: a meta-analysis. Can J Anaesth 2006;53:461–9.

124. Zhang J, Ho KY, Wang Y. Efficacy of pregabalin in acute postoperative pain: a meta-analysis. Br J Anaesth 2011;106:454–62.

125. Siddiqui NT, Fischer H, Guerina L, et al. Effect of a preoperative gabapentin on postoperative analgesia in patients with inflammatory bowel disease following major bowel surgery: a randomized, placebo-controlled trial. Pain Pract 2014; 14:132–9.

126. Verret M, Lauzier F, Zarychanski R, et al. Canadian Perioperative Anesthesia Clinical Trials G: Perioperative Use of Gabapentinoids for the Management of Postoperative Acute Pain: A Systematic Review and Meta-analysis. Anesthesiology 2020;133:265–79.

127. Jessen Lundorf L, Korvenius Nedergaard H, Moller AM. Perioperative dexmedetomidine for acute pain after abdominal surgery in adults. Cochrane Database Syst Rev 2016;2:CD010358.

128. Abdallah FW, Dwyer T, Chan VW, et al. IV and Perineural Dexmedetomidine Similarly Prolong the Duration of Analgesia after Interscalene Brachial Plexus

Block: A Randomized, Three-arm, Triple-masked, Placebo-controlled Trial. Anesthesiology 2016;124:683–95.

129. Das B, Lakshmegowda M, Sharma M, et al. Supraclavicular brachial plexus block using ropivacaine alone or combined with dexmedetomidine for upper limb surgery: A prospective, randomized, double-blinded, comparative study. Rev Esp Anestesiol Reanim 2016;63:135–40.

130. Blaudszun G, Lysakowski C, Elia N, et al. Effect of perioperative systemic alpha2 agonists on postoperative morphine consumption and pain intensity: systematic review and meta-analysis of randomized controlled trials. Anesthesiology 2012;116:1312–22.

131. Garg AX, Kurz A, Sessler DI, et al. Perioperative aspirin and clonidine and risk of acute kidney injury: a randomized clinical trial. JAMA 2014;312:2254–64.

132. Choi YY, Park JS, Park SY, et al. Can intravenous patient-controlled analgesia be omitted in patients undergoing laparoscopic surgery for colorectal cancer? Ann Surg Treat Res 2015;88:86–91.

133. Lloyd GM, Kirby R, Hemingway DM, et al. The RAPID protocol enhances patient recovery after both laparoscopic and open colorectal resections. Surg Endosc 2010;24:1434–9.

134. Brouquet A, Cudennec T, Benoist S, et al. Impaired mobility, ASA status and administration of tramadol are risk factors for postoperative delirium in patients aged 75 years or more after major abdominal surgery. Ann Surg 2010;251: 759–65.

135. Inturrisi CE, Colburn WA, Kaiko RF, et al. Pharmacokinetics and pharmacodynamics of methadone in patients with chronic pain. Clin Pharmacol Ther 1987; 41:392–401.

136. Gottschalk A, Durieux ME, Nemergut EC. Intraoperative methadone improves postoperative pain control in patients undergoing complex spine surgery. Anesth Analg 2011;112:218–23.

137. Gourlay GK, Willis RJ, Lamberty J. A double-blind comparison of the efficacy of methadone and morphine in postoperative pain control. Anesthesiology 1986; 64:322–7.

138. Richlin DM, Reuben SS. Postoperative pain control with methadone following lower abdominal surgery. J Clin Anesth 1991;3:112–6.

139. Kharasch ED. Intraoperative methadone: rediscovery, reappraisal, and reinvigoration? Anesth Analg 2011;112:13–6.

140. D'Souza RS, Gurrieri C, Johnson RL, et al. Intraoperative methadone administration and postoperative pain control: a systematic review and meta-analysis. Pain 2020;161:237–43.

141. Murphy GS, Avram MJ, Greenberg SB, et al. Postoperative Pain and Analgesic Requirements in the First Year after Intraoperative Methadone for Complex Spine and Cardiac Surgery. Anesthesiology 2020;132:330–42.

142. Murphy GS, Szokol JW. Intraoperative Methadone in Surgical Patients: A Review of Clinical Investigations. Anesthesiology 2019;131:678–92.

Fluid and Hemodynamics

W. Brenton French, MD[a], Michael Scott, MBChB, FRCP, FRCA, FFICM[b],*

KEYWORDS

- Fluid therapy • Goal-directed therapy • Cardiac output monitoring
- Enhanced recovery

KEY POINTS

- Enhanced Recovery After Surgery (ERAS) pathways can improve perioperative fluid and hemodynamic therapy by avoiding preoperative dehydration and reducing postoperative dependence on intravenous fluids.
- Perioperative fluid management practices have changed over time, shifting away from liberal fluid therapy toward more restrictive or goal-directed approaches.
- Goal-directed hemodynamic therapy (GDHT) which uses cardiac output monitoring to optimize volume status and avoid perioperative hypotension has been shown to improve outcomes.
- Intraoperative mean arterial pressure is increasingly important, with hypotension in the operating room associated with worse postoperative outcomes.
- Within ERAS programs, high-risk patients are most likely to benefit from perioperative GDHT, and institution-specific approaches are likely ideal during the implementation of such programs.

INTRODUCTION

Appropriate hemodynamic management is a critical component of care in the perioperative patient. Surgery induces a significant inflammatory response which may vary based on the condition of the patient, the urgency of surgical intervention, the type of procedure, and the volume of blood loss. Physiologic changes in the perioperative period can lead to capillary leakage and redistribution of fluids, activation of fluid and sodium retention pathways, and significant metabolic changes.[1,2] Anesthesia induces hypotension due to peripheral vasodilation and altered cardiac function, and the use of neuraxial blockades may lead to vasoplegia and venodilation.[3,4] Although a complicated subject, appropriate hemodynamic optimization of the patient during surgery is key to managing the potentially harmful effects of the surgical stress response. Over the years there has been a multitude of studies evaluating various fluid administration practices in the operating room (OR), leading to changes in the practice of perioperative care. Changing fluid management practices in the OR and clinical evidence,

[a] Department of Surgery, Virginia Commonwealth University Health System, 1250 E Marshall Street, Richmond, VA 23219, USA; [b] Department of Anesthesiology and Critical Care Medicine, University of Pennsylvania, 3400 Spruce Street, Philadelphia, PA 19104, USA
* Corresponding author.
E-mail address: Michael.Scott@Pennmedicine.Upenn.edu

Anesthesiology Clin 40 (2022) 59–71
https://doi.org/10.1016/j.anclin.2021.11.002   anesthesiology.theclinics.com

particularly in the setting of Enhanced Recovery After Surgery (ERAS) pathways, have created questions and debate surrounding the optimal intraoperative fluid and hemo-dynamic management strategies for the surgical patient.

Hemodynamic management refers to interventions or therapy that aim to maintain certain levels of cardiovascular blood flow and pressure. The intended result is adequate tissue perfusion and oxygenation in the presence of the surgical stress response. Hypovolemia and hypotension lead to reduced organ perfusion and post-operative complications.[5] On the other hand, excessive volume administration can lead to equally poor outcomes, and the effects of hypervolemia on postoperative com-plications are well-described.[6–9] Thus, the goal for the anesthesia provider is to find the proper balance between hypovolemia and excessive fluid volume administration (**Fig. 1**). However, fluid requirements may be somewhat different in ERAS settings when compared with more traditional perioperative care. The two key concepts in perioperative fluid and hemodynamic therapy, and the overarching focus of this chap-ter, are the maintenance of circulatory "flow" and "pressure" in the surgical patient.

FLUID REQUIREMENTS IN AN ENHANCED RECOVERY AFTER SURGERY PATHWAY

In an ERAS setting, the preoperative elements of the pathway aim to bring the patient to surgery when they are at or near a euvolemic state. Emergency settings, in contrast, involve patients in a state of physiologic stress, typically via infection, systemic inflam-matory response syndrome (SIRS), or hemorrhage. Elective or scheduled surgery rep-resents a more controlled environment for perioperative management. Traditionally,

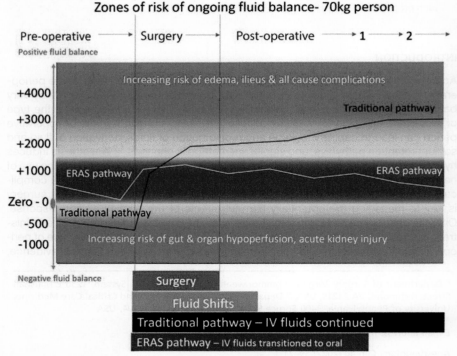

Fig. 1. Comparison of fluid management between ERAS pathways and traditional perioper-ative care.

however, elective patients were expected to have a prolonged period of *nil per os* (NPO) starting the night before surgery.[10] This would lead to the patient becoming dehydrated, which would then necessitate aggressive, high-volume fluid therapy during surgery.[11] As advanced hemodynamic or cardiac output monitoring was lacking in the typical patient, the volume of fluid administered in surgery was typically determined using traditional vital signs monitoring, urine output, blood loss, and clinical judgment. ERAS pathways operate differently. Rather than prolonged preoperative dehydration followed by excessive perioperative fluid administration, certain elements of ERAS work to improve and simplify fluid and hemodynamic management in the perioperative period:

- Preoperative oral fluid intake: patients are allowed to drink clear liquids up until 2 hours before the start of surgery, avoiding preoperative dehydration.
- Carbohydrate loading: preoperative carbohydrate drinks counteract the catabolism of preoperative fasting and serve to maintain hydration.
- Preference for minimally invasive surgical techniques: laparoscopic surgery and the avoidance of open procedures, when possible, help to reduce physiologic derangement and insensible fluid losses.
- Correction of anemia: patients with anemia at baseline are referred for intravenous iron infusions to improve the oxygenation of tissues during the surgical stress response.

These elements act as a continuum of care across the preoperative, intraoperative, and postoperative periods.[12] Each phase of the process is critical. The preoperative elements of ERAS, when appropriately applied, help to ensure the patient arrives without significant physiologic derangement or hypovolemia. This in turn lowers the threshold to avoid under-perfusion and simplifies hemodynamic management. Improved perioperative fluid therapy and hemodynamics, without excessive intravascular volume administration, improve organ and tissue perfusion. This leads to fewer complications such as acute kidney injury (AKI), infections, pulmonary complications, and various other morbidities (see **Fig. 1**). This in turn can achieve the reductions in length of stay (LOS) and costs that are associated with ERAS pathways in various studies.

APPROACHES TO INTRAOPERATIVE FLUID THERAPY

A critical component to maintaining perfusion is to ensure adequate volume in the vasculature, as this is the first step to ensuring optimized circulatory "flow." Various approaches to intraoperative IV fluid therapy have developed over the years, but the overarching strategies are "fixed volume" versus "goal-directed" or individualized therapy. In the literature on intraoperative fluid therapy, there are many studies and clinical reviews which use a variety of vague and poorly defined terms such as "restrictive" and "liberal" fluid plans and various "goal-directed fluid" or "hemodynamic" therapies. Thus, a detailed review of these concepts is necessary.

Fixed Volume Strategies

With the increasing awareness of the consequences of hypervolemia, modern perioperative practice moved toward intraoperative fluid administration that was more "restrictive" than older, traditional therapies.[12,13] In the past it was common for patients to receive 4 to 5L of crystalloid during surgery.[13–15] This was done with the assumption that the patient was experiencing severe physiologic stress by the nature of the surgical procedure and thus had high volume requirements. Clinical evidence, however, began to show evidence toward more restrictive fluid administration plans improving outcomes.[14,16,17] The concept involves giving the patient only the amount of fluid that is physiologically necessary to both maintain perfusion and avoid volume overload. The "restrictive" approach, though, has never been clearly defined, and this term is used with a high degree of subjectivity. "Zero balance" approaches, which aim to keep the patient at a net-even level of fluid during their surgical admission, have also been advocated, but their relation to "restrictive" plans, or if they are different, remain unclear in the literature.[18,19]

There is a generalized belief that ERAS protocols advocate for a "zero-balance" or "restrictive" approach to intraoperative fluid therapy. This is a misconception. ERAS pathways advocate a balance between fluid "restriction" and volume overload, in full awareness of the complications of both. Some recent evidence has shown that ERAS pathway implementation is associated with a higher incidence of postoperative AKI, and an association with overly-restrictive approaches should not be ignored.[20–22] Myles and colleagues demonstrated this phenomenon in the RELIEF trial. In this study of nearly 3000 patients undergoing major abdominal surgery, they randomized patients to a "restrictive" plan, which aimed to achieve a net "zero-balance" of fluid and a "liberal" fluid plan. The restrictive group received a bolus of 5 cc/kg at the start of surgery and 5 cc/kg/h of maintenance fluid during surgery. The liberal group received a 10 cc/kg bolus and 8 cc/kg/h of maintenance fluid. This resulted in the restrictive patients receiving 1.7 L of crystalloid versus 3.0 L in the liberal group. Postoperative median fluid balance was +1.38 L in the restrictive group than +3.09 L in the liberal group. The study identified no difference in 1-year disability-free survival between the groups but found the restrictive group to have a higher incidence of AKI (8.6% vs 5.0%, $P<.001$). The results of the trial underscore the importance of avoiding approaches that overly-restrict fluid administration, particularly given the well-described association of AKI with mortality and costs.

Given the current evidence, fluid approaches within ERAS that rely on clinical judgment and protocolized, weight-based fluid administration, as opposed to goal-directed or individualized therapies, should likely target a weight gain of 1 to 2 kg of fluid by postoperative day 1.

Goal-Directed Therapies

Goal-directed approaches in the OR have been studied for over 30 years. This concept was initially studied by Shoemaker and colleagues, who in 1988 demonstrated that targeting supra-normal values for cardiac index and oxygenation dramatically improved rates of postoperative mortality in major surgery patients.[23] In the following years, there have been a multitude of clinical trials that evaluated different forms of goal-directed approaches within various patient populations.[24,25] Regarding intraoperative fluid management, goal-directed fluid therapy (GDFT) is defined as the use of cardiac output monitoring to guide the administration of fluid. The concept behind GDFT is the optimization of stroke volume to ensure optimal "flow" and perfusion of tissues.[26] Optimized perfusion ensures adequate organ function and aids in wound healing in the perioperative patient.[27,28] Typically, GDFT entails fluid administration in response to the stroke volume, and it aims to determine the patient's position on the Frank–Starling curve (**Fig. 2**). Following a fluid challenge, if the stroke volume does not increase by at least 10%, then the patient is considered not volume-responsive and additional fluid, in this case, is not likely to benefit. Various protocols and procedures have been studied, and no single methodology or "protocol" for GDFT is recommended. Some study protocols used maintenance fluid, typically 1 to 5 cc/kg/h depending on the type of surgery, whereas some mandated only fluid boluses that are administered in response to a drop in stroke volume.[12,29,30] For practical use of these approaches, a provider's level of comfort or experience will likely dictate

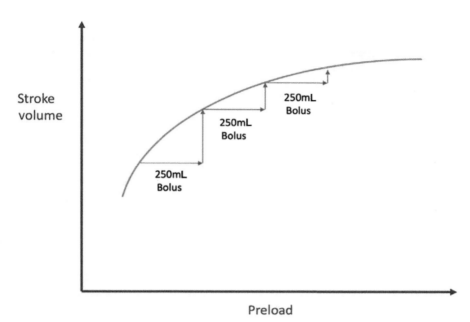

Fig. 2. Frank–Starling curve demonstrating concept behind goal-directed fluid therapy. Small fluid blouses are used to determine the patient's position on the curve.

the use, type, and amount of maintenance fluid. However, the key concept is to avoid excessive fluid administration at baseline and to give additional fluid as dictated by cardiac output monitoring.

CARDIAC OUTPUT MONITORING TECHNIQUES

Several devices monitor cardiac output with varying degrees of invasiveness and monitors exist for each potential setting. Each device has its benefits and drawbacks, but the choice of device is ultimately left to provider preference and familiarity. Some of the frequently used methodologies are reviewed here.

Pulmonary Artery Catheter

In the past, monitoring of cardiac output required a pulmonary artery catheter (PAC) and thermodilution. This technique involves cold fluid intermittently injected into the right atrium while the resulting temperature change is calculated in the pulmonary artery. This is then used to calculate the cardiac output.[31] Devices that provide continuous cardiac output monitoring via the PAC are available.[32] Given its invasiveness and the complications associated with the PAC, its use in modern practice is limited. It is mainly used at provider discretion for those with major cardiac disease, right ventricular dysfunction, or in those who are otherwise extremely high risk for surgery. While the PAC with thermodilution is still considered by some as the standard for cardiac output monitoring, newer and farless invasive technologies have been developed for use in modern perioperative care.

Esophageal Doppler Monitor

The esophageal Doppler monitor (EDM) is well-validated and has been used in many clinical trials on GDFT. This probe is similar in size to a nasogastric tube and is inserted into the esophagus following the induction of anesthesia. When directed at the aorta, the device tracks the velocity of blood flow through the aorta in relation to time. Using the estimated aortic cross-sectional area, it can derive stroke volume and cardiac output.[33] The EDM does have some limitations: the patient must first be asleep before insertion, and the probe must be adjusted occasionally to track aortic blood flow should the probe or patient change position.

Arterial Waveform Analysis

Multiple platforms use arterial waveform analysis technology to determine stroke volume and cardiac output. These devices require an arterial line. Using the stroke volume, blood pressure, systemic vascular resistance, and arterial compliance, the arterial line probe can generate stroke volume and cardiac output. In simple terms, the stroke volume can be calculated when arterial compliance is known by the expected change in arterial blood volume between systole and diastole.[34] These devices have also been well-validated and used in certain GDFT studies.

Thoracic Bioimpedance and Bioreactance

Bioimpedance is a technology that uses the circulating fluid volume in the thoracic cavity to derive cardiac output. This relies on the difference in electrical conduction between the fluid/liquid and solid components of the body. By emitting an alternating current from multiple skin pads and utilizing the changes in electrical conductance or impedance through the thoracic cavity, the circulating blood volume can be calculated. This in turn is related to the stroke volume and cardiac output.[35,36] Bioreactance uses the same principle but was developed to improve the signal-to-noise ratio and usability of bioimpedance. It uses the phase shift of the electrical signal, which is related to the thoracic blood flow.[37,38] A benefit of these devices is that they are completely noninvasive, using the placement of electrodes on the skin that are similar to electrocardiogram leads.

AVOIDANCE OF HYPOTENSION

A second key concept in hemodynamic therapy is the maintenance of adequate mean arterial pressure (MAP). Hypotension in the OR is associated with adverse outcomes, and maintaining adequate MAP is a key component of perioperative care. This was illustrated in a retrospective cohort analysis of intraoperative vital signs data by Salmasi and colleagues of more than 57,000 patients.[39] Postoperative myocardial injury and AKI were strongly associated with intraoperative MAPs below the absolute threshold of 65 mm Hg. This risk was increased with lower blood pressures and a longer duration of hypotension. Other studies similarly showed a significant increase in myocardial injury, AKI, and mortality following perioperative hypotension. Sun and colleagues reviewed more than 5000 noncardiac surgical patients and showed odds ratios of 2.34 and 3.53 for AKI with 11 to 20 min and greater than 20-min exposures to a MAP of less than 55 mm Hg respectively.[40] Monk and colleagues showed increased 30-day mortality risk with a similar pattern concerning the duration and depth of intraoperative hypotension.[41] Other studies have shown the same associations, which reiterate the critical importance of maintaining adequate arterial pressure during surgery.[42–44]

COMBINING FLOW AND PRESSURE: GOAL-DIRECTED HEMODYNAMIC THERAPY

Incorporation of the control of MAP with a GDFT approach is defined as goal-directed *hemodynamic* therapy (GDHT). While sometimes used interchangeably with GDFT, GDHT incorporates the avoidance of hypotension into these protocols (**Fig. 3**). This

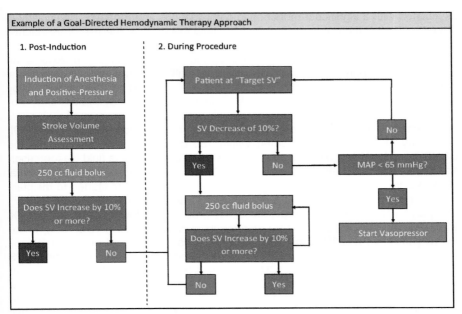

Fig. 3. Goal-directed hemodynamic therapy: a practical guide. • The concept of stroke volume optimization aims to ensure adequate but not excessive circulating blood volume to maintain tissue perfusion. • When cardiac output monitoring is available, small fluid challenges or boluses are given to patients while their stroke volume is monitored. These are typically 100 to 250 cc boluses given rapidly over 5 to 10 minutes with the patient supine. The stroke volume is then monitored for 5 additional minutes following completion of the bolus, and a 10% increase in SV is generally considered "volume-responsive."[27,45] • The approach signals the general location of the patient on the Frank–Starling curve. The intent is to have the patient on the "flat" part of the curve, which signifies normovolemia. If the SV does not rise at least 10%, then additional fluid is not likely to benefit. • The SV is typically "optimized" just after induction of anesthesia and before the start of surgery. Fluid boluses are given until the stroke volume does not increase by 10%. However, typically a maximum of 500 to 750 cc are used for this to prevent excessive volume administration in patients with normal cardiac function. • The SV is then maintained during surgery. If the stroke volume drops 10% or more, then a fluid challenge is given. If the patient responds to this fluid bolus, additional fluid is given until the SV does not rise 10%. • Several surgical factors may affect the stroke volume, including (1) patient positioning, (2) peritoneal insufflation for laparoscopic surgery, and (3) ventilation changes. When SV changes of 10% or more occur in relation to these factors, a fluid challenge while monitoring SV can ensure the patient remains euvolemic. • Alternatively, dynamic indices such as stroke volume variation (SVV) or pulse pressure variation (PPV) may also be used in place of or in addition to SV. These indices use change in intrathoracic pressure during positive pressure ventilation to "simulate" small fluid challenges. Large variations in arterial pressure or stroke volume are attributed to hypovolemia. Typically an SVV of 10% to 12% is considered volume-responsive. Before using these variables, however, certain conditions must be met: (1) the patient cannot be spontaneously breathing, (2) tidal volumes must be greater than 8 mL/kg, (3) no cardiac arrhythmias are present, and (4) the thoracic cavity is not open.

ensures adequate "flow" or circulatory volume while maintaining adequate "pressure" to help ensure adequate organ and tissue perfusion. However, in the literature the two are typically discussed as the same, given the differences of various hemodynamic endpoints of the methodologies studied in clinical trials. GDHT has historically been associated with a significant reduction in complications and mortality, particularly in studies following the principle of optimizing flow followed by the use of vasoactive drugs to achieve a target MAP.[24,30,46]

The FEDORA trial published by Calvo-Vecino and colleagues[30] in 2018 is an example of such principles. It was a prospective, multicenter randomized control trial studying 420 patients assigned to intraoperative goal-directed hemodynamic therapy (GDHT) versus traditional therapy. Eligible patients underwent major abdominal, urologic, gynecologic, or orthopedic surgery with both laparoscopic and open surgical approaches. The primary outcome was moderate or severe complications (AKI, SSI, pulmonary edema, ARDS) occurring within 180 days of surgery. Patients in the GDHT group had hemodynamic monitoring with an EDM to guide fluid, vasopressor, and inotrope administration. Fluid boluses of 250 cc were given to achieve an optimal stroke volume, after which either vasopressors or inotropes were started to maintain MAP of greater than 65 mm Hg and a cardiac index of greater than 2.5 L/min/m^2. Compared with traditional therapy, the GDHT group had a lower risk of AKI (1.44% vs 8.53%) ARDS (0.48% vs 5.69%), cardiopulmonary edema (0% vs 6.16%), pneumonia (1.91% vs 8.53%), superficial SSI (0.96% vs 4.74%), and deep SSI (1.91% vs 8.06%). Secondary outcomes also demonstrated shorter average hospital LOS (5 vs 7 days) and shorter average ICU LOS (16h vs 24h) in the GDHT group than traditional therapy. The OPTIMISE trial published in 2014 was a randomized, multicenter trial in the United Kingdom of 734 patients over age 50 undergoing major gastrointestinal surgery.[29] Patients were randomized to a cardiac output-guided hemodynamic algorithm versus standard therapy. The intervention group protocol maximized stroke volume and maintained a continuous infusion of dopexamine, and the patients were to maintain a MAP of greater than 60 mm Hg with vasopressor support as needed. Results showed the intervention group achieved a reduction in the primary outcome (moderate or severe complication or mortality within 30 days of surgery) and improvement in mortality at 180 days despite the trial reporting nonsignificance for the primary endpoint. In a meta-analysis incorporating 95 randomized trials, goal-directed therapy was associated with a lower risk of mortality (odds ratio (OR): 0.66, 95% confidence interval (CI): 0.50–0.87), AKI (OR: 0.73; 95% CI: 0.58–0.92), and pneumonia (OR: 0.69; 95% CI: 0.51–0.92) and led to shorter hospital LOS (−0.90; 95% CI: −1.32 to −0.48) when compared to standard fluid management.[24] In their analysis, the authors excluded older studies that used a PAC to monitor cardiac output, as they believed the clinical practice of GDHT has changed significantly with the incorporation of novel cardiac output monitoring devices.

In goal-directed therapy studies, some evidence suggests that the timing of fluid administration may be a key factor in improving outcomes. Studies, such as FEDORA, have shown that the volume of fluid administered between patients was not significantly different between GDHT and control groups.[30,47] A hypothesis is that occult instances of hypoperfusion, which would not be identified by traditional monitoring techniques, may be apparent by the drop in cardiac output. Studies on intraoperative hypotension, as mentioned previously, that show an association with increased complications with brief periods of intraoperative hypotension lend evidence to this.[39,41,42]

Overall, GDHT has been shown to reduce perioperative organ dysfunction and improve outcomes. However, while many studies show benefit, the heterogeneity of the trials in their populations, endpoints, and methodologies make specific conclusions difficult to establish from meta-analyses on this topic. In addition, the control groups from older studies represent what was considered usual care at the time, which was typically liberal intraoperative fluid therapy. Thus, some studies which have evaluated GDHT against the modern perioperative practice have shown less benefit, likely due to an improvement in our understanding of the consequences of excessive volume administration and the prevalence of carefully monitored fluid management within ERAS pathways.

THE ROLE OF GOAL-DIRECTED HEMODYNAMIC THERAPY IN ENHANCED RECOVERY AFTER SURGERY PATHWAYS AND PRACTICAL IMPLEMENTATION

The role of GDHT within ERAS pathways has been debated, as there is some evidence that ERAS programs may "blunt" the benefits of GDHT in certain populations. Lobo and Rollins demonstrated this in a meta-analysis in 2016 evaluating studies of goal-directed therapy specifically within ERAS programs.[48] They found no statistical difference in postoperative morbidity, mortality, or overall LOS when intervention and control patients were both managed within an ERAS pathway. Given advances in modern practice and the improvements seen in ERAS, one can conclude that not all patients should be managed with intraoperative GDHT. On this point, the World ERAS Society recommends that GDHT be used in high-risk patients or procedures with an anticipated high intravascular volume shift or loss.[49] Patients undergoing short procedures or who lack significant comorbidities are less likely to benefit from a GDHT program. While benefits may be questionable in some populations, when appropriately executed GDHT does not result in patient harm.[12] However, there is some evidence of an association of ERAS programs with AKI.[21] Weiner and colleagues evaluated the incidence of AKI in colorectal surgery patients following the implementation of an ERAS pathway and found that the incidence of AKI, by the Kidney Disease Improving Global Outcomes definition, nearly doubled.[20] This finding was mirrored in similar studies.[21,22] Higher ASA status, the presence of comorbidities, and reduced preoperative renal function are known risk factors for the development of perioperative AKI.[50] Paired with the lack of harm associated with intraoperative GDHT, there is a strong argument in favor of GDHT approaches to intraoperative fluid therapy in such high-risk patients. As has been emphasized, not all patients are expected to benefit, as low-risk patients undergoing low-risk procedures likely require a very large number to treat before any benefit is observed. However, those at high risk of postoperative complications, or patients undergoing highly morbid procedures, are expected to benefit based on the current evidence and societal guidelines.

Implementation of intraoperative GDHT is a complex subject. Based on existing evidence, it is wise for institutions to approach GDHT implementation based on their patient populations and the prevalence of comorbidities. Health systems serving a surgical population with high rates of comorbidities or who routinely perform high-risk surgeries are likely to see the most benefits. Inevitably it relies on resource allocation and availability of minimally or noninvasive cardiac output monitoring. Regarding which specific patients should have GDHT during surgery, this is likely best left at the discretion of the institution or physician group. A multidisciplinary team of surgeons and anesthesiologists should set clear institutional recommendations on which patients will be managed with GDHT. Given the marginal benefits, as demonstrated in the literature, in low-risk patients already managed with an ERAS pathway, including all patients in GDHT is likely not feasible or a wise allocation of resources. One approach would be to classify certain planned operation types, such as all major colonic or rectal resections, all liver resections, multi-level spinal surgery, and others, as cases where GDHT should be used. Additionally, patients who are high-risk by certain criteria, such as ASA status, baseline renal function, or other comorbidities, should also receive GDHT, but again this would be determined by the patient population served. Complications such as AKI, infections, or prolonged ileus should be tracked and reviewed by a multidisciplinary team, and changes to the GDHT protocol or the institutional inclusion criteria should be considered when appropriate. As in any clinical guidance, however, it is essential to maintain provider autonomy regarding patient care. While GDHT in high-risk patients, avoidance of hypotension, and careful monitoring of fluid needs are recommended as components of ERAS pathways, each patient is different and perioperative therapy should be tailored appropriately with clinical judgment.

SUMMARY

Many of the principles in ERAS pathways act to improve and simplify perioperative fluid and hemodynamic therapy. With the rising popularity of ERAS, perioperative fluid management over the last several years has shifted away from liberal fluid therapy to more restrictive and goal-directed approaches. Alongside this, there is an increased awareness of the relationship between intraoperative hypotension and increased postoperative complications, and maintaining adequate intraoperative MAP is a critical component of care. GDHT, made possible for most patients by minimally or noninvasive cardiac output monitoring, has shown an ability to improve outcomes. However, within ERAS pathways its role is likely best suited to high-risk patients or those undergoing high-risk procedures. Health systems or providers seeking to implement GDHT and other perioperative therapies should pursue institutional-specific practices tailored to their respective populations. By using an integrated approach that incorporates the preoperative, intraoperative, and postoperative components of ERAS, modern surgical care can move toward a reduction in both perioperative complications and health care costs.

CLINICS CARE POINTS

- ERAS pathways improve preoperative volume status, aiming to keep the patient at or near a euvolemic state on arrival to the operating room.

- Overly restrictive intraoperative fluid administration practices have shown increased rates of acute kidney injury within ERAS pathways. Providers should also be aware that the definition of "restrictive" fluid therapy has changed over time.

- Hypotension during surgery should be avoided given its strong association with postoperative complications such as renal and myocardial injury.

- Individualized intraoperative GDHT protocols, through optimizing volume status and avoiding hypotension, have demonstrated an ability to improve outcomes in high-risk surgical patients.

- When guided by cardiac output monitoring, the timing of fluid administration during surgery is likely a key factor in improving organ perfusion.

- Institutions implementing goal-directed approaches within their ERAS pathways should tailor these programs to their patient populations. Implementation and auditing of such programs should be managed by multidisciplinary teams of surgeons and anesthesiologists.

REFERENCES

1. Desborough JP. The stress response to trauma and surgery. Br J Anaesth 2000; 85(1):109–17.
2. Finnerty CC, Mabvuure NT, Ali A, et al. The surgically induced stress response. JPEN J Parenter Enteral Nutr 2013;37(5 Suppl):21S, 9S.

3. Akata T. General anesthetics and vascular smooth muscle: direct actions of general O on cellular mechanisms regulating vascular tone. Anesthesiology 2007; 106(2):365–91.

4. Gould TH, Grace K, Thorne G, et al. Effect of thoracic epidural anaesthesia on colonic blood flow. Br J Anaesth 2002;89(3):446–51.

5. Chappell D, Jacob M, Hofmann-Kiefer K, et al. A rational approach to perioperative fluid management. Anesthesiology 2008;109(4):723–40.

6. Strunden MS, Heckel K, Goetz AE, et al. Perioperative fluid and volume management: physiological basis, tools and strategies. Ann Intensive Care 2011;1(1):2.

7. Holte K, Sharrock NE, Kehlet H. Pathophysiology and clinical implications of perioperative fluid excess. Br J Anaesth 2002;89(4):622–32.

8. Grocott MPW, Mythen MG, Gan TJ. Perioperative fluid management and clinical outcomes in adults. Anesth Analg 2005;100(4):1093–106.

9. Lowell JA, Schifferdecker C, Driscoll DF, et al. Postoperative fluid overload: not a benign problem. Crit Care Med 1990;18(7):728–33.

10. Maltby JR. Fasting from midnight–the history behind the dogma. Best Pract Res Clin Anaesthesiol 2006;20(3):363–78.

11. Ljungqvist O, Scott M, Fearon KC. Enhanced recovery after surgery: a review. JAMA Surg 2017;152(3):292–8.

12. Miller TE, Roche AM, Mythen M. Fluid management and goal-directed therapy as an adjunct to enhanced recovery after surgery (ERAS). Can J Anesth 2015;62(2): 158–68. https://doi.org/10.1007/s12630-014-0266-y.

13. Myles PS, Bellomo R, Corcoran T, et al. Restrictive versus liberal fluid therapy for major abdominal surgery. N Engl J Med 2018;378(24):2263–74.

14. Brandstrup B, Tønnesen H, Beier-Holgersen R, et al. Effects of intravenous fluid restriction on postoperative complications: comparison of two perioperative fluid regimens: a randomized assessor-blinded multicenter trial. Ann Surg 2003; 238(5):641–8.

15. Tambyraja AL, Sengupta F, MacGregor AB, et al. Patterns and clinical outcomes associated with routine intravenous sodium and fluid administration after colorectal resection. World J Surg 2004;28(10):1046–51 [discussion 1051–2].

16. Nisanevich V, Felsenstein I, Almogy G, et al. Effect of intraoperative fluid management on outcome after intraabdominal surgery. Anesthesiology 2005;103(1): 25–32.

17. Voldby AW, Brandstrup B. Fluid therapy in the perioperative setting—a clinical review. J Intensive Care Med 2016;4(1):1–12.

18. Miller TE, Myles PS. Perioperative fluid therapy for major surgery. Anesthesiology 2019;130(5):825–32.

19. Brandstrup B, Svendsen PE, Rasmussen M, et al. Which goal for fluid therapy during colorectal surgery is followed by the best outcome: near-maximal stroke volume or zero fluid balance? Br J Anaesth 2012;109(2):191–9.

20. Wiener JGD, Goss L, Wahl TS, et al. The association of enhanced recovery pathway and acute kidney injury in patients undergoing colorectal surgery. Dis Colon Rectum 2020;63(2):233–41.

21. Marcotte JH, Patel K, Desai R, et al. Acute kidney injury following implementation of an enhanced recovery after surgery (ERAS) protocol in colorectal surgery. Int J Colorectal Dis 2018;33(9):1259–67.

22. Koerner CP, Lopez-Aguiar AG, Zaidi M, et al. Caution: increased acute kidney injury in enhanced recovery after surgery (ERAS) protocols. Am Surg 2019; 85(2):156–61.

23. Shoemaker WC, Appel PL, Kram HB, et al. Prospective trial of supranormal values of survivors as therapeutic goals in high-risk surgical patients. Chest 1988;94(6):1176–86.

24. Chong MA, Wang Y, Berbenetz NM, et al. Does goal-directed haemodynamic and fluid therapy improve peri-operative outcomes?: a systematic review and meta-analysis. Eur J Anaesthesiol 2018;35(7):469–83.

25. Cecconi M, Corredor C, Arulkumaran N, et al. Clinical review: goal-directed therapy-what is the evidence in surgical patients? The effect on different risk groups. Crit Care 2013;17(2):209.

26. Meng L, Heerdt PM. Perioperative goal-directed haemodynamic therapy based on flow parameters: a concept in evolution. Br J Anaesth 2016;117(suppl 3): iii3–17.

27. Marik PE, Monnet X, Teboul J-L. Hemodynamic parameters to guide fluid therapy. Ann Intensive Care 2011;1(1):1.

28. Gottrup F. Oxygen in wound healing and infection. World J Surg 2004;28(3): 312–5.

29. Pearse RM, Harrison DA, MacDonald N, et al. Effect of a perioperative, cardiac output-guided hemodynamic therapy algorithm on outcomes following major gastrointestinal surgery: a randomized clinical trial and systematic review. JAMA 2014;311(21):2181–90.

30. Calvo-Vecino JM, Ripollés-Melchor J, Mythen MG, et al. Effect of goal-directed haemodynamic therapy on postoperative complications in low-moderate risk surgical patients: a multicentre randomised controlled trial (FEDORA trial). Br J Anaesth 2018;120(4):734–44.

31. Alhashemi JA, Cecconi M, Hofer CK. Cardiac output monitoring: an integrative perspective. Crit Care 2011;15(2):1–9.

32. Vincent J-L, Rhodes A, Perel A, et al. Clinical review: update on hemodynamic monitoring - a consensus of 16. Crit Care 2011;15(4):1–8.

33. Funk DJ, Moretti EW, Gan TJ. Minimally invasive cardiac output monitoring in the perioperative setting. Anesth Analg 2009;108(3):887–97.

34. Montenij LJ, de Waal EEC, Buhre WF. Arterial waveform analysis in anesthesia and critical care. Curr Opin Anaesthesiol 2011;24(6):651–6.

35. Khalil SF, Mohktar MS, Ibrahim F. The theory and fundamentals of bioimpedance analysis in clinical status monitoring and diagnosis of diseases. Sensors 2014; 14(6):10895–928.

36. Jensen L, Yakimets J, Teo KK. A review of impedance cardiography. Heart Lung 1995;24(3):183–93.

37. Keren H, Burkhoff D, Squara P. Evaluation of a noninvasive continuous cardiac output monitoring system based on thoracic bioreactance. Am J Physiol Heart Circ Physiol 2007;293(1):H583–9.

38. Squara P, Denjean D, Estagnasie P, et al. Noninvasive cardiac output monitoring (NICOM): a clinical validation. Intensive Care Med 2007;33(7):1191–4.

39. Salmasi V, Maheshwari K, Yang D, et al. Relationship between intraoperative hypotension, defined by either reduction from baseline or absolute thresholds, and acute kidney and myocardial injury after noncardiac surgery a retrospective cohort analysis. Anesthesiology 2017;126(1):47–65.

40. Sun LY, Wijeysundera DN, Tait GA, et al. Association of intraoperative hypotension with acute kidney injury after elective noncardiac surgery. Anesthesiology 2015; 123(3):515–23.

41. Monk TG, Bronsert MR, Henderson WG, et al. Association between intraoperative hypotension and hypertension and 30-day postoperative mortality in noncardiac surgery. Anesthesiology 2015;123(2):307–19.

42. Walsh M, Devereaux PJ, Garg AX, et al. Relationship between intraoperative mean arterial pressure and clinical outcomes after noncardiac surgery. Toward an empirical definition of hypotension. Anesthesiology 2013;119(3):507–15.

43. van Waes JAR, van Klei WA, Wijeysundera DN, et al. Association between intra-operative hypotension and myocardial injury after vascular surgery. Anesthesiology 2016;124(1):35–44.

44. Mascha EJ, Yang D, Weiss S, et al. Intraoperative mean arterial pressure variability and 30-day mortality in patients having noncardiac surgery. Anesthesiology 2015;123(1):79–91.

45. Thiel SW, Kollef MH, Isakow W. Non-invasive stroke volume measurement and passive leg raising predict volume responsiveness in medical ICU patients: an observational cohort study. Crit Care 2009;13(4):R111.

46. Arulkumaran N, Corredor C, Hamilton MA, et al. Cardiac complications associated with goal-directed therapy in high-risk surgical patients: a meta-analysis. Br J Anaesth 2014;112(4):648–59.

47. Noblett SE, Snowden CP, Shenton BK, et al. Randomized clinical trial assessing the effect of Doppler-optimized fluid management on outcome after elective colorectal resection. Br J Surg 2006;93(9):1069–76.

48. Rollins KE, Lobo DN. Intraoperative goal-directed fluid therapy in elective major abdominal surgery: a meta-analysis of randomized controlled trials. Ann Surg 2016;263(3):465–76.

49. Gustafsson UO, Scott MJ, Hubner M, et al. Guidelines for perioperative care in elective colorectal surgery: enhanced recovery after surgery (ERAS®) society recommendations: 2018. World J Surg 2019;43(3):659–95.

50. Zorrilla-Vaca A, Mena GE, Ripolles-Melchor J, et al. Risk factors for acute kidney injury in an enhanced recovery pathway for colorectal surgery. Surg Today 2021;51(4):537–44.

Hip and Knee Arthroplasty

Ellen M. Soffin, MD, PhD[a],*, Thomas W. Wainwright, PT[b]

KEYWORDS

- Enhanced recovery after surgery • ERAS • Total joint arthroplasty
- Total hip arthroplasty • Total knee arthroplasty • Pathways • Analgesia
- Peripheral nerve blocks

KEY POINTS

- Clinical care elements included in enhanced recovery pathways for total joint arthroplasty vary widely between institutions and geographic practice settings despite favorable outcomes.
- Provided care is rigorously defined, delivered, and assessed, variation in details of core elements is reasonable and may be associated with successful local outcomes.
- Multimodal analgesia, tranexamic acid, and early mobilization form the basis of effective pathways for total hip and total knee arthroplasty.
- There remain difficulties agreeing on absolute consensus on universal enhanced recovery pathways for total hip and total knee arthroplasty.

INTRODUCTION

Enhanced recovery pathways for total joint arthroplasty (TJA) combine best evidence with best practice to improve outcomes and reduce health care costs. Classically, clinical pathways for total hip arthroplasty (THA) and total knee arthroplasty (TKA) bundle multidisciplinary care elements into pre-, intra-, and postoperative phases (**Box 1**). When organized and delivered as a package of care, enhanced recovery pathways show consistent evidence of benefit for reducing morbidity, improving clinical outcomes, and shortening length of hospital stay.[1] The gains that may be achieved via enhanced recovery pathways for TJA are attributed to reducing variation in pathway content (clinical care elements) and process (delivery of care elements). Accordingly, much of the research into enhanced recovery efficacy for TJA has been devoted to linking standardization of care with better outcomes.

It is evident that process and content variation are viewed differently in enhanced recovery research and practice. Whereas variation in process is classically regarded

[a] Department of Anesthesiology, Critical Care & Pain Management, Hospital for Special Surgery, 535 East 70th Street, New York, NY 10021, USA; [b] Orthopaedic Research Institute, Bournemouth University, 89 Holdenhurst Road, Bournemouth, Dorset BH8 8FT, UK
* Corresponding author. .
E-mail address: soffine@hss.edu

Anesthesiology Clin 40 (2022) 73–90
https://doi.org/10.1016/j.anclin.2021.11.003
1932-2275/22/© 2021 Elsevier Inc. All rights reserved.

anesthesiology.theclinics.com

Box 1
Standard care elements for total joint arthroplasty pathways

Preoperative
- Patient education and expectation setting
- Optimization of modifiable risk factors (detect and correct anemia, smoking cessation, nutritional support, cardiopulmonary and physical optimization where indicated)
- Avoid prolonged fasting
- Pre-emptive analgesia (see **Fig. 2**)

Intraoperative
- Short-acting anesthetics (neuraxial or total intravenous anesthesia-based general anesthetic)
- Multimodal analgesia (local infiltration analgesia, peripheral nerve blocks and continuous catheters; neuraxial and intrathecal analgesia; maximize use of nonopioid intravenous agents)
- Goal: euvolemia
- Goal: normothermia
- Timely antibiotic administration
- Timely antifibrinolytic administration (see **Fig. 1**)
- Postoperative nausea and vomiting prophylaxis

Postoperative
- Continue nonopioid-based multimodal analgesia
- Early mobilization
- Early intravenous/arterial line removal
- Early oral nutrition
- Bowel regimen
- Delirium prevention: screening and early intervention

Enhanced recovery pathways for TJA comprise evidence-based, multidisciplinary, multimodal components of care.[7–11]

---

as an opportunity to improve outcomes, variation in clinical content is frequently interpreted as evidence of uncertainty regarding optimal practice.[2] Enhanced recovery for TJA serves as a salient example of the tension between these 2 types of variation. Major gains have been made in minimizing variation in care processes to reduce length of hospital stay and readmission after TJA. However, in parallel, significant heterogeneity and complexity in clinical content have evolved within reported protocols. Ironically, this has occurred on a background of applying standardization to the process of creating the pathways themselves.[3]

Despite this complexity, positive outcomes after TJA continue to be reported. This raises a series of pragmatic questions:

Which elements are necessary?
Which ones are sufficient?
How can one reconcile variation in clinical content with the goal of standardized care?

These questions are occurring in the current climate in which calls for a return to fundamental ERAS principles based on targeted modulation of procedure-specific physiology are being made.[4,5]

To address these issues, the authors consider recent evidence suggesting that variation within a set of core protocol elements may be less important than providing the core elements themselves within pathways for TJA. They then update the literature surrounding variation in care delivery. Finally, the authors highlight differences in a selection of THA and TKA pathways from a range of international practice settings, each of which is associated with favorable outcomes after TJA. The authors speculate that provided care is rigorously defined, delivered, and assessed, variation in details of some content elements is reasonable and may be associated with successful local outcomes.

CONTENT VARIATION: ESSENTIAL ELEMENTS WITHIN CARE PATHWAYS FOR TOTAL JOINT ARTHROPLASTY

Over recent decades, clinical pathways and care programs for THA and TKA have undergone significant evolution as enhanced recovery has become standard of care.[6,7] A wealth of evidence has accumulated to inform clinical and society guidelines for pathway content, which in turn have been developed to guide creation and implementation of TJA protocols worldwide.[8–11] Despite these advances, society guidelines that evaluate the same or similar evidence make different recommendations for care elements, and the details of recommended elements are not always clearly defined. These disparate recommendations present challenges not only for implementing or refining a TJA protocol, but also for directly comparing results and outcomes of published studies that include different care elements.[12,13]

There are approximately 20 clinical care elements with high-quality evidence to support inclusion in a TJA pathway (see **Box 1**).[7–10] Despite the wealth and strength of evidence, to date, there is no consensus on which care elements and combinations thereof are the most important to achieve optimal outcomes after TJA. Until such time as this is clear, attempts to develop universally accepted, fully standardized enhanced recovery pathways for TJA will be limited. Moreover, as highlighted by the differences found in guidelines and society recommendations, one may never reach a fully standardized protocol that is suitable for all TJA patients and practice settings. In lieu of this, it may be possible – indeed, preferable – to derive the essential care elements associated with optimal outcomes after TJA and leave room for variation in care based on local circumstances and patient-individualized care (until future research provides conclusive guidance for the currently undefined care elements).

In an early analysis of this question, Khan and colleagues demonstrated that an enhanced recovery protocol including a few core components was associated with reductions in complications, length of stay (LOS), and 30-day mortality.[14] The pathway featured patient education, multimodal analgesia with local anesthetic infiltration, standardized anesthesia, tranexamic acid (TXA), and early mobilization. In the most recent affirmation of these early results, the POWER2 trial concluded that optimal outcomes and the lowest incidence of complications after TJA were among patients who received regional anesthesia, (TXA), and early mobilization.[15] Likewise, in a US-based population analysis of enhanced recovery elements and outcomes, multimodal analgesia, TXA, antiemetics on the day of surgery, and early mobilization had the strongest individual effects on reducing complications and LOS.[16] A similar population-based study subsequently confirmed these results, and further concluded that the incidence of complications differed minimally with different combinations of care elements.[17]

As the preceding discussion suggests, the 3 core elements that are consistently associated with improved outcomes after TJA are: TXA, multimodal analgesia with locoregional techniques, and early mobilization and rehabilitation.[18] Despite this evidence, there is considerable variation in how these elements are integrated into TJA pathways. Further, each represents an exemplar of how variation in the mode of provision may be less important than providing the element itself.

Tranexamic Acid

Of all the antifibrinolytic medications, TXA has been the best characterized agent for minimizing perioperative blood loss and transfusion requirements after THA and

TKA.[19] Two recent network meta-analyses both concluded that all TXA formulations were statistically superior to placebo for the outcomes of blood loss and transfusion after THA or TKA.[20,21] These benefits were found irrespective of whether intravenous, topical, oral, or combined intravenous/topical TXA regimens were provided.

Despite the publication of more than 2000 studies on TXA and outcomes after TJA, there is no consensus regarding the most effective and safest route, dose, and timing of administration (**Fig. 1**). Although all routes and formulations of TXA are effective,[19–23] emerging data support oral TXA as noninferior to the intravenous route for minimizing bleeding, transfusion, and infection, without increasing the risk of deep vein thrombosis.[22,23] Of particular relevance for value-based care, oral TXA is significantly less expensive than intravenous or topical formulations, and arguably easier for perioperative staff to access and administer.[22,23] These benefits would be expected to

Oral

- Reported doses range from 1-4 g, given 1-8 hours prior to surgery.[19-23]
- The most common dose is 2g, given 2 hours prior to surgery.[19,23]
- The optimal dose and timing are unclear, but a minimum dose of 2g is recommended.[20]

Topical

- Reported doses range from 0.5-3g, given at the end of surgery.[19]

Intravenous

- The most common regimen is 10-20 mg/kg, administered as a single dose prior to surgical incision.[20,21]

Combination

- Combinations of oral, intravenous and topical TXA are effective, compared to placebo or no TXA.[19-21]
- The optimal combinations are unclear.[19-23]

Fig. 1. Tranexamic acid options for total joint arthroplasty pathways. Controversy persists regarding the optimal regimen and formulation of TXA to protect against blood loss and transfusion. There is consensus that TXA should be included in THA and TKA pathways, where not contraindicated.[8–10,19–23] Irrespective of route and formulation, higher doses and multiple doses are not recommended.[19–21]

decrease direct and indirect costs of care (via reduced workload of perioperative personnel) and translate into cost-saving benefits for health care systems. Oral TXA may also represent a patient safety advantage over intravenous formulations by eliminating inadvertent intrathecal administration, as has been described in case reports in patients undergoing spinal anesthesia for TJA.[24]

Multimodal Analgesia with Locoregional Techniques

Providing effective, opioid-sparing multimodal analgesia with 2 or more classes of analgesic agent is associated with improved outcomes after TJA. Although expert guidelines consistently recommend multimodal analgesia, the specific choice and combination of agents have historically been left to local stakeholders (**Fig. 2**). Typically, unless precluded by patient risk factors and comorbidities, acetaminophen, a nonsteroidal anti-inflammatory drug (NSAID), or a cyclo-oxygenase-2-selective inhibitor and a gabapentinoid form the basis of the analgesic regimen within TJA pathways.[8–11,25] Notably, although no new analgesic agents have been added to the formulary in recent years, considerable evidence has accumulated to support removing gabapentinoids from TJA pathways in gabapentinoid-naïve patients.[11,26,27] This is based on years of accumulating data suggesting minimal evidence of benefit for acute pain, and significant risk of harm, particularly when coadministered with opioids.[26,27] Indeed, the latest PROSPECT guidelines specifically recommend against providing gabapentinoid therapy as part of the analgesic management of THA.[11]

Peripheral nerve blocks (PNBs), local infiltration analgesia, and periarticular injection of local anesthetics have assumed a central role in pathways for THA and TKA in many centers.[28] There is evidence that single injection and continuous catheter techniques improve analgesia, minimize opioid consumption, conserve hospital resources, and reduce cardiac, pulmonary and renal complications after TJA.[29] Currently, reports of novel blocks and regional analgesic strategies are outpacing capacity to assess the relative value and benefits when added to pathways for TJA.[30–33] Nonetheless, most clinical guidelines recommend routine use of PNBs for TJA.[8,9,11,29] A notable exception to this is the 2019 guideline on TJA from the Enhanced Recovery After Surgery Society, which did not find compelling evidence for recommending routine use of PNB for TJA.[10] Rather, simple multimodal opioid-sparing regimens including high-dose preoperative steroid administration plus high-volume local anesthetic infiltration have been proposed as an alternative strategy.[34,35]

Early Mobilization

It is unsurprising that good analgesic control leads to early mobilization, which in turn is associated with globally improved outcomes following TJA. Early mobilization in the first 24 hours after THA or TKA is consistently effective for reducing LOS, acute early complications, thromboembolic events, morbidity, and mortality, and improving patient satisfaction.[36–39] Despite widespread endorsement of early mobilization as part of enhanced recovery guidelines in many surgical subspecialities,[10,40] it has previously been reported that less than 10% of TJA patients ambulate on the day of surgery.[41] Reasons for this are speculative but have been proposed to include patient-, structural-, and cultural-related issues.[42] For example, the ideal time to initiate mobilization is undefined, and often left to the discretion of nurses and physical therapists.[43] Delayed mobilization may also be related to institutional practice and local protocols, where some units encourage early mobilization, and others do not. Patient motivation is likely to be a key driver of time-to-mobilization, and a factor that is not modifiable by anesthetic or surgical technique, but which may be increased following the COVID-19 pandemic. It has been proposed that patients are likely to be strongly motivated to get

Pre-emptive analgesia

- Acetaminophen, NSAIDs, COX-2 selective inhibitors, steroids
- Gabapentinoids for appropriate patients[26,27]

Loco-regional techniques (TKA)

- Peripheral nerve blocks/continuous catheters (femoral, sciatic, adductor canal, IPACK, genicular), LIA, PAI, epidural catheter, intrathecal opioids.

Loco-regional techniques (THA)

- Peripheral nerve blocks/continuous catheters (QLB, fascia iliaca, SIFI, PENG, ESPB, lumbar plexus), LIA, PAI, epidural catheter, intrathecal opioids

Systemic analgesia and adjuncts

- Opioids, dexmedetomidine, dexamethasone, lidocaine, ketamine, antidepressants.

Fig. 2. Analgesic options for total joint arthroplasty pathways. Controversy persists regarding the optimal analgesic regimen. There is consensus that opioid-sparing multimodal analgesia should be included in THA and TKA pathways. A reasonable strategy includes combinations of nonopioid agents, locoregional techniques and opioids as needed (at the lowest dose/shortest duration required).[8–10] COX, cyclo-oxygenase; ESPB, erector spinae plane block; IPACK, interspace between the popliteal artery and posterior capsule of the knee; LIA, local infiltration analgesia; NSAID, nonsteroidal anti-inflammatory; PAI, periarticular injection; PENG, pericapsular nerve group; QLB, quadratus lumborum block; SIFI, suprainguinalfascia iliaca; THA, total hip arthroplasty; TKA, total knee arthroplasty.

home sooner following surgery to distance themselves from possible exposure to COVID-19.[44] In addition, the recent increase in the number of TJAs performed within ambulatory surgical centers, and the growing trend toward outpatient TJA surgery will further necessitate the structural and cultural changes needed to facilitate early mobilization and achievement of independent mobility so that discharge requirements are achieved on the day of surgery.

OUTCOME VARIATION: STANDARDIZING MEASUREMENT OF PATHWAY EFFICACY

Interestingly, debates regarding the optimal selection of pathway elements have not necessarily focused on outcomes. Health care systems may not value pain, opioid-consumption, opioid-related adverse effects except in so far as they affect LOS, and there is rarely an incentive to return TJA patients more quickly to normal function and everyday activities. Patient-focused outcomes have largely been missing from evaluations of interventions directed toward reducing LOS. Most studies evaluating pathway efficacy are restricted to traditional outcomes, such as LOS, readmission, mortality, and complications, and may not be sufficiently sensitive to detect benefits of individual clinical interventions, like PNBs, which would not be expected to influence mid-to long-term outcomes.[45] More recently, studies have considered patient-reported outcome measures and system-wide cost savings as indices of pathway efficacy.[46] These have increased the complexity of effectiveness analyses, but also the relevance of study findings, and are required for comparative evaluation of published studies.

A complete review of methods to standardize outcomes assessment is out with the scope of this article, but calls have been made to derive a core set of outcomes and measurements for enhanced recovery programs. In addition to process evaluation, these should ideally reflect the different perspectives of key stakeholders (patients and practitioners) as well as the stage of recovery, and assessment of procedure-specific clinical improvement[45,46] In the case of TJA, it should also be acknowledged that although patient-reported outcome measures (PROMs) show improvement in most patients, discrepancies are seen when compared with measures of physical performance, both in the early and later recovery phase.[47,48]

PROCESS VARIATION: QUANTIFIABLE AND UNQUANTIFIABLE ASPECTS OF CARE PATHWAY DELIVERY

Enhanced recovery efficacy cannot be considered in isolation from pathway adherence. Along with minimizing variation in care, strict pathway adherence has long been advocated as an effective strategy to reduce complications after surgery.[40] Ample evidence to support this concept can also be found for patients undergoing THA and TKA where adherence above a minimum threshold or minimum number of care elements within a pathway has been associated with reductions in any complication (eg, cardiopulmonary, stroke, acute kidney injury, thromboembolic event, and infection),[15–17,49] major complications (eg, cardiopulmonary,[16,17] in-hospital mortality,[16] infection,[15] transfusion,[15–17] and need for revision surgery[15]), and LOS,[15–17,49] in both clinical and population-based studies.[15–17,49]

Early data to support this concept associated lower costs of care and shorter LOS after TJA with a pathway adherence threshold of 80%.[49] Recent population-based and large clinical studies evaluating the impact of increasing the number of care components in TJA pathways have similarly associated higher numbers of components with incremental decreases in any complication rates.[15–17] Interestingly, in these studies, overall adherence approximated 70%, and greater adherence to classic protocol care elements was generally associated with better outcomes, shorter LOS, and reductions in mild, moderate and severe postoperative complications.[15–17,49]

Individual complications may also be more reliably minimized when a pathway is provided en bloc compared with delivering individual targeted interventions. A recent systematic review and meta-analysis on prevention of postoperative pulmonary complications found that the greatest protective benefits were among patients cared for under an enhanced recovery pathway, compared with those who received single or combined pulmonary or respiratory interventions.[50]

It is unclear why the whole is greater than the sum of the parts, but emerging data suggest this may be attributed, at least partially, to staff experiences of delivering care. This is likely to be a key aspect of successful outcomes, but one which is subject to great variability and is difficult to quantify. Nonetheless, a recent systematic review of care delivery by enhanced recovery teams concluded that evidence-based guidelines were useful for improving patient care, but outcomes mainly improved over time, as staff attitudes toward enhanced recovery became more favorable and practices became progressively ingrained.[51] Further, an ethnographic study on enhanced recovery for TJA implementation found that care was viewed as a message that had to be accepted and communicated consistently by staff, but ultimately, successful implementation requires empowering patients to work toward their own recovery.[52]

REAL-WORLD EXAMPLES: VARIABLE PATHWAYS, SIMILAR OUTCOMES AFTER TOTAL JOINT ARTHROPLASTY

This discussion illustrates a current tension in selecting care elements for TJA pathways: some elements (eg, optimal TXA route, timing, and dosing) have a wealth of options for delivery and reasonable evidence to support any of them for inclusion in a TJA pathway. Others (eg, PNBs) are associated with gaps in knowledge that preclude straightforward selection. Unquantifiable local aspects of care organization and delivery and patient factors also clearly impact outcomes but cannot be directly incorporated into the pathways themselves. Each results in the requirement to make choices in the face of uncertainty. How should one decide which elements to include? Individual selection is likely to be based on practitioner experience, local resource availability, and patient population.

The authors propose that provided the outcomes of interest are standardized, the pathway includes the core elements associated with favorable outcomes and optimal outcomes are achieved for the local practice setting, the individual details of the core elements provided to the patient probably matter less than ensuring care is organized and delivered according to core enhanced recovery principles. To explore this, the authors considered components of TKA and THA pathways from a range of international practice settings and compared measured outcomes achieved according to each pathway. This comparison is intended to be illustrative and to identify gaps in consensus and variation in chosen outcomes that assess pathway efficacy. The authors emphasize that **Table 1** is based on details available in the published literature and may not represent the complete, up-to-date practice within the included institutions at the time of writing. This highlights the dynamic nature of care pathways, and the fact that real-world practice will often lag (and sometimes lead) the published evidence.

The authors included pathways from 5 enhanced recovery centers for TJA: one from the United Kingdom (Healthcare NHS Foundational Trust, Northumbria), one from Denmark (Copenhagen University Hospital, Hvidovre), one from Canada (Hôpital Maisonneuve-Rosemont, Montreal), and two from the United States, of which one was a Veteran's Administration Hospital (VA Palo Alto Health Care System, Palo Alto, California), and one was a tertiary care academic medical center (Mayo Clinic, Rochester, Minnesota).

Of the 3 core care elements with the most evidence to support inclusion in TJA pathways, day-of-surgery mobilization was the only component with 100% agreement between the centers. Although all centers include TXA for THA and TKA, there was no consensus regarding dosing strategy, timing, or route of administration, and none included oral TXA. All centers included prophylaxis against postoperative nausea and vomiting, although details of the individual agents provided, and whether agents

Table 1
Selected pathways for total hip arthroplasty and total knee arthroplasty

	United Kingdom[38]	Denmark[6,53]	Canada[54]	United States (Palo Alto)[55,56]	United States (Minnesota)[57–59]
Preoperative multimodal analgesia	• Paracetamol (1g) • Oxycodone can be given on an individual, as-needed basis	• Paracetamol (1g) • Celecoxib (400 mg)	• Acetaminophen (1 g) • Celecoxib (400 mg) • Pregabalin (150 mg) • Oxycodone ER (10 mg)	• Acetaminophen (1g) • celecoxib (400 mg) • Gabapentin (600 mg) for opioid tolerant patients • TKA: continuous adductor canal catheter placed ± IPACK block (by surgeon request) • THA: continuous erector spinae plane catheter placed	• Acetaminophen (1 g) • Celecoxib (400 mg) • Oxycodone IR 5–10 mg or oxycodone CR 10–20 mg can be given
Intraoperative anaesthetic	• Spinal anesthesia with sedation	• General anesthesia with LMA and TIVA.	• Epidural anesthesia with sedation • Epidural catheter removed at the end of surgery	• Spinal anesthesia with sedation	• Spinal anesthesia with sedation

(continued on next page)

Table 1
(continued)

	United Kingdom[38]	Denmark[6,53]	Canada[54]	United States (Palo Alto)[55,56]	United States (Minnesota)[57–59]
Intraoperative multimodal and locoregional analgesia	• Surgeon administered local infiltration analgesia (100 mL levobupivacaine, 1.25 mg/mL) ketamine (5 mg boluses, up to a total dose of 0.5 mg/kg) on an individual, as needed basis • Paracetamol 1 g intravenously ± parecoxib 40 mg intravenously if not given preoperatively	• Surgeon administered periarticular infiltration	• Surgeon administered periarticular infiltration (ropivacaine 400 mg, ketorolac 30 mg, and epinephrine)	• As above; regional analgesic techniques performed prior to surgery start	• Fentanyl up to 250 µg intravenously, +/− hydromorphone up to 1 mg intravenously as needed • Options include: adductor canal block, continuous catheter, periarticular infiltration, IPACK block.
Blood management	• Intravenous tranexamic acid (up to 30 mg/kg) and • Topical tranexamic acid (total combined dose 3g)	• Tranexamic acid (1 g) before incision and • Tranexamic acid (1 g) 3 h postoperatively	• Intravenous tranexamic acid (up to 15 mg/kg) before incision and • Intravenous tranexamic acid (1g) prior to closing	• Intravenous tranexamic acid (1. g) before tourniquet inflation and • 1g tranexamic acid before tourniquet release	• Intravenous tranexamic acid (1 g) before incision
PONV and antibiotic prophylaxis & other intra-operative medications	• Intravenous ondansetron (4 mg) • Intravenous dexamethasone (8 mg) • Teicoplanin and gentamicin, dosed according to patient weight.	• Intravenous methylprednisolone (125 mg) • Selected prophylactic antibiotic provided before incision	• Aprepitant (125 mg) • Scopolamine patch (1.5 mg) • Selected prophylactic antibiotic provided before incision	• Intravenous ondansetron (4 mg) • First line: cefazolin	• Intravenous ondansetron (4 mg) • Intravenous dexamethasone (4 mg) • First line: cefazolin

Post-operative multimodal analgesia	• Paracetamol (1g four times daily) • Diclofenac PR for up to 48 h • Gabapentin (300 mg twice daily for up to 10 d) as needed • Oxycodone (5–20 mg twice daily for 2 d) followed by Codeine phosphate (30–60 mg 4 times daily) • Additional rescue analgesia options include oxycodone (5–10 mg every 2 hours); morphine sulfate 10 mg/5 mL oral solution 5–10 mg every 4 hours); intravenously morphine (1–10 mg)	• Paracetamol (1 g 4 times daily for 7 d) • Celecoxib (200 mg twice daily) • Oral morphine (10 mg) as needed for rescue analgesia	• Acetaminophen (1 g 3 times daily) • Celecoxib (100 mg twice daily) • Pregabalin (75 mg at bedtime) • Tramadol (50–100 mg every 4–6 h as needed) • If insufficient pain control, add oxycodone (5–7.5 mg every 3 h)	• Acetaminophen (1g every 6 h) • Celecoxib (200 mg twice daily) • Oxycodone (5–10 mg every 6 h) • Additional rescue analgesia options include oxycodone 5–10 mg every 4 h as needed; intravenous hydromorphone or morphine every 4 h as needed • Perineural infusion of ropivacaine 0.2% (adductor canal catheter)	PACU: • Acetaminophen (1 g every 6 h) • Letamine (10 mg intravenously, once as needed for pain score $\geq$ 4) • Additional rescue analgesia options include: intravenous fentanyl (25 µg) or hydromorphone (0.2 mg) for pain $\geq$ 4 • Oxycodone IR (5 mg for pain $\leq$ 4 or 10 mg orally for pain $\geq$ 5; 1 dose prior to discharge to the floor) Floor: • Acetaminophen (1 g every 6 h) • Ketorolac (15 mg every 6 h for 4 doses) • Tramadol (50–100 mg) or • Oxycodone (5–10 mg) or • Hydromorphone 2–4 mg • For breakthrough pain ($\geq$7) fentanyl (25 µg pain; up to 3 doses)
Mobilization	• Goal: day of surgery	• Goal: day of surgery	• Goal: day of surgery	• Goal: day of surgery	• Goal: day of surgery

(continued on next page)

Table 1
(continued)

	United Kingdom[38]	Denmark[6,53]	Canada[54]	United States (Palo Alto)[55,56]	United States (Minnesota)[57-59]
Outcomes	• Decrease in LOS • Reduction in 30-d and 90-d mortality • Conservation of hospital resources (bed days) • Reduction in requirement for blood transfusion • Reduction in morbidity (myocardial infarction, CVA, PE/DVT) • No change in readmission rate	• Decrease in LOS • High patient satisfaction scores • Lower incidence of complications (myocardial infarction) • No adverse effects on patient readmission	• Decrease in LOS • Reduction in grade 1–2 complications (events requiring no therapy) but no effects on grade 3–5 complications (events requiring intervention) • Reduction in direct health care costs	• Increased use of spinal anesthesia • Increased use of continuous peripheral nerve catheters • No differences in 30-d postoperative complications • No differences in hospital readmission, emergency department visits, or blood transfusions between patients who received spinal or general anesthesia • Increased early ambulation after THA in patients who received continuous erector spinae plane block	• Decrease in LOS • Reduction in patient-reported pain • Reduction in postoperative confusion • Improved participation with physical therapy • Reduction in total direct hospital costs

Abbreviations: IPACK, interspace between the popliteal artery and posterior capsule of the knee; LMA, laryngeal mask airway; LOS, length of stay; TIVA, total intravenous anesthesia.

were given pre- or intraoperatively varied across centers. Only Copenhagen University Hospital included high-dose methylprednisolone as an intraoperative agent.

There was reasonable agreement in terms of combinations of oral and intravenous analgesics, with all centers providing acetaminophen or paracetamol, and all including an NSAID. Celecoxib was the most commonly chosen NSAID. There was poor agreement in choice, dose, and route of opioid administration, although all centers included opioids with administration parameters (usually according to pain score and with progression from weak to strong opioids). Likewise, choice, dose and duration of gabapentinoid were not uniform between the centers. Differences in each of these elements may be influenced by local regulatory and prescribing practices, as well as by different patient expectations and demands.

Although all centers included a source of locoregional analgesia, the details of individual techniques represented a prominent source of variation. Some centers restricted local anesthetic delivery to surgeon-administered periarticular injection, while others included anesthesiologist-administered fascial plane blocks, continuous catheter techniques, and combinations of blocks and injections. Given that each center published compelling data to support their choice(s) of locoregional technique, variation in the details between centers is likely to reflect, at least in part, differences in institutional expertise and culture. These aspects are likely to be crucial to overall pathway success at the local level, but may not be generalizable to other geographic and practice settings.

Choice of outcomes was likewise variable, with most centers reporting their experiences with traditional enhanced recovery outcomes and when evaluating the pathways as a whole: LOS, complications, readmission, and resource consumption. In contrast, patient-relevant outcomes like pain and satisfaction were more frequently found when studies focused on optimizing individual care elements within a defined pathway. Despite these points of variation, the global effect of pathways was similar, with consistent results found for standard enhanced recovery outcomes.

FUTURE DIRECTIONS

One of the major successes of enhanced recovery has been to translate large variations in care into standardized practice. However, it has become evident that no 2 pathways for THA or TKA are the same. According to fundamental enhanced recovery principles, this would be considered a shortcoming. Conversely, as presented here, evidence suggests that optimal outcomes can be achieved by allowing some variation in detail, provided the core elements of care are delivered. Effective pathways rely on translating best evidence into practice; yet they also require individual tailoring according to local experience and resources. Likewise, greater adherence to enhanced recovery elements improves outcomes, but what are the proper elements to which one should adhere? Evidence continues to support TJA pathways, which include blood management, multimodal analgesia, and early mobilization, as the basis of the care trajectory. Consequently, the emphasis should be on providing these essential elements of care, rather than on perfecting the details thereof. In this sense, adaptation of enhanced recovery care to local culture becomes more important than defining all details of each care element. For example, providing opioid-sparing analgesia via locoregional techniques assumes more global importance than the individual peripheral nerve or field block selected for the pathway. On the other hand, minimizing variation within the institution may be more important than seeking to create a single pathway suitable for all settings and patients. To this end, pathways should be kept simple (including the fewest number of active and proven care elements) so that they are reproducible, and all care elements can be delivered as intended to every patient (and monitored via local compliance audit).

Now that enhanced recovery for TJA has largely been integrated into health care systems worldwide, the future task for anesthesia and enhanced recovery care teams is to achieve the pain- and risk-free procedure. Adding to the challenge, this will need to be achieved in conjunction with rising patient demand and medical complexity. Logically, as patient-specific risks are evaluated and incorporated into care pathways, further variation and individualization of care may be expected. Indeed, as care and outcomes continue to improve, TJA is increasingly being offered to patients who were formerly considered to be poor surgical candidates. Key demographics for optimization and risk reduction include the patient with diabetes mellitus, obesity, advanced age, frailty, and/or cognitive dysfunction. At the other end of the spectrum, shifts in practice patterns and reimbursement mandate more TJA procedures will be performed in the ambulatory setting and on a same-day discharge basis. A balance between standardization and permissive variation is likely to be key to successful translation of TJA from hospital to ambulatory settings and to the future of enhanced recovery for THA and TKA.

CLINICS CARE POINTS

- Ensure the TJA-enhanced recovery pathway includes tranexamic acid, multimodal analgesia, and early mobilization.
- Remove institutional process variation, then regularly audit compliance to each care component of the institutional enhanced recovery care pathway.
- Examine local clinical outcomes in parallel with changes to the evidence base to identify gaps in care and opportunities to improve defined outcomes.

DISCLOSURE

The authors have no relevant financial disclosures.

REFERENCES,

1. Petersen PB, Kehlet H, Jørgensen CC. Lundbeck Foundation Centre for Fast-track Hip and Knee Replacement Collaborative Group. Improvement in fast-track hip and knee arthroplasty: a prospective multicentre study of 36,935 procedures from 2010 to 2017. Sci Rep 2020;10(1):21233.
2. Urbach DR, Baxter NN. Reducing variation in surgical care. Br Med Jl 2005; 330(7505):1401–2.
3. Brindle M, Nelson G, Lobo DN, et al. Recommendations from the ERAS® Society for standards for the development of enhanced recovery after surgery guidelines. BJS Open 2020;4:157–63.
4. Kehlet H. ERAS implementation—time to move forward. Ann Surg 2018;267: 998–9.
5. Memtsoudis SG, Poeran J, Kehlet H. Enhanced recovery after surgery in the United States: from evidence-based practice to uncertain science? JAMA 2019;321(11):1049–50.
6. Husted H. Fast-track hip and knee arthroplasty: clinical and organizational aspects. Acta Orthop Suppl 2012;83(346):1–39.
7. Soffin EM, YaDeau JT. Enhanced recovery after surgery for primary hip and knee arthroplasty: a review of the evidence. Br J Anaesth 2016;117(suppl 3):iii62–72.

8. Soffin EM, Gibbons MM, Ko CY, et al. Evidence review conducted for the agency for healthcare research and quality safety program for improving surgical care and recovery: focus on anesthesiology for total hip arthroplasty. Anesth Analg 2019;128(3):454–65.

9. Soffin EM, Gibbons MM, Ko CY, et al. Healthcare research and quality safety program for improving surgical care and recovery: focus on anesthesiology for total knee arthroplasty. Anesth Analg 2019;128(3):441–53.

10. Wainwright TW, Gill M, McDonald DA, et al. Consensus statement for perioperative care in total hip replacement and total knee replacement surgery: Enhanced Recovery After Surgery (ERAS®) Society recommendations. Acta Orthop 2020; 91(3):363.

11. Anger M, Valovska T, Beloeil H, et al, PROSPECT Working Group* and the European Society of Regional Anaesthesia and Pain Therapy. PROSPECT guideline for total hip arthroplasty: a systematic review and procedure-specific postoperative pain management recommendations. Anaesthesia 2021. https://doi.org/10.1111/anae.15498.

12. Deng Q-F, Gu H-Y, Peng W-Y, et al. Impact of enhanced recovery after surgery on postoperative recovery after joint arthroplasty: results from a systematic review and meta-analysis. Postgrad Med J 2018;94(1118):678–93.

13. Zhu S, Qian W, Jiang C, et al. Enhanced recovery after surgery for hip and knee arthroplasty: a systematic review and meta-analysis. Postgrad Med J 2017; 93(1106):736–42.

14. Khan SK, Malviya A, Muller SD, et al. Reduced short-term complications and mortality following Enhanced Recovery primary hip and knee arthroplasty: results from 6000 consecutive procedures. Acta Orthop 2014;85(1):26–31.

15. Ripollés-Melchor J, Abad-Motos A, Díez-Remesal Y, et al. Postoperative Outcomes Within Enhanced Recovery After Surgery Protocol in Elective Total Hip and Knee Arthroplasty (POWER2) Study Investigators Group for the Spanish Perioperative Audit and Research Network (REDGERM). Association between use of enhanced recovery after surgery protocol and postoperative complications in total hip and knee arthroplasty in the Postoperative Outcomes Within Enhanced Recovery After Surgery Protocol in Elective Total Hip and Knee Arthroplasty Study (POWER2). JAMA Surg 2020;155(4):e196024.

16. Memtsoudis SG, Fiasconaro M, Soffin EM, et al. Enhanced recovery after surgery components and perioperative outcomes: a nationwide observational study. Br J Anaesth 2020;124(5):638–47.

17. Chen KK, Chan JJ, Zubizarreta NJ, et al. Enhanced recovery after surgery protocols in lower extremity joint arthroplasty: using observational data to identify the optimal combination of components. J Arthroplasty 2021;36(8):2722–8.

18. Johnson RL, Kopp SL. Optimizing perioperative management of total joint arthroplasty. Anesthesiol Clin 2014;32(4):865–80.

19. Fillingham YA, Ramkumar DB, Jevsevar DS, et al. Tranexamic acid in total joint arthroplasty: the endorsed clinical practice guides of the American Association of Hip and Knee Surgeons, American Society of Regional Anesthesia and Pain Medicine, American Academy of Orthopaedic Surgeons, Hip Society, and Knee Society. Reg Anesth Pain Med 2019;44(1):7–11.

20. Fillingham YA, Ramkumar DB, Jevsevar DS, et al. The efficacy of tranexamic acid in total knee arthroplasty: a network meta-analysis. J Arthroplasty 2018;33(10): 3090–8.e1.

21. Fillingham YA, Ramkumar DB, Jevsevar DS, et al. The efficacy of tranexamic acid in total hip arthroplasty: a network meta-analysis. J Arthroplasty 2018;33(10): 3083–9.e4.
22. Ye W, Liu Y, Liu WF, et al. Comparison of efficacy and safety between oral and intravenous administration of tranexamic acid for primary total knee/hip replacement: a meta-analysis of randomized controlled trial. J Orthop Surg Res 2020; 15(1):21.
23. Sun C, Zhang X, Chen L, et al. Comparison of oral versus intravenous tranexamic acid in total knee and hip arthroplasty: a GRADE analysis and meta-analysis. Medicine (Baltimore) 2020;99(44):e22999.
24. Patel S, Robertson B, McConachie I. Catastrophic drug errors involving tranexamic acid administered during spinal anaesthesia. Anaesthesia 2019;74(7): 904–14.
25. American Society of Anesthesiologists Task Force on Acute Pain Management. Practice guidelines for acute pain management in the perioperative setting: an updated report by the American Society of Anesthesiologists Task Force on Acute Pain Management. Anesthesiology 2012;116:248–73.
26. Kharasch ED, Clark JD, Kheterpal S. Perioperative Gabapentinoids: Deflating the Bubble. Anesthesiology 2020;133(2):251–4.
27. Verret M, Lauzier F, Zarychanski R, et al. Perioperative use of gabapentinoids for the management of postoperative acute pain: a systematic review and meta-analysis. Anesthesiology 2020;133(2):265–79.
28. Soffin EM, Wu CL. Regional and multimodal analgesia to reduce opioid use after total joint arthroplasty: a narrative review. HSS J 2019;15(1):57–65.
29. Memtsoudis SG, Cozowicz C, Bekeris J, et al. Peripheral nerve block anesthesia/ analgesia for patients undergoing primary hip and knee arthroplasty: recommendations from the International Consensus on Anesthesia-Related Outcomes after Surgery (ICAROS) group based on a systematic review and meta-analysis of current literature. Reg Anesth Pain Med 2021. https://doi.org/10.1136/rapm-2021-102750. rapm-2021-102750.
30. Terkawi AS, Mavridis D, Sessler DI, et al. Pain management modalities after total knee arthroplasty: a network meta-analysis of 170 randomized controlled trials. Anesthesiology 2017;126(5):923–37.
31. Bugada D, Bellini V, Lorini LF, et al. Update on selective regional analgesia for hip surgery patients. Anesthesiol Clin 2018;36(3):403–15.
32. Hussain N, Brull R, Sheehy B, et al. Does the addition of iPACK to adductor canal block in the presence or absence of periarticular local anesthetic infiltration improve analgesic and functional outcomes following total knee arthroplasty? A systematic review and meta-analysis. Reg Anesth Pain Med 2021;46(8):713–21.
33. Guay J, Johnson RL, Kopp S. Nerve blocks or no nerve blocks for pain control after elective hip replacement (arthroplasty) surgery in adults. Cochrane Database Syst Rev 2017;10(10):CD011608.
34. Andersen LO, Kehlet H. Analgesic efficacy of local infiltration analgesia in hip and knee arthroplasty: a systematic review. Br J Anaesth 2014;113:360–74.
35. Kehlet H, Lindberg-Larsen V. High-dose glucocorticoid before hip and knee arthroplasty: to use or not to use-that's the question. Acta Orthop 2018;89:477–9.
36. Schneider M, Kawahara I, Ballantyne G, et al. Predictive factors influencing fast track rehabilitation following primary total hip and knee arthroplasty. Arch Orthop Trauma Surg 2009;129(12):1585–91.
37. Husted H, Otte KS, Kristensen BB, et al. Low risk of thromboembolic complications after fast-track hip and knee arthroplasty. Acta Orthop 2010;81(5):599–605.

38. Malviya A, Martin K, Harper I, et al. Enhanced recovery program for hip and knee replacement reduces death rate. Acta Orthop 2011;82(5):577–81.
39. Guerra ML, Singh PJ, Taylor NF. Early mobilization of patients who have had a hip or knee joint replacement reduces length of stay in hospital: a systematic review. Clin Rehabil 2015;29(9):844–54.
40. Ljungqvist O, Scott M, Fearon KC. Enhanced recovery after surgery: a review. JAMA Surg 2017;152(3):292–8.
41. Chua MJ, Hart AJ, Mittal R, et al. Early mobilisation after total hip or knee arthroplasty: a multicentre prospective observational study. PLoS One 2017;12(6): e0179820.
42. Wainwright TW, Burgess L. Early ambulation and physiotherapy after surgery. In: Ljungqvist O, Francis N, Urman R, editors. Enhanced recovery after surgery. Cham: Springer; 2020. https://doi.org/10.1007/978-3-030-33443-7_23. October 9, 2021.
43. Tayrose G, Newman D, Slover J, et al, Rapid mobilization decreases length-of-stay in joint replacement patients. Bull Hosp Jt Dis 2013;71(3):222-226.
44. Wainwright TW. Enhanced recovery after surgery (ERAS) for hip and knee replacement—why and how it should be implemented following the COVID-19 pandemic. Medicina 2021;57:81. https://doi.org/10.3390/medicina57010081. October 9, 2021.
45. Etges APBS, Stefani LPC, Vrochides D, et al. A standardized framework for evaluating surgical enhanced recovery pathways: a recommendations statement from the TDABC in Health-care Consortium. J Health Econ Outcomes Res 2021;8(1):116–24.
46. Feldman LS, Lee L, Fiore J Jr. What outcomes are important in the assessment of enhanced recovery after surgery (ERAS) pathways? Can J Anaesth 2015;62(2): 120–30.
47. Luna IE, Kehlet H, Peterson B, et al. Early patient-reported outcomes versus objective function after total hip and knee arthroplasty: a prospective cohort study. Bone Joint J 2017;99-B(9):1167–75.
48. Luna IE, Kehlet H, Wede HR, et al. Objectively measured early physical activity after total hip or knee arthroplasty. J Clin Monit Comput 2019;33(3):509–22.
49. Stowers MD, Manuopangai L, Hill AG, et al. Enhanced recovery after surgery in elective hip and knee arthroplasty reduces length of hospital stay. ANZ J Surg 2016;86:475–9.
50. Odor PM, Bampoe S, Gilhooly D, et al. Perioperative interventions for prevention of postoperative pulmonary complications: systematic review and meta-analysis. BMJ 2020;368:m540.
51. Cohen R, Gooberman-Hill R. Staff experiences of enhanced recovery after surgery: systematic review of qualitative studies. BMJ Open 2019;9(2):e022259.
52. Drew S, Judge A, Cohen R, et al. Enhanced recovery after surgery implementation in practice: an ethnographic study of services for hip and knee replacement. BMJ Open 2019;9(3):e024431.
53. Husted H, Holm G. Fast track in total hip and knee arthroplasty–experiences from Hvidovre University Hospital, Denmark. Injury 2006;37(Suppl 5):S31–5.
54. Vendittoli PA, Pellei K, Desmeules F, et al. Enhanced recovery short-stay hip and knee joint replacement program improves patients outcomes while reducing hospital costs. Orthop Traumatol Surg Res 2019;105(7):1237–43.
55. Tamboli M, Leng JC, Hunter OO, et al. Five-year follow-up to assess long-term sustainability of changing clinical practice regarding anesthesia and regional

analgesia for lower extremity arthroplasty. Korean J Anesthesiol 2020;73(5): 401–7.

56. Xu L, Leng JC, Elsharkawy H, et al. Replacement of fascia iliaca catheters with continuous erector spinae plane blocks within a clinical pathway facilitates early ambulation after total hip arthroplasty. Pain Med 2020;21(10):2423–9.

57. Duncan CM, Moeschler SM, Horlocker TT, et al. A self-paired comparison of perioperative outcomes before and after implementation of a clinical pathway in patients undergoing total knee arthroplasty. Reg Anesth Pain Med 2013;38(6): 533–8.

58. Johnson RL, Amundson AW, Abdel MP, et al. Continuous posterior lumbar plexus nerve block versus periarticular injection with ropivacaine or liposomal bupivacaine for total hip arthroplasty: a three-arm randomized clinical trial. J Bone Joint Surg Am 2017;99(21):1836–45.

59. Amundson AW, Johnson RL, Abdel MP, et al. A three-arm randomized clinical trial comparing continuous femoral plus single-injection sciatic peripheral nerve blocks versus periarticular injection with ropivacaine or liposomal bupivacaine for patients undergoing total knee arthroplasty. Anesthesiology 2017;126(6): 1139–50.

Anaesthesia for Hepatic Resection Surgery

Anton Krige, MBChB, DIMC, FRCA, FFICM[a],*, Leigh J.S. Kelliher, MBBS, BSc, FRCA, MD[b]

KEYWORDS

- ERAS • Enhanced recovery • Hepatic resection surgery
- Pancreatic resection surgery • Whipple's procedure

KEY POINTS

- There has been significant improvement in outcomes after liver resection in the last 20 years
- Improved outcomes are due to a combination of patient selection, prehabilitation, techniques to increase functional liver remnant, anesthetic and surgical technique, refinement of ERAS pathways, and neoadjuvant chemotherapy,
- The role of minimally invasive surgery and robotically assisted surgery continues to expand and be impactful in improving outcomes
- Analgesia techniques to facilitate rapid restoration of function while minimizing opioids are evolving as are techniques to minimize intraoperative hemorrhage

Abbreviations	
ERAS	Enhanced Recovery After Surgery

INTRODUCTION

Approximately 150,000 individuals are expected to experience colorectal cancer (CRC) in the United States in 2020 and over half of these patients will go on to develop liver metastases in the future. Although only 20% of these will be suitable for curative hepatic resection there has been a tremendous improvement in overall outcomes following CLRMs in the past 2 decades with a doubling in 5-year overall survival (OS) rates from 30% in the 1980s and 1990s to 60% in the 21st century.[1]

These advances have been a combination of improvements in patient selection, operative procedures, and perioperative management.[2]

Hepatic resection remains the only curative option for CLRMs and current perioperative mortality rates are less than 5% and as low as 1% in high-volume centers. The highest

[a] Department of Anaesthesia and Critical Care, Royal Blackburn Teaching Hospital, Haslingden Road, Blackburn BB2 3HH, UK; [b] Department of Anaesthetics, Royal Surrey County Hospital NHS Foundation Trust, Egerton Road, Guildford, Surrey GU2 7AS, UK
* Corresponding author.
E-mail address: Anton.Krige@elht.nhs.uk

Anesthesiology Clin 40 (2022) 91–105
https://doi.org/10.1016/j.anclin.2021.11.004   **anesthesiology.theclinics.com**
1932-2275/22/Crown Copyright © 2021 Published by Elsevier Inc. All rights reserved.

mortality is seen in those with underlying liver dysfunction. Morbidity ranges widely—reported between 16% and 67%—with a recent systematic review demonstrating an association between postoperative complications and shorter overall, as well as disease-free, survival (DFS).[3] The incidence and severity of postoperative complications are highest in cirrhotic patients. Major complications in this group include bile leak, coagulopathy, postoperative bleeding, and liver failure. Effective preoperative assessment, risk stratification, and optimization are vital in reducing morbidity and mortality.

Treatment options for isolated CLRMs comprise regional approaches with or without systemic chemotherapy. The regional approaches range from potentially curative surgical resection to several other options when surgical resection is unsuitable that is, thermal ablation, regional hepatic intraarterial chemotherapy, chemoembolization, radioembolization, and radiation therapy (RT), including stereotactic RT.

INDICATIONS FOR HEPATIC RESECTION SURGERY

Resection of isolated CRLMs is the most common indication—two-thirds of patients' CRLMs will already have extra-hepatic spread at presentation. Other indications are for primary benign and malignant hepatobiliary tumors and occasionally for hepatic trauma although the latter is usually managed conservatively.

HISTORY OF SURGICAL TECHNIQUES

The first partial hepatectomy was performed by Luis in 1886 for a large adenoma in a female patient who unfortunately died from hemorrhage 6 hours after surgery. Paquelin's cautery—consisting of burning flammable liquids such as benzene at high temperatures within the operative site—had been used to resect and cauterize the tumor site.

In 1889, Keen reported a series of 73 cases involving wedge excisions of the liver with a mortality of 15% and in 1908 Dr Pringle, a surgeon in Glasgow, reported the use of obstruction of the portal vein and hepatic artery to control bleeding during surgery for trauma of the liver with one of the 4 operated patients surviving. Wendell followed this in 1911 with the first reported successful right hepatic lobe resection. Although credited to a French team in 1951—due to publication timing in English-speaking journals—it seems the first known case of right hepatic lobectomy with hilar dissection may have been by the Japanese surgeon Hondo in 1949. It was not until the 1950's that Couinaud among others developed the current concept of segmental anatomy of the liver which formed the basis for segmental hepatectomy. The rapid reductions in mortality seen in the 1980s are credited to a better understanding of the safe limits of resection regarding liver function using indocyanine green (ICG) clearance, intraoperative ultrasound allowing real-time assessment of hepatic vascular anatomy and the development of portal vein embolization (PVE) to prevent liver failure after large resections. The 21st century has seen the development and growth of laparoscopic hepatectomy from 1991, when Reich reported the first case, through to 2011 when a large registry of hepatectomies from Japan reported 63% as laparoscopic, with 90-day mortality rates as low as 0.67%. Recent years have seen the advent of robotic surgery with some reports indicating it may be better suited to right hepatectomy than laparoscopic surgery regarding the duration of surgery and conversion rate, although this remains controversial.[4]

ANATOMY

The highly vascular nature of the liver—receiving 25% of cardiac output with 80% supplied by the portal vein and 20% by the hepatic artery—provides the greatest

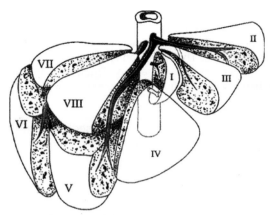

Fig. 1. Couinard's segmental picture of the liver. The representative appearance of the hepatic segments separated within the liver.

intraoperative challenge to hepatic resection surgery. The porta hepatis contains all the structures entering the liver.

Fig.1 depicts the 2 lobar segments (left and right) subdivided into 5 liver sectors with further subdivision into the 8 liver segments defined by their blood supply and biliary drainage as described by Couinaud. These segments are contiguous regarding blood supply and biliary drainage allowing resection without disruption or damage to neighboring segments.

Unique to the liver is its ability to regenerate. This phenomenon starts within 48 hours of resection reaching a significant volume within weeks to months and allows for large resections without consequent liver failure via hyperplasia of the liver remnant. The same principle leads to the increase in FLR when PVE is used preoperatively.

PREOPERATIVE MANAGEMENT
Patient Selection

This involves the assessment of the following:

1. *Patient factors*: patients must have an appropriate biological age and adequate cardiopulmonary function to endure the considerable inflammatory and neuroendocrine response. Additionally, the impact of comorbid diseases and recovery from any neoadjuvant chemotherapy all need to be taken into account.
2. *Tumor factors*: the biology of the tumor provides important prognostic information and various clinicopathologic based scoring systems have been validated with 4 in current use for predicting recurrence.[5] These help to guide whether surgery is the appropriate treatment and whether the patient might benefit from neoadjuvant chemotherapy.[6,7] The biology of the primary colon cancer also influences the prognosis in CLRM.[8]
3. *Anatomic factors*: resectable CLRMs have been defined by modern consensus as tumors that can be completely resected while leaving a functional volume of residual liver or functional liver remnant (FLR). Imaging studies define the location of the lesions, the resectable margin (ideally >1 cm), and the FLR. An FLR of less than 20% is unsuitable due to the high rate of postoperative liver failure and mortality. The FLR threshold required is greater than 30% if preoperative chemotherapy has been administered and greater than 40% if preexisting liver dysfunction

(NASH or cirrhosis) is present. These patients could be considered for PVE in an attempt to increase their FLR to meet the necessary threshold for resection. There is evidence for reduced rates of postoperative liver failure and improved survival following preoperative PVE. The American Hepato-Pancreato-Biliary Association, the Society for Surgery of the Alimentary Tract, and the Society of Surgical Oncology published consensus guidelines covering FLR and PVE in 2006.[9]

Assessment of Cardiopulmonary Function

Cardiopulmonary exercise testing (CPET) is widely used in the United Kingdom (UK) to provide an objective assessment of exercise capacity along with useful diagnostic information regarding likely causes of any exercise intolerance. There have been multiple studies validating the association between the measurement of peak oxygen consumption (peak Vo_2), oxygen consumption at anaerobic threshold (AT), and ventilatory efficiency (Ve/VCO2) including a systematic review by Smith and colleagues in 2009.[10] Specific to assessment for hepatic resection surgery Junejo and colleagues reported that an AT less than 10 mLs O2/kg/min predicted in-hospital death with 100% sensitive and 76% specificity.[11]

Some centers favor the use of the Carlisle model[12–14] which starts with baseline mortality risk using actuarial data (in the UK, based on the latest Office of National Statistics data) and then individualizing this prediction of baseline mortality risk and median survival by the weighting of any key comorbidities and biochemical markers that are independently associated with lifespan, the peak Vo_2 (which is a validated predictor of lifespan) and the VeVCO2. This model does not account for the 5-year survival in different types of cancer (including the effect of individual tumor biology, cancer volume, and staging) and, in the case of hepatic resection surgery, the liver function, hence the CPET result needs to be combined with the surgical team's knowledge of the latter 2 factors to enable a complete risk stratification. Once complete, this allows informed and shared decision making with the patient as well as better planning, preparation, and optimization.

Alternative options for the objective assessment of cardiopulmonary function in the absence of CPET include the "Six-Minute Walk Test" and the "Incremental Shuttle Walk Test."

Identifying and assessing frailty is increasingly being recognized as an important factor when predicting both postoperative and long-term survival[15] with both validated subjective scoring systems and objective surrogates, for example, the "Get up and go" test (time standing up from sitting in a chair) and handgrip strength measurement in use.[16]

Assessment of Liver Function

The presence of severe underlying liver disease (cirrhosis or nonalcoholic steatohepatitis (NASH)—the latter possibly as a complication of neoadjuvant chemotherapy) is a contraindication. If the underlying liver disease is less severe the surgery could be considered depending on the anticipated FLR and other comorbidities. This requires imaging-based volumetric assessment of the FLR together with an estimation of liver synthetic function. The Child–Pugh score is generally used for the latter (**Table1.**). Child–Pugh A and Child–Pugh B cases with an FLR greater than 40% can be considered.

In some centers, ICG clearance is used to assess liver function with normal clearance at 15 minutes (ICG_{15}) of 90%. A clearance of less than 60% indicates a high likelihood of postoperative liver failure and mortality. ICG is a dye dilution that is selectively taken up by hepatocytes following intravenous injection in an ATP-dependent process

Table 1
Child–Pugh classification of severity of cirrhosis

Parameter	1 Point	2 Points	3 Points
Ascites	Absent	Slight	Moderate
Bilirubin	<2 mg/dL (<34.2 micromol/L)	2–3 mg/dL (34.2–51.3 micromol/L)	>3 mg/dL (>51.3 micromol/L)
Albumin	>3.5 g/dL (35 g/L)	2.8–3.5 g/dL (28–35 g/L)	<2.8 g/dL (<28 g/L)
Prothrombin time:			
Seconds over control	<4	4–6	>6
INR	<1.7	1.7–2.3	>2.3
Encephalopathy	None	Grade 1–2	Grade 3–4

Modified Child–Pugh classification of the severity of liver disease according to the degree of ascites, the serum concentrations of bilirubin and albumin, the prothrombin time, and the degree of encephalopathy. A total Child–Turcotte–Pugh score of 5 to 6 is considered Child–Pugh class A (well-compensated disease); 7 to 9 is class B (significant functional compromise); and 10 to 15 is class C (decompensated disease). These classes correlate with one- and 2-year patient survival: class A: 100% and 85%; class B: 80% and 60%; and class C: 45% and 35%.
Abbreviation: INR, international normalized ratio.

and is not metabolized or undergo enterohepatic recirculation therefore its rate of disappearance from the plasma (measured by transcutaneous pulse-densitometry within 6–8 minutes) represents liver blood flow, parenchymal cellular function, and biliary excretion.

Models using machine learning algorithms are an exciting development and are likely to further refine the accuracy of risk prediction in the future, comparing outcomes with all the data mentioned above along with liver function data and relevant preoperative biochemistry. A recent study from Washington University demonstrated accuracy for predicting postoperative complications using a combination of preoperative test results, comorbidities, and intraoperative variables input into a deep learning algorithm.[17]

Prehabilitation and Optimization

These are programs involving generic preoperative lifestyle interventions such as nutritional supplements, exercise programs, stress reduction, and smoking cessation before surgery.

It has been estimated by the American Society for Enhanced Recovery and Perioperative Quality that 2 out of 3 patients undergoing GI surgery are malnourished and have a threefold greater risk of perioperative complication and fivefold greater risk of death.[18]

A 2018 systematic review of preoperative nutrition (whey protein) either alone or in combination with an exercise program in colorectal surgery patients reported a 2-day reduction in hospital stay in the prehabilitation group.[19]

A further enhancement to correcting malnourishment and sarcopenia is the concept of immunonutrition (IM) usually consisting of combinations of the amino acid arginine, omega-3 fatty acids, and sometimes further protein enhancement via BCAAs (branched-chain amino acids). There have been 3 recent systematic reviews of perioperative IM for hepatic resection with Wong and colleagues[20] concluding from ten RCTs that IM reduces wound infection rates and hospital stay, recommending it be included as a component in ERAS for liver surgery; McKay et al[21] reported large heterogeneity in results with one cohort study showing a 26.9% reduction in postoperative complications using BCAAs and another showing a 25.4% reduction in postoperative ascites with preoperative IM. Guan and colleagues[22] included 11 RCTs with 1136 patients in a metanalysis concluding that IM is safe and feasible significantly reducing overall postoperative complications, postoperative liver failure, and hospital stay. Currently, IM is not widely implemented but seems worth consideration within ERAS guidelines for hepatic resection.

An RCT from 2016 investigating prehabilitation in hepatic resection surgery demonstrated an improvement in cardiopulmonary function and quality of life with CPET plus a 4-week high-intensity exercise program.[23] The same research group had previously demonstrated a significant reduction in exercise capacity following neoadjuvant chemotherapy (NACR) for CRC comparing CPET variables at baseline and following NACR. The intervention group in this RCT experienced a significant increase in CPET measured exercise capacity following a 6-week high-intensity exercise program with the control group still not recovering to their pre-NACR fitness.[24] This may be relevant in hepatic resection whereby many patients undergo NACR and a 3 to 4-week window exists before their surgery to implement such a program.

Preoperative hemoglobin optimization, largely via intravenous iron infusion, has been implemented widely in the UK as a prehabilitation component in major surgery. While the recently published PREVENTT study[25] reported no outcome improvements in anemic patients receiving intravenous iron therapy preoperatively this study did not include hepatic resection surgery patients and did not reflect current anemia pathways, with the intervention delivered too close to surgery and limited to one treatment dose and thus few patients achieved target hemoglobin. Munoz and colleagues[26] previously reported the incidence of preoperative hemoglobin less than $130g.L^{-1}$ in patients undergoing hepatic resection for CRLMs as 37%. As this is surgery whereby the major intraoperative risk is blood loss and any consequent blood transfusion significantly worsens perioperative outcomes, preoperative optimization of hemoglobin is crucial. This may also allow safer normovolemic hemodilution intraoperatively for larger resections.

An issue specific to hepatic resection surgery is the impact of intrahepatic fat (either NAFLD or NACR-induced) which may be further worsened by inflammation that is, steatohepatitis (NASH)—termed chemotherapy-associated steatohepatitis (CASH) if new and deemed secondary to NACR. These conditions have been independently associated with postoperative morbidity but may be rapidly modifiable using dietary interventions in the window between NACR and surgery.[27]

INTRAOPERATIVE MANAGEMENT
Surgical Technique

Surgical approaches include open surgery, laparoscopic-assisted surgery, and robotic-assisted surgery and there is a large variation between surgeons, centers, and countries regarding the preferred approach. Laparoscopic approaches remain largely limited to minor resections that is, involving less than 3 Couinaud segments. To date several large propensity score-matched cohort comparisons have shown longer or similar operative time, less intraoperative blood loss or transfusion requirement, shorter hospital stays, lower or comparable morbidity, and equivalent mortality compared with open surgery.[28–30] The first RCT comparing open and laparoscopic-assisted hepatic resection conducted at the Oslo University Hospital[31] reported a lower complication rate (19% vs 31%) and a shorter hospital stay in the laparoscopic group with similar blood loss, operative time and resection models. Mortality was low and not significantly different between groups. The perceived advantages of laparoscopy are better-magnified views and less bleeding due to the pneumoperitoneum compressing low-pressure vessels during transection. Although the latter is borne out in the cohort studies this advantage was not seen in the RCT.

There are three phases to the operation with differing anesthesia goals:

1. Initial phase:
   a. mobilization of the liver,
   b. ultrasound localization of the lesions with confirmation of resectability,
   c. if confirmed, followed by cholecystectomy and dissection of the porta hepatis.
2. Resection phase.
3. Hemostasis and closure.

Anesthetic Technique

Anesthesia for hepatic resection surgery has some unique aspects primarily focused on strategies to limit blood loss during the resection alongside minimizing reperfusion injury to the liver to reduce the risk of postoperative liver failure.

Monitoring Recommendations

- Large bore venous access
  - optional placement of a pulmonary artery catheter introducer alongside a central venous catheter (CVC) could be considered for large complex resections to aid rapid volume loading if necessary and for easy venesection if performing normovolemic hemodilution
- Availability of a rapid infusion system
- Arterial line (also aids regular blood sugar and lactate monitoring)
- CVC – allows CVP targeting and norepinephrine infusion
- Minimally invasive CO monitoring using esophageal Doppler or arterial pressure-based systems—primarily for goal-directed fluid therapy during the postresection phase of surgery

Anesthesia

- Avoid halothane due to hepatotoxicity
- Atracurium/cisatracurium preferred as they are unaffected by liver dysfunction
- Intravenous fluid administration is limited until the posttransection phase—vasopressor infusions are titrated to maintain optimal perfusion pressure
- Ensure normothermia throughout for optimal coagulation using intravenous fluid warmers, forced air warming blankets, or warming gel mats

Analgesia Options

Administration of simple analgesia perioperatively is limited due to the hepatotoxicity of paracetamol. It may be considered for smaller resections with good underlying liver function following endorsement from the surgical team.

As this group is at risk of renal dysfunction and impaired coagulation the use of nonsteroidal anti-inflammatory drugs is discouraged.

Several metanalyses have found an opioid-sparing effect for perioperative gabapentinoids and low dose ketamine (eg, 0.5 mg/kg)—with the latter also leading to lower pain scores and these may comprise one of the elements of a multimodal package.[32]

In open liver resection, thoracic epidural analgesia (TEA) remains the mainstay of analgesia (and may also reduce bleeding via lowering the CVP). However, more recently continuous wound infusion catheters (CWIC) have shown potential to become the standard approach. There have been 3 recent RCTs comparing TEA to CWIC with Revie and colleagues[33] reporting a shorter hospital stay for CWIC despite superior analgesia in the TEA group; Hughes and colleagues[34] also found shorter recovery times in CWIC and the multi-centre POP-UP study[35] which included hepatic and pancreatic resections found CWIC noninferior to TEA within an ERAS protocol with significantly less vasopressor consumption perioperatively and shorter infusion duration postoperatively in the CWIC group. CWIC also avoids the concern around epidural catheter removal if postoperative coagulopathy develops.

For laparoscopic surgery, intrathecal opiate (morphine or diamorphine) is effective with a recent metanalysis including 40 studies (2500 patients) examining the use of intrathecal opioids in abdominal surgery[36] finding a reduced consumption of postoperative intravenous opiate, lower pain scores, longer time to first analgesic request, and shorter hospital stay with intrathecal opioids. The only adverse events were an increase in pruritis in the intrathecal opiate group and a dose-dependent increase in respiratory depression which disappeared when 2 outlying studies which used excessive doses (greater than 800mcg) were removed. Apart from 6 studies the doses used ranged from 100mcg to 400mcg with 300mcg being the most common. The authors recommend for safety using less than 500mcg. The metanalysis included several hepatic resection studies which all showed safety and benefit for intrathecal opiate.[37–39] Indeed intrathecal opiate may even be adequate for open liver resection with a 2020 study reporting reduced opiate requirements and improved analgesia compared with conventional multimodal analgesia alone.[40]

Anecdotally and requiring research this author finds a hybrid approach for open liver resection which combines the benefits of intrathecal opiate and CWIC very effective.

Intrathecal opiate analgesia may be further enhanced by combining it with intravenous lidocaine infusions perioperatively with evidence for suggesting it may reduce opiate requirements, improve analgesia, shorten hospital stay and reduce ileus rates along with ameliorating postoperative inflammation.[41–50] This approach is routinely used in our institution for laparoscopic approaches whereby CWIC or TEA is not required. Caution is required and intravenous lidocaine either avoided or the dose reduced if there is any underlying liver dysfunction or a large resection with a higher risk of postoperative liver failure is planned.

Strategies for Reducing Bleeding

There is a paucity of high-quality evidence for the efficacy of the different techniques for reducing blood loss, transfusion requirements, and consequent mortality as concluded by a 2016 COCHRANE review.[51]

Several older observational studies indicated that maintaining a CVP < 5 mm Hg was associated with reduced blood loss, length of stay, morbidity, and mortality.[52–55] This must be balanced against the risks of cardiovascular compromise and air embolus. Despite a COCHRANE review[56] not finding any effect on outcomes when analyzing randomized trials, it remains a standard practice in most units.

The following have been used in isolation or together, depending on local practice and individual cases, to achieve low CVP targets:

- Anti-Trendelenburg 15°[57]
- Fluid restriction to 1 mL/kg/h
- TEA or intrathecal analgesia
- GTN infusion at 5 to 15 mcg/min[58]
- Minimization of PEEP/reduced ventilation
- Mannitol 0.5 g/kg and furosemide 10 mg

Acute normovolemic hemodilution is a technique whereby the patient undergoes venesection following induction of anesthesia—the volume removed depending on preoperative hemoglobin and cardiovascular stability—and normovolemia is reestablished with albumin administration. The blood removed is then retransfused during the postresection phase. The COCHRANE review reported less blood loss during resection when combining this with low CVP than low CVP alone.[51]

Surgical options for reducing blood loss comprise the vascular occlusion techniques depicted in **Fig. 2** which isolate the hepatic circulation from the systemic circulation and may be broadly divided into temporary hepatic inflow occlusion (Pringle maneuver) and total vascular exclusion (TVE). The Pringle maneuver can be applied continuously or intermittently with a limit of an hour or less. It results in a 10% decrease in cardiac output, a 40% increase in SVR, and a 40% increase in mean arterial pressure. It carries an increased risk of air embolus, which may be reduced by positioning the patient at 15° Trendelenburg. Repeated intermittent 5 to 10-minute occlusions with several minutes of reperfusion in between are favored. There is growing evidence for a reduction in blood loss, transfusion risk, and associated reperfusion injury and postoperative liver failure using a Pringle maneuver.[59–63]

Prophylactic tranexamic acid may be considered to reduce bleeding and transfusion rates. While the evidence for its use largely extrapolated from other settings[64–66] one study randomizing over 200 liver resection cases between tranexamic acid and placebo demonstrated reduced blood loss and transfusion rates in the treatment group.[67]

Intraoperative Strategies to Minimize Postoperative Liver Failure

The incidence of postoperative liver failure may be reduced by avoiding the administration of any hepatotoxic drugs perioperatively, minimizing intraoperative bleeding, and consequent blood transfusion, minimizing vascular occlusion times thereby reducing reperfusion injury to the liver and maintaining an optimal hemodynamic

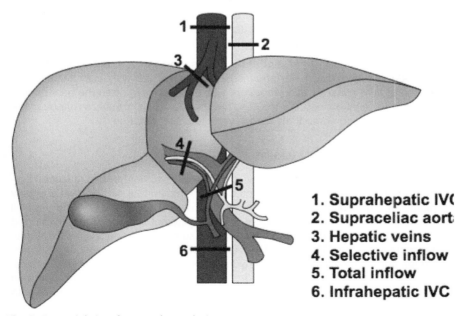

1. Suprahepatic IVC
2. Supraceliac aort
3. Hepatic veins
4. Selective inflow
5. Total inflow
6. Infrahepatic IVC

Fig. 2. Potential sites for vascular occlusion.

balance that is, providing a low CVP, while avoiding excessive hypovolemia and ensuring an adequate perfusion pressure. Good communication between surgical and anesthesia teams regarding surgical manipulation and filling status is crucial to ensuring good outcomes. Individualized targets and planned surgical manipulation should be discussed at the WHO team brief before surgery.

Preoperative glucocorticoids can be considered although the evidence is conflicting with 2 meta-analyses both analyzing the same 5 RCTs reaching different conclusions.[68,69] Reductions in IL6 and bilirubin levels were statistically significant on day one postoperatively and nonsignificant trends toward lower prothrombin times however this did not translate into lower overall complication rates, or a shorter hospital stay. Therefore, it seems to be a safe intervention that reduces short-term inflammation, however, the clinical benefit seems to be limited.

POSTOPERATIVE MANAGEMENT

The majority of hepatic resections with normal underlying liver function have an uneventful postoperative course, without the high ileus rates and difficulty reestablishing enteral feeding seen in other types of major abdominal surgery. The focus should be on ERAS with early mobilization and nutrition and a short hospital stay.

Cases with underlying liver dysfunction or very large resections have greater risks of postoperative complications that is, bile leak, ascites, liver failure, pulmonary complications, and thrombotic complications.

Ascites is common leading to increased fluid shifts and complicating fluid and electrolyte management. Hypophosphatemia is common and occasionally sodium and water retention with edema formation secondary to hyperaldosteronism are seen.

The most concerning complication are liver failure which may be complicated by:

- Hypoglycemia - requiring glucose infusion.
- Encephalopathy - supported by lactulose and minimizing opiates.
- Coagulopathy is usually corrected with FFP as required; larger volume blood loss may require targeted blood product and/or tranexamic acid administration guided by thromboelastographic monitoring.

The nature of the electrolyte disturbance, glucose requirement, and amount of ascites and edema together with the intravascular volume status will determine the type and volume of fluid administration required, with 20% albumin often the best option.

N-acetylcysteine infusions are often used until liver function normalizes although the evidence is mixed, and some trials report worsened liver function.[70–72]

ENHANCED RECOVERY AFTER SURGERY

The ERAS society published perioperative care guidelines[73] for hepatic resection surgery in 2016 although the 23 items selected for the multimodal pathway were largely transplanted from existing ERAS guidelines for colorectal surgery and may not all apply to liver surgery. Encouragingly, a recent systematic review[74] demonstrated that these pathways are effective in this type of surgery for reducing hospital stay (2.2-day reduction in the ERAS group), complications (only in the laparoscopic surgery sub-group), and hospital cost without any increase in mortality or readmission rates. Only 4 of the 27 studies included compared compliance rates which were greater in the ERAS groups (65% to 73.8% vs 20% to 48.7%). Further research is required to determine which ERAS elements are the most important for achieving improved outcomes.

FUTURE DIRECTIONS

Likely future developments will be in the areas of machine learning algorithms and AI to improve patient selection, interventions to address hepatic steatosis preoperatively within effective prehabilitation programs, three-dimensional simulation, and navigation technology,[4] improved intraoperative imaging, and refinement of laparoscopic-assisted and robotic approaches.

SUMMARY

Outcomes for liver resection surgery have improved significantly in the past decade due to better patient selection, patient preparation, improved anesthetic and surgical techniques to reduce intraoperative bleeding and the implementation of ERAS programs.

CLINICS CARE POINTS

- Patient selection, optimization of medical conditions, and prehabilitation.
- Reducing blood loss during resection.
- Opioid sparing analgesia approach that restores function.
- Avoidance and management of postoperative liver failure.
- Mobilization and early nutrition for most patients.

DISCLOSURE

The authors have no conflicts of interest to disclose.

REFERENCES

1. Siegel RL, Miller KD, Jemal A. Cancer statistics, 2020. Ca Cancer J Clin 2020; 70:7–30.
2. Yamazaki S, Takayama T. Current topics in liver surgery. Ann Gastroenterological Surg 2019;3:146–59.
3. Dorcaratto D, Mazzinari G, Fernandez M, et al. Impact of postoperative complications on survival and recurrence after resection of colorectal liver metastases. Ann Surg 2019;270(6):1018–27.
4. Kokudo N, Takemura N, Ito K, et al. The history of liver surgery: achievements over the past 50 years. Ann Gastroenterological Surg 2020;4:109–17.
5. Roberts KJ, White A, Cockbain A, et al. Performance of prognostic scores in predicting long-term outcome following resection of colorectal liver metastases. Br J Surg 2014;101:856–66.
6. Fong Y, Fortner J, Sun RL, et al. Clinical score for predicting recurrence after hepatic resection for metastatic colorectal cancer. Ann Surg 1999;230:309.
7. Konopke R, Kersting S, Distler M, et al. Prognostic factors and evaluation of a clinical score for predicting survival after resection of colorectal liver metastases. Liver Int 2009;29:89–102.
8. Yamashita S, Brudvik KW, Kopetz SE, et al. Embryonic origin of primary colon cancer predicts pathologic response and survival in patients undergoing resection for colon cancer liver metastases. Ann Surg 2018;267:514–20.
9. Charnsangavej C, Clary B, Fong Y, et al. Selection of patients for resection of hepatic colorectal metastases: expert consensus statement. Ann Surg Oncol 2006; 13:1261–8.

10. Smith TB, Stonell C, Purkayastha S, et al. Cardiopulmonary exercise testing as a risk assessment method in non cardio-pulmonary surgery: a systematic review. Anaesthesia 2009;64:883–93.

11. Junejo MA, Mason JM, Sheen AJ, et al. Cardiopulmonary exercise testing for pre-operative risk assessment before hepatic resection. Br J Surg 2012;99:1097–104.

12. Carlisle JB. Assessing fitness, predicting outcome, and the missing axis. Br J Anaesth 2012;109:35–9.

13. Carlisle J. Pre-operative co-morbidity and postoperative survival in the elderly: beyond one lunar orbit. Anaesthesia 2014;69:17–25.

14. Carlisle J, Danjoux G, Kerr K, et al. Validation of long-term survival prediction for scheduled abdominal aortic aneurysm repair with an independent calculator using only pre-operative variables. Anaesthesia 2015;70:654–65.

15. Lin H-S, Watts JN, Peel NM, et al. Frailty and post-operative outcomes in older surgical patients: a systematic review. BMC Geriatr 2016;16:157.

16. Clegg A, Young J, Iliffe S, et al. Frailty in elderly people. Lancet 2013;381:752–62.

17. Fritz BA, Cui Z, Zhang M, et al. Deep-learning model for predicting 30-day post-operative mortality. Br J Anaesth 2019;123:688–95.

18. Wischmeyer PE, Carli F, Evans DC, et al. Workgroup PQI (POQI) 2: American Society for Enhanced Recovery and Perioperative Quality Initiative Joint Consensus Statement on Nutrition Screening and Therapy Within a Surgical Enhanced Recovery Pathway. Anesth Analg 2018;126:1883–95.

19. Gillis C, Buhler K, Bresee L, et al. Effects of nutritional prehabilitation, with and without exercise, on outcomes of patients who undergo colorectal surgery: a systematic review and meta-analysis. Gastroenterology 2018;155:391–410.e4.

20. Wong CS, Liau S-S. Perioperative immunonutrition in major hepatic resection: a systematic review and meta-analysis. Hpb 2018;20:S369–70.

21. McKay BP, Larder AL, Lam V. Pre-Operative vs. Peri-Operative Nutrition Supplementation in Hepatic Resection for Cancer: A Systematic Review. Nutr Cancer 2019;71:1–20.

22. Guan H, Huang Q, Liu C, et al. Clinical efficacy of immunonutrition support in perioperative period of hepatectomy: a Meta analysis. Chin J Dig Surg 2019;18:951–9.

23. Dunne DFJ, Jack S, Jones RP, et al. Randomized clinical trial of prehabilitation before planned liver resection. Br J Surg 2016;103:504–12.

24. West M, Loughney L, Lythgoe D, et al. Effect of prehabilitation on objectively measured physical fitness after neoadjuvant treatment in preoperative rectal cancer patients: a blinded interventional pilot study. Br J Anaesth 2014;114:244–51.

25. Richards T, Baikady RR, Clevenger B, et al. Preoperative intravenous iron to treat anaemia before major abdominal surgery (PREVENTT): a randomised, double-blind, controlled trial. Lancet 2020. https://doi.org/10.1016/s0140-6736(20)31539-7.

26. Muñoz M, Laso-Morales MJ, Gómez-Ramírez S, et al. Pre-operative haemoglobin levels and iron status in a large multicentre cohort of patients undergoing major elective surgery. Anaesthesia 2017;72:826–34.

27. Doherty DT, Coe PO, Rimmer L, et al. Hepatic steatosis in patients undergoing resection of colorectal liver metastases: A target for prehabilitation? A narrative review. Surg Oncol 2019;30:147–58.

28. DelPiccolo N, Onkendi E, Nguyen J, et al. Outcomes of minimally invasive versus open major hepatic resection. J Laparoendosc Adv S 2020;30:790–6.

29. Lewin JW, O'Rourke NA, Chiow AKH, et al. Long-term survival in laparoscopic vs open resection for colorectal liver metastases: inverse probability of treatment weighting using propensity scores. Hpb 2016;18:183–91.

30. Brough D, O'Rourke N. Laparoscopic hepatic resection. Laparosc Surg 2020; 4:18.

31. Chan AKC, Jamdar S, Sheen AJ, et al. The OSLO-COMET randomized controlled trial of laparoscopic versus open resection for colorectal liver metastases. Ann Surg 2018;268:e69.

32. Kumar K, Kirksey MA, Duong S, et al. A review of opioid-sparing modalities in perioperative pain management: methods to decrease opioid use postoperatively. Anesth Analg 2017;125:1749.

33. Revie EJ, McKeown DW, Wilson JA, et al. Randomized clinical trial of local infiltration plus patient-controlled opiate analgesia vs. epidural analgesia following liver resection surgery. HPB 2012;14:611–8.

34. Hughes MJ, Harrison EM, Peel NJ, et al. Randomized clinical trial of perioperative nerve block and continuous local anaesthetic infiltration via wound catheter versus epidural analgesia in open liver resection (LIVER 2 trial). Br J Surg 2015;102:1619–28.

35. Mungroop TH, Veelo DP, Busch OR, et al. Continuous wound infiltration versus epidural analgesia after hepato-pancreato-biliary surgery (POP-UP): a randomised controlled, open-label, non-inferiority trial. Lancet Gastroenterol Hepatol 2016;1:105–13.

36. Koning MV, Klimek M, Rijs K, et al. Intrathecal hydrophilic opioids for abdominal surgery: a meta- analysis, meta-regression, and trial sequential analysis. Br J Anaesth 2020;125:358–72.

37. Dichtwald S, Ben-Haim M, Papismedov L, et al. Intrathecal morphine versus intravenous opioid administration to impact postoperative analgesia in hepato-pancreatic surgery: a randomized controlled trial. J Anesth 2017;31:237–45.

38. Kang R, Chin KJ, Gwak MS, et al. Bilateral single-injection erector spinae plane block versus intrathecal morphine for postoperative analgesia in living donor laparoscopic hepatectomy: a randomized non-inferiority trial. Reg Anesth Pain Med 2019;44:1059.

39. Roy J-D, Massicotte L, Sassine M-P, et al. A comparison of intrathecal morphine/fentanyl and patient-controlled analgesia with patient-controlled analgesia alone for analgesia after liver resection. Anesth Analg 2006;103:990–4.

40. Tang J, Churilov L, Tan CO, et al. Intrathecal morphine is associated with reduction in postoperative opioid requirements and improvement in postoperative analgesia in patients undergoing open liver resection. Bmc Anesthesiol 2020;20:207.

41. Terkawi AS, Tsang S, Kazemi A, et al. A clinical comparison of intravenous and epidural local anesthetic for major abdominal surgery. Reg Anesth pain Med 2016;41:28–36.

42. Weibel S, Jokinen J, Pace NL, et al. Efficacy and safety of intravenous lidocaine for postoperative analgesia and recovery after surgery: a systematic review with trial sequential analysis † †This review is an abridged version of a Cochrane Review previously published in the Cochrane. Database Syst Rev 2015;Issue 7: CD009642 (see www.thecochranelibrary.com for information).1 Cochrane Reviews are regularly updated as new evidence emerges and in response to feedback, and Cochrane Database of Systematic Reviews should be consulted for the most recent version of the review. British Journal of Anaesthesia 2016; 116: 770–783.

43. McCarthy GC, Megalla SA, Habib AS. Impact of Intravenous Lidocaine Infusion on Postoperative Analgesia and Recovery from Surgery. Drugs 2010;70:1149–63.

44. Yon J, Choi G, Kang H, et al. Intraoperative systemic lidocaine for pre-emptive analgesics in subtotal gastrectomy: a prospective, randomized, double-blind, placebo-controlled study. Can J Surg 2014;57:175182.

45. Eipe N, Gupta S, Penning J. Intravenous lidocaine for acute pain: an evidence-based clinical update. BJA Education 2016;16:292–8.

46. Tikuišis R, Miliauskas P, Samalavičius NE, et al. Intravenous lidocaine for post-operative pain relief after hand-assisted laparoscopic colon surgery: a random-ized, placebo-controlled clinical trial. Tech Coloproctol 2014;18:373–80.

47. Greenwood E, Nimmo S, Paterson H, et al. Intravenous lidocaine infusion as a component of multimodal analgesia for colorectal surgery—measurement of plasma levels. Perioper Med 2019;8:1.

48. Kaba A, Laurent S, Detroz B. Intravenous lidocaine infusion facilitates acute reha-bilitation after laparoscopic colectomy. Anesthesiology 2007;106(1):11–8.

49. Vigneault L, Turgeon A, Côté D, et al. Perioperative intravenous lidocaine infusion for postoperative pain control: a meta-analysis of randomized controlled trials. Can J Anaesth 2011;58(1):22–37.

50. Sun Y, Li T, Wang N, et al. Perioperative systemic lidocaine for postoperative anal-gesia and recovery after abdominal surgery: a meta-analysis of randomized controlled trials. Dis Colon Rectum 2012;55(11):1183–94.

51. Moggia E, Rouse B, Simillis C, et al. Methods to decrease blood loss during liver resection: a network meta-analysis. Cochrane Db Syst Rev 2016. https://doi.org/10.1002/14651858.cd010683.pub3.

52. Jones RMcL, Moulton CE, Hardy KJ. Central venous pressure and its effect on blood loss during liver resection. Br J Surg 1998;85:1058–60.

53. Bhattacharya S, Jackson DJ, Beard CI, et al. Central venous pressure and its ef-fects on blood loss during liver resection. Br J Surg 1999;86:282–3.

54. Chen H, Merchant NB, Didolkar MS. Hepatic resection using intermittent vascular inflow occlusion and low central venous pressure anesthesia improves morbidity and mortality. J Gastrointest Surg 2000;4:162–7.

55. Smyrniotis V, Kostopanagiotou G, Theodoraki K, et al. The role of central venous pressure and type of vascular control in blood loss during major liver resections. Am J Surg 2004;187:398–402.

56. Gurusamy KS, Li J, Vaughan J, et al. Cardiopulmonary interventions to decrease blood loss and blood transfusion requirements for liver resection. Cochrane Db Syst Rev 2012;5:CD007338.

57. Soonawalla ZF, Stratopoulos C, Stoneham M, et al. Role of the reverse-Trendelenberg patient position in maintaining low-CVP anaesthesia during liver resections. Langenbeck's Arch Surg 2008;393:195–8.

58. SAND L, LUNDIN S, RIZELL M, et al. Nitroglycerine and patient position effect on central, hepatic and portal venous pressures during liver surgery. Acta Anaesthe-siol Scand 2014;58:961–7.

59. Man K, Fan S-T, Ng IOL, et al. Prospective Evaluation of Pringle Maneuver in Hep-atectomy for Liver Tumors by a Randomized Study. Ann Surg 1997;226:704–13.

60. Kim Y-I, Chung H-J, Song K-E, et al. Evaluation of a protease inhibitor in the pre-vention of ischemia and reperfusion injury in hepatectomy under intermittent Prin-gle maneuver. Am J Surg 2006;191:72–6.

61. Clavien P-A, Yadav S, Sindram D, et al. Protective Effects of Ischemic Precondi-tioning for Liver Resection Performed Under Inflow Occlusion in Humans. Ann Surg 2000;232:155–62.

62. Lentsch AB, Kato A, Yoshidome H, et al. Inflammatory mechanisms and therapeutic strategies for warm hepatic ischemia/reperfusion injury. Hepatology 2000;32:169–73.
63. Kim YI, Ishii T, Aramaki M, et al. The Pringle maneuver induces only partial ischemia of the liver. Hepato-gastroenterol 1995;42:169–71.
64. Crescenti A, Borghi G, Bignami E, et al. Intraoperative use of tranexamic acid to reduce transfusion rate in patients undergoing radical retropubic prostatectomy: double blind, randomised, placebo controlled trial. BMJ (Clinical research ed) 2011;343:d5701.
65. collaborators C-2 trial, Shakur H, Roberts I, Bautista R, et al. Effects of tranexamic acid on death, vascular occlusive events, and blood transfusion in trauma patients with significant haemorrhage (CRASH-2): a randomised, placebo-controlled trial. Lancet 2010;376:23–32.
66. Ker K, Edwards P, Perel P, et al. Effect of tranexamic acid on surgical bleeding: systematic review and cumulative meta-analysis. BMJ (Clinical research ed) 2012;344:e3054.
67. Wu C-C, Ho W-M, Cheng S-B, et al. Perioperative Parenteral Tranexamic Acid in Liver Tumor Resection. Ann Surg 2006;243:173–80.
68. Richardson AJ, Laurence JM, Lam VWT. Use of pre-operative steroids in liver resection: a systematic review and meta-analysis. Hpb 2014;16:12–9.
69. Li N, Gu W, Weng J, et al. Short-term administration of steroids does not affect postoperative complications following liver resection: Evidence from a meta-analysis of randomized controlled trials. Hepatol Res 2015;45:201–9.
70. Kemp R, Mole J, Gomez D. Group on behalf of the NHS: Current evidence for the use of N-acetylcysteine following liver resection. Anz J Surg 2018;88:E486–90.
71. Grendar J, Ouellet JF, McKay A, et al. Effect of N-acetylcysteine on liver recovery after resection: A randomized clinical trial. J Surg Oncol 2016;114:446–50.
72. Yassen K: Intravenous Infusion of N-acetylcysteine in cirrhotic patients undergoing liver resection attenuates the postoperative increase in liver enzymes, C reactive protein and intercellular adhesion molecule 1. A randomized controlled trial 2020 doi:10.26226/morressier.58f5b030d462b80296c9e6a0
73. Melloul E, Hübner M, Scott M, et al. Guidelines for Perioperative Care for Liver Surgery: Enhanced Recovery After Surgery (ERAS) Society Recommendations. World J Surg 2016;40:2425–40.
74. Noba L, Rodgers S, Chandler C, et al. Enhanced Recovery After Surgery (ERAS) Reduces Hospital Costs and Improve Clinical Outcomes in Liver Surgery: a Systematic Review and Meta-Analysis. J Gastrointest Surg 2020;24:918–32.

Anaesthesia for Pancreatic Surgery

Leigh J.S. Kelliher, MBBS, BSc, FRCA, MD[a],*, Anton Krige, MBChB, DIMC, FRCA, FFICM[b]

KEYWORDS

- ERAS • Enhanced recovery • Fast track • Pancreaticoduodenectomy
- Whipple's procedure • Pancreatic cancer

KEY POINTS

- Pancreatic cancer is a leading cause of cancer death globally and pancreatic resection remains the only curative treatment option.
- Pancreatic resection is complex and is itself associated with a significant risk of morbidity and mortality.
- Careful patient selection and optimization alongside perioperative care based on current enhanced recovery guidance may reduce postoperative morbidity and facilitate further oncological treatment, thereby improving long-term outcomes.
- Future efforts to improve outcomes must focus on the earlier detection of malignancy, advances in surgical and anesthetic techniques, and the development of more effective adjuvant therapies.

INTRODUCTION

The anatomy and physiology of the pancreas and its location within the body mean pancreatic surgery is often complicated and high risk. The most common pancreatic surgical procedures are pancreaticoduodenectomy and distal pancreatectomy. The indications for surgery are varied but this article will principally focus on pancreaticoduodenectomy within the setting of pancreatic cancer.

PANCREATIC CANCER

Despite advances in treatment and improved survival times for many different types of cancer, the prognosis for those diagnosed with pancreatic cancer remains poor. Globally there are almost half a million new cases of pancreatic cancer (mainly adenocarcinoma) diagnosed every year, giving an age-standardized incidence rate of 4.8 per

Declarations/conflicts of interest: I have no declarations/conflicts of interest.
[a] Department of Anaesthetics, Royal Surrey County Hospital NHS Foundation Trust, Egerton Road, Guildford, Surrey, GU2 7AS, UK; [b] Department of Anaesthesia and Critical Care, Royal Blackburn Teaching Hospital, Haslingden Road, Blackburn BB2 3HH, UK
* Corresponding author.
E-mail address: lkelliher@nhs.net

Anesthesiology Clin 40 (2022) 107–117
https://doi.org/10.1016/j.anclin.2021.11.005
anesthesiology.theclinics.com

100,000.[1] These rates are 3 to 4 times higher in the developed world with north America, Europe, and Australasia topping the list. It is estimated that the overall 1-year survival for all patients diagnosed is approximately 25%, dropping to 5% at 5 years.[2] Surgical removal of the primary tumor is the only curative treatment and one major determinant of survival is the stage of cancer at presentation. This may be divided into 4 categories—resectable, borderline resectable, locally advanced unresectable, and metastatic.[3] Only 10% to 15% of patients present with resectable disease. 5-year survival may be as high as 25% for those whereby surgery is possible, compared with a median survival of 6 months in those whereby it is not.[2] As a result, while the incidence of pancreatic cancer is far smaller than that of lung, breast, colon, prostate, skin, and others it is the seventh leading cause of cancer death globally.[1]

PANCREATICODUODENECTOMY

Pancreaticoduodenectomy is a complex surgical procedure involving *en-bloc* resection of the head of the pancreas, gallbladder, duodenum, distal stomach (pylorus), and proximal jejunum followed by reconstruction via gastrojejunostomy, hepaticojejunostomy, and pancreaticojejunostomy (**Fig. 1**). The principle indication for this surgery is cancer of the pancreatic head but it is also used for the treatment of other periampullary cancers—duodenal and cholangiocarcinoma—as well as benign tumors, chronic pancreatitis affecting the head of the pancreas, and neuroendocrine tumors. The procedure was pioneered in the 1930s by an American surgeon named Allen Oldfather Whipple[4] and hence is widely known as the Whipple procedure. Historically it has been associated with significant postoperative mortality and morbidity, reported as high as 25% and 60%, respectively, in the 1960s.[5] With advances in surgical technique, perioperative care, and patient selection these figures have reduced, and the current mortality is estimated at approximately 4% with some high-volume centers reporting mortality as low as 1%.[6,7] Postoperative morbidity remains a significant issue with the principal problems being surgical site infections, pulmonary complications, anastomotic leaks, fistulas and delayed gastric emptying.[8] In an attempt to reduce some of these complications, alternatives to the classical pancreaticoduodenectomy have been developed. Primary among these is the pylorus-preserving

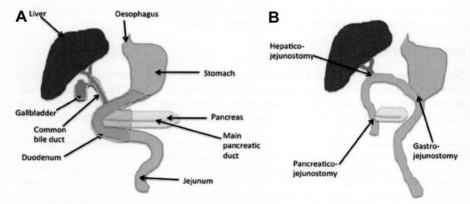

Fig. 1. The anatomy of the classical pancreaticoduodenectomy (Whipple procedure). (*A*) Anatomy resected (shaded area). (*B*) Reconstruction. (*From* Gall, T. M. H., Tsakok, M., Wasan, H., & Jiao, L. R. (2015). Pancreatic cancer: current management and treatment strategies. *Postgraduate Medical Journal*, *91*(1080), 601–607. https://doi.org/10.1136/postgradmedj-2014-133222)

pancreaticoduodenectomy (PPPD) (**Fig. 2**) whereby the distal stomach is not resected. Proponents of this approach assert it is associated with shorter operative times and less intraoperative bleeding as well as better long-term gastrointestinal function, fewer peptic ulcers, and lower incidence of dumping syndrome[9] but critics point to its association with delayed postoperative gastric emptying and that, as the resection is less radical, the chance of incomplete tumor removal/positive margins is increased.[10] A recent Cochrane review of comparing pancreaticoduodenectomy with PPPD found no differences in mortality, morbidity or survival between the 2 procedures although the authors also commented on the relatively poor quality of available data.[11]

OPEN VERSUS MINIMALLY INVASIVE SURGERY

Classically, pancreaticoduodenectomy is an open procedure. A variety of incisions are used including chevron, straight transverse, and curved transverse and with no current evidence/consensus for the superiority of one over another the choice often depends on surgical preference. In common with many other surgical procedures, minimally invasive techniques (both laparoscopic and robotically assisted) have been developed with the goal of reducing postoperative morbidity and recovery times. Several meta-analyses have examined the evidence comparing minimally invasive with open pancreaticoduodenectomy the results of which indicate that while the minimally invasive approach may be associated with less intraoperative blood loss, lower transfusion rates, and shorter hospital stays, there is no difference in major morbidity or mortality and operative times are longer.[12-14] All point to the need for further high-quality evidence. Currently, the use of minimally invasive pancreaticoduodenectomy depends on the available surgical expertise and careful patient selection.

ADJUVANT/NEOADJUVANT CHEMORADIOTHERAPY

With high rates of early cancer recurrence and poor one- and 5-year survival following pancreaticoduodenectomy alone, the use of adjuvant chemotherapy ± radiotherapy to improve outcomes has been a subject of investigation over the past 4 decades.

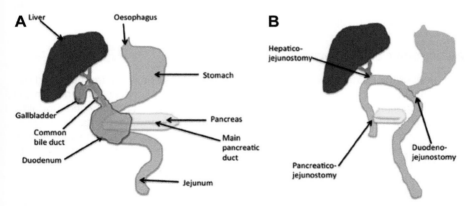

Fig. 2. The anatomy of the pylorus-preserving pancreaticoduodenectomy (PPPD). (*A*) Anatomy resected (shaded area). (*B*) Reconstruction. (*From* Gall, T. M. H., Tsakok, M., Wasan, H., & Jiao, L. R. (2015). Pancreatic cancer: current management and treatment strategies. *Postgraduate Medical Journal, 91*(1080), 601–607. https://doi.org/10.1136/postgradmedj-2014-133222)

By the late 1980s evidence was emerging that surgery followed by adjuvant chemo-radiotherapy with 5-Fluorouracil led to improved survival versus surgery alone.[15] Over the decades as there has been a great deal of research into finding the optimal chemotherapeutic agents and treatment protocol and at this current time practice varies across the globe. Some centers advocate the use of combined radiotherapy and chemotherapy, whereas others favor chemotherapy alone as first-line adjuvant treatment following pancreaticoduodenectomy. Agents commonly utilized are gemci-tabine, S1 (tegafur/gimeracil/oteracil), FOLFIRINOX (folinic acid, 5-fluorouracil, irinote-can, oxaliplatin), or combinations of these, all of which have been shown to improve survival.[16]

Despite the demonstrable survival benefits associated with adjuvant therapy, a sig-nificant proportion of patients are not eligible/unable to receive it. Approximately 25% of patients are found to have unresectable cancer (either due to local invasion or metastasis) at the time of surgery[17] and do not, therefore, receive adjuvant therapy. Accurate staging is essential and this statistical just illustrates how challenging it can be. Patients suspected of having pancreatic cancer first undergo investigation in the form of CT or MRI imaging with resectability being assessed via the size and invasiveness of the primary tumor and whether or not metastases/lymphatic spread is present. The sensitivity of CT/MRI for detecting micrometastases is poor and many centers utilize FDG PET scanning to enhance this. While more invasive, the development of endoscopic ultrasound (EUS) assessment has further enhanced the accuracy of diagnosis and staging, particularly in cases whereby a tissue diagnosis is required as EUS facilitates the sampling of the tumor via fine-needle aspiration (FNA). Even when the resectability of the tumor is predicted accurately, 20% of pa-tients undergoing a successful resection do not recover adequately from the surgery to commence adjuvant therapy. This has led researchers to examine the role of neo-adjuvant therapy (as opposed to the traditional approach of surgery first) not only as a way of ensuring more patients are able to receive chemo/radiotherapy but also for potentially reducing the number of patients found to be inoperable at the time of sur-gery, increasing the chance of clear resection margins and preventing early cancer recurrence. To date the benefits of neoadjuvant therapy remain hypothetical with most studies finding no overall survival benefit;[16,18,19] however, the search for the optimal protocol continues and several RCT's compare neoadjuvant therapy with surgery-first are ongoing.

PREOPERATIVE CONSIDERATIONS

The preoperative issues encountered when treating these patients are many and de-cision making can be extremely complex. As discussed, pancreaticoduodenectomy is major abdominal surgery associated with a significant risk of morbidity and mortality. Most of the patients present with obstructive jaundice and will have marked physio-logic derangement. In addition, they are often elderly, cachectic, immunosuppressed, and with poor nutritional status. Anemia and diabetes are common and with advancing age come many other chronic comorbidities. The emotional impact of this diagnosis must not be underestimated either—many patients will require coun-seling/treatment of anxiety. Management is based on staging and given the prognosis without surgery is so dismal, it is essential that this is done as accurately as possible. Finally, for patients deemed to have resectable disease, the time between diagnosis and surgery is critical, meaning the time-frame for preoperative assessment, coun-seling, risk-stratification, and optimization is limited. A multi-disciplinary team approach comprising experienced and expert health care professionals is essential.

RISK STRATIFICATION

Given the high-risk nature of the surgery and patient population, many centers choose to assess patients' cardiovascular, respiratory, and skeletal muscle systems with cardiopulmonary exercise testing (CPET) in addition to routine preoperative tests. CPET variables have been shown to correlate with adverse postoperative outcomes following a variety of noncardiopulmonary surgeries, including pancreaticoduodenectomy[20,21] and it is used widely for risk stratification and to inform decision-making.

NUTRITION

Perioperative malnutrition is common in patients with pancreaticoduodenectomy and is associated with a higher incidence of postoperative complications.[22] Patients nutritional status should be assessed preoperatively and those found to be significantly malnourished should receive supplementation to increase calorie and protein intake and replace minerals and vitamins either orally (via sip feeds) or enterally (via tube feeds). Equally, postoperative nutrition should be supplemented orally or enterally. The routine use of parenteral nutrition has not been shown to be beneficial and is associated with complications, and therefore, should be avoided.[23,24]

PREOPERATIVE BILIARY DRAINAGE

For many patients, the first symptom of pancreatic cancer is jaundice. Compression of the common bile duct by tumor in the head of the pancreas causes obstructive jaundice which in turn can result in renal impairment, liver dysfunction, cardiac dysfunction, immune dysfunction, and abnormalities of blood clotting.[25] Drainage of the biliary system either percutaneously or endoscopically will correct the obstruction and ameliorate these risks but is associated with procedure-specific complications including hemorrhage, sepsis, and localized inflammation[26] which may delay, or worsen, overall outcome following pancreaticoduodenectomy. A systematic review examining the practice of preoperative biliary drainage found insufficient evidence to support or refute its use, with the authors concluding that routine use of preoperative biliary drainage should be avoided.[25] Current ERAS guidelines indicate that it may still be considered for patients with serum bilirubin greater than 250 μmol/L.[24]

ERAS RECOMMENDATIONS

Originating in colorectal surgery with the purpose of improving postoperative outcomes via minimizing the stress of anesthesia and surgery, fast-track programs have shown to be beneficial for a variety of surgical procedures.[27–30] The Enhanced Recovery After Surgery (ERAS) Society produced consensus guidelines for the perioperative care of patients with pancreaticoduodenectomy in 2013.[24] These are summarized in **Table 1**. A number of systematic reviews have examined the evidence for the use of fast-track programs in pancreaticoduodenectomy concluding that it is feasible, safe, and may be associated with reduced length of hospital stay and postoperative morbidity.[31–35] However, the majority of the evidence comes from retrospective cohort studies with no RCTs identified. A study from 2019 attempted to identify factors associated with early discharge following pancreaticoduodenectomy by retrospectively examining the records of more than 10,000 patients from the ACS-NSQIP database. They found that early discharge (LOS 5 days or less) was significantly associated with younger age, absence of obesity, COPD and hypertension, neoadjuvant chemotherapy, shorter operative time, and minimally invasive surgery. Patients that received

Table 1
ERAS society perioperative care recommendations for pancreaticoduodenectomy

Recommendation	Strength
Routine perioperative counseling	Strong
Avoid routine preoperative biliary drainage if serum bilirubin <250 μmol/L	Weak
Stop smoking and alcohol consumption for 1 mo before surgery	Strong
Oral or enteral preoperative nutritional supplements only for patients who are significantly malnourished	Weak
Consider immuno-nutrition 5–7 d preoperatively	Weak
Avoid bowel preparation	Strong
Preoperative oral carbohydrate load – except in diabetics	Strong
Avoid preoperative sedatives	Weak
LMWH continued for 4 wk postoperatively	Strong
Routine antimicrobial prophylaxis	Strong
Epidural analgesia (open surgery)	Weak
Multimodal approach to PONV prevention	Strong
Avoid hypothermia	Strong
Postoperative glycaemic control	Strong
Aim for near-zero fluid balance with goal-directed fluid therapy using balanced crystalloid solution	Strong
Early removal of surgical drains (72 h)	Strong
Early removal of urinary catheter (48 h)	Strong
Consider artificial nutrition in patients with delayed gastric emptying	Strong
Allow early oral intake, building to normal diet over 3–4 d.	Strong
Early and scheduled mobilization from the morning of the first postoperative day	Strong
Audit compliance and outcomes	Strong

From Lassen, K., Coolsen, M. M. E., Slim, K., Carli, F., de Aguilar-Nascimento, J. E., Schäfer, M., Parks, R. W., Fearon, K. C. H., Lobo, D. N., Demartines, N., Braga, M., Ljungqvist, O., & Dejong, C. H. C. (2012). Guidelines for Perioperative Care for Pancreaticoduodenectomy: Enhanced Recovery After Surgery (ERAS®) Society Recommendations. *World Journal of Surgery, 37*(2), 240–258. https://doi.org/10.1007/s00268-012-1771-1.

an epidural, jejunostomy tube, abdominal drain, or who required adhesiolysis were significantly less likely to be discharged early.[36] A number of these factors are potentially modifiable and may indicate areas of focus for future enhanced recovery programs.

ANESTHETIC TECHNIQUE

Pancreaticoduodenectomy is a high-risk intrabdominal surgery and the anesthetic technique should reflect this. Tracheal intubation, wide bore peripheral and central iv access, invasive blood pressure monitoring, regular blood gas sampling, active warming, glycemic control, VTE, and antimicrobial prophylaxis are all standard. Massive hemorrhage is among the potential intraoperative complications and should be prepared for. The use of cardiac output monitoring to guide fluid and vasopressor management has been shown to reduce complications in major gastrointestinal surgery and should be considered.[36] Depth of anesthesia monitoring minimizing effective dosing of anesthetic agent, perhaps making hemodynamic management simpler while reducing the incidence of postoperative delirium both of which may be of benefit in this high-risk population.[37,38]

Fluid management and analgesia are 2 particularly challenging aspects of anesthetic care in this setting. Prolonged surgery, inflammatory mediators, anesthesia/epidural induced hypotension, and blood loss can all complicate the estimation of fluid requirements. Fluid overload is associated with increased morbidity following pancreaticoduodenectomy[39] and ERAS guidelines recommend targeting a near-zero fluid balance using a balanced crystalloid solution and cardiac output monitoring to help guide fluid bolus administration.[24]

Analgesic modality will depend on the surgical approach adopted and local expertise and practice. For open surgery, current ERAS guidelines advocate the use of thoracic epidural analgesia[24] and while an effective, well-managed epidural offers excellent resting and dynamic pain relief epidural analgesia can be associated with hypotension and fluid overload[40] and failure rates as high as 30% have been reported.[41] They are not recommended in the context of minimally invasive surgery. There are many alternatives that might be considered including the use of local anesthetic wound catheters, abdominal field blocks, intrathecal opioids, lidocaine infusions, and of course parenteral opioids. There is no consensus evidence for any particular technique/combination and analgesic regimens should be tailored to fit with local expertise and surgical practice. ERAS recommends in general that analgesia should be multimodal, opioid-sparing with the aim of providing effective pain relief, allowing early mobilization while minimizing the risks of ileus, PONV, drowsiness, hallucination, and respiratory depression.

POSTOPERATIVE CARE

The high-risk nature of this surgery alongside the frequent occurrence of complications necessitates that these patients are managed postoperatively in an ICU/HDU setting. Alongside the general risks that come with major intraabdominal surgery such as bleeding, sepsis, pulmonary complications, ileus, wound infection, and venous thromboembolism are some procedure-specific complications that frequently arise.

DELAYED GASTRIC EMPTYING

Occurring in approximately 10% to 25%[42] delayed gastric emptying causes significant discomfort for patients, prolongs recovery time, and prevents a return to the normal oral diet. An underlying cause such as a collection or anastomotic leak must be excluded but most delayed gastric emptying resolves with time.[6] A proportion of patients will require naso-gastric drainage and nutritional supplementation. Clear evidence to support the prophylactic use of prokinetic agents such as metoclopramide to reduce the incidence and duration of DGE has yet to emerge.

PANCREATIC LEAK/FISTULA

The incidence of pancreatic leak (anastomotic breakdown of the pancreaticojejunostomy and leakage of pancreatic secretions) is estimated between 8% and 13%.[43] Diagnosis may be confirmed by the presence of amylase (>100 IU/L) in the perianastomotic drain. Most leaks may be managed conservatively by keeping the drain in place until the leak stops.[6,43] However, a proportion may develop abscess formation and sepsis, pseudo-aneurysm, or a major gastrointestinal hemorrhage. Pancreatic leak-associated mortality may be as high as 5%.[44]

FUTURE DIRECTIONS

Pancreatic cancer remains a challenge to cure due to often late presentation and invasiveness of treatment. Surgery is the only curative treatment, but it is associated with significant morbidity and mortality and only a small proportion of cancers are resectable. Future efforts must be directed toward increasing this number, either by earlier detection and screening or by developing more effective neoadjuvant treatment.

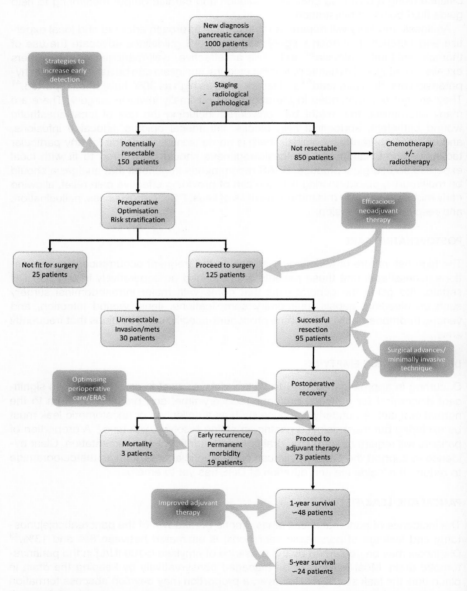

Fig. 3. The cancer journey for 1000 patients diagnosed with pancreatic cancer and areas which may lead to improvement in oncological outcomes.

Prognosis is poor even following successful surgery and with morbidity rates of 20% to 40% a significant number of patients never recover adequately enough to proceed with further treatment. Efforts to reduce postoperative morbidity through the continuing development of minimally invasive techniques and perioperative care pathways are essential (**Fig. 3**).

CLINICS CARE POINTS

- Perioperative malnutrition is common in patients with pancreaticoduodenectomy and associated with postoperative morbidity. All patients should be routinely screened and those found to be significantly malnourished, treated with oral or enteral supplementation. The routine use of parenteral nutritional support should be avoided.
- Perioperative fluid management can be extremely challenging in this group of patients and is complicated by prolonged surgery, the magnitude of the inflammatory response, anesthesia/epidural-induced hypotension, and blood loss. A tailored approach using a balanced crystalloid solution and cardiac output monitoring to guide fluid boluses is recommended with the goal of maintaining adequate end-organ perfusion while avoiding fluid overload, targeting a near-zero fluid balance.
- Delayed-gastric emptying occurs frequently following pancreaticoduodenectomy and will often resolve with conservative management and time. It is important to exclude significant underlying pathology such as an abdominal collection or anastomotic leak

DISCLOSURE

The authors have no conflicts of interest to disclose.

REFERENCES

1. Available at: https://gco.iarc.fr/. Accessed September 26, 2020
2. Available at: https://www.cancerresearchuk.org/ Accessed September 26, 2020
3. Tempero MA, Malafa MP, Al-Hawary M, et al. Pancreatic adenocarcinoma, version 2.2017, NCCN Clinical Practice Guidelines in Oncology. J Natl Compr Canc Netw 2017;15(8):1028–61.
4. Whipple AO, Parsons WB, Mullins CR, et al. Treatment of carcinoma of the ampulla of Vater. Ann Surg 1935;102:763–79.
5. Stojadinovic A, Brooks A, Hoos A, et al. An evidence-based approach to the surgical management of resectable pancreatic adenocarcinoma. J Am Coll Surg 2003;196(6):954–64.
6. Ho CK, Kleeff J, Friess H, et al. Complications of pancreatic surgery. HPB (Oxford) 2005;7:99–108.
7. Fernandez-del Castillo C, Morales-Oyarvide V, McGrath D, et al. Evolution of the Whipple procedure at the Massachusetts General Hospital. Surgery 2012;152(3 Suppl 1):S56–63.
8. Kumar SV, Prasad JS. A Postoperative morbidity following Whipple's procedure for periampullary carcinoma: a retrospective study spanning 5 years. Int J Res Med Sci 2019;7:4314–9.
9. Traverso LW, Longmire WP Jr. Preservation of the pylorus in pancreaticoduodenectomy: a follow-up evaluation. Ann Surg 1980;192:306–10.
10. Tran K, Smeenk H, Eijck C, et al. Pylorus preserving pancreaticoduodenectomy versus standard whipple procedure. Ann Surg 2004;240:738–45.

11. Hüttner FJ, Fitzmaurice C, Schwarzer G, et al. Pylorus-preserving pancreatico-duodenectomy (pp Whipple) versus pancreaticoduodenectomy (classic Whipple) for surgical treatment of periampullary and pancreatic carcinoma. Cochrane Database Syst Rev 2016;2:CD006053.

12. Wang S, Shi N, You L, et al. Minimally invasive surgical approach versus open procedure for pancreaticoduodenectomy: A systematic review and meta-analysis. Medicine (Baltimore) 2017;96(50):e8619.

13. Zhang H, Lan X, Peng B, et al. Is total laparoscopic pancreaticoduodenectomy superior to open procedure? A meta-analysis. World J Gastroenterol 2019; 25(37):5711–31.

14. Peng L, Lin S, Li Y, et al. Systematic review and meta-analysis of robotic versus open pancreaticoduodenectomy. Surg Endosc 2017;31:3085–97. https://doi.org/10.1007/s00464-016-5371-2.

15. Further evidence of effective adjuvant combined radiation and chemotherapy following curative resection of pancreatic cancer. Gastrointestinal Tumor Study Group. Cancer 1987;59:2006–10.

16. Motoi F, Unno M. Adjuvant and neoadjuvant treatment for pancreatic adenocarcinoma. Jpn J Clin Oncol 2020;50(5):483–9.

17. Papalezova KT, Tyler DS, Blazer DG 3rd, et al. Does preoperative therapy optimize outcomes in patients with resectable pancreatic cancer? J Surg Oncol 2012;106:111–8.

18. Liu W, Fu XL, Yang JY, et al. Efficacy of neo-adjuvant chemoradiotherapy for resectable pancreatic adenocarcinoma: a PRISMA-compliant meta-analysis and systematic review. Medicine (Baltimore) 2016;95(15):e3009.

19. Cools KS, Sanoff HK, Kim HJ, et al. Impact of neoadjuvant therapy on postoperative outcomes after pancreaticoduodenectomy. J Surg Oncol 2018;118(3): 455–62.

20. Hennis PJ, Meale PM. Grocott MPWCardiopulmonary exercise testing for the evaluation of perioperative risk in non-cardiopulmonary surgery. Postgrad Med J 2011;87:550–7.

21. Junejo MA, Mason JM, Sheen AJ, et al. Cardiopulmonary exercise testing for pre-operative risk assessment before pancreaticoduodenectomy for cancer. Ann Surg Oncol 2014;21(6):1929–36.

22. Nygren J, Thorell A, Ljungqvist O. New developments facilitating nutritional intake after gastrointestinal surgery. Curr Opin Clin Nutr Metab Care 2003;6:593–7.

23. Goonetilleke KS, Siriwardena AK. Systematic review of peri-operative nutritional supplementation in patients undergoing pancreaticoduodenectomy. JOP 2006; 7(1):5–13.

24. Lassen K, Coolsen MM, Slim K, et al. Guidelines for perioperative care for pancreaticoduodenectomy: Enhanced Recovery After Surgery (ERAS®) Society recommendations. World J Surg 2013;37(2):240–58.

25. Fang Y, Gurusamy KS, Wang Q, et al. Pre-operative biliary drainage for obstructive jaundice. Cochrane Database Syst Rev 2012;9(9):CD005444.

26. Lynskey GE, Banovac F, Chang T. Vascular complications associated with percutaneous biliary drainage: a report of three cases. Semin Intervent Radiol 2007; 24(3):316–9.

27. Rawlinson A, Kang P, Evans J, et al. A systematic review of enhanced recovery protocols in colorectal surgery. Ann R Coll Surg Engl 2011;93(8):583–8.

28. Elsarrag M, Soldozy S, Patel P, et al. Enhanced recovery after spine surgery: a systematic review. Neurosurg Focus 2019;46(4):E3.

29. Zhu S, Qian W, Jiang C, et al. Enhanced recovery after surgery for hip and knee arthroplasty: a systematic review and meta-analysis. Postgrad Med J 2017; 93(1106):736–42.
30. Scheib SA, Thomassee M, Kenner JL. Enhanced Recovery after Surgery in Gynecology: A Review of the Literature. J Minim Invasive Gynecol 2019;26(2): 327–43.
31. Spelt L, Ansari D, Sturesson C, et al. Fast-track programmes for hepatopancreatic resections: where do we stand? HPB (Oxford) 2011;13(12):833–8.
32. Hall TC, Dennison AR, Bilku DK, et al. Enhanced recovery programmes in hepatobiliary and pancreatic surgery: a systematic review. Ann R Coll Surg Engl 2012; 94(5):318–26.
33. Coolsen MME, van Dam RM, van der Wilt AA, et al. Systematic Review and Meta-analysis of Enhanced Recovery After Pancreatic Surgery with Particular Emphasis on Pancreaticoduodenectomies. World J Surg 2013;37:1909–18.
34. Kagedan DJ, Ahmed M, Devitt KS, et al. Enhanced recovery after pancreatic surgery: a systematic review of the evidence. HPB (Oxford) 2015;17(1):11–6.
35. Mahvi DA, Pak LM, Bose SK, et al. Fast-Track Pancreaticoduodenectomy: Factors Associated with Early Discharge. World J Surg 2019;43(5):1332–41.
36. Pearse RM, Harrison DA, MacDonald N, et al. Effect of a perioperative, cardiac output-guided hemodynamic therapy algorithm on outcomes following major gastrointestinal surgery: a randomized clinical trial and systematic review. JAMA 2014;311(21):2181–90 [published correction appears in JAMA. 2014 Oct 8;312(14):1473].
37. Punjasawadwong Y, Phongchiewboon A, Bunchungmongkol N. Bispectral index for improving anaesthetic delivery and postoperative recovery. Cochrane Database Syst Rev 2014;2014(6):CD003843.
38. Radtke FM, Franck M, Lendner J, et al. Monitoring depth of anaesthesia in a randomized trial decreases the rate of postoperative delirium but not postoperative cognitive dysfunction. Br J Anaesth 2013;110(Suppl 1):i98–105.
39. Wright GP, Koehler TJ, Davis AT, et al. The drowning whipple: Perioperative fluid balance and outcomes following pancreaticoduodenectomy. J Surg Oncol 2014; 110:407–11.
40. Pratt WB, Steinbrook RA, Maithel SK, et al. Epidural analgesia for pancreatoduodenectomy: a critical appraisal. J Gastrointest Surg 2008;12(7):1207–20. https://doi.org/10.1007/s11605-008-0467-1.
41. Hermanides J, Hollmann MW, Stevens MF, et al. Failed epidural: causes and management. Br J Anaesth 2012;109(Issue 2):144–54.
42. Wente MN, Bassi C, Dervenis C, et al. Delayed gastric emptying (DGE) after pancreatic surgery: a suggested definition by the International Study Group of Pancreatic Surgery (ISGPS). Surgery 2007;142:761–8.
43. Cullen J, Sarr M, Ilstrup D. Pancreatic anastomotic leak after pancreaticoduodenectomy: Incidence, significance, and management. Am J Surg 1994;168(4): 295–8.
44. American Gastroenterological Association. American Gastroenterological Association medical position statement: epidemiology, diagnosis, and treatment of pancreatic ductal adenocarcinoma. Gastroenterology 1999;117:1463–84.

Anesthesia and Enhanced Recovery After Surgery in Bariatric Surgery

Christa L. Riley, MD[a,b],*

KEYWORDS

- Enhanced recovery • ERAS • Bariatric surgery • Multimodal analgesia
- Prehabilitation • Fluid management
- Postoperative nausea and vomiting (PONV) prophylaxis • Preoperative fasting

KEY POINTS

- Enhanced recovery after surgery pathways incorporate evidence-based strategies into care plans with the goal decreasing reducing patient surgical stress response and accelerating functional recovery through aggregation of incremental improvements.
- Anesthesiologists are integral to the implementation of perioperative enhanced recovery after surgery elements to facilitate recovery from bariatric surgery.
- Implementation of enhanced recovery after surgery pathways in bariatric surgery reduces hospital length of stay and the incidence of postoperative nausea and vomiting.
- Multimodal, opioid-sparing pain control strategies are key elements of the enhanced recovery after surgery pathways and integral to obtaining quick functional recovery.
- Anesthesia considerations for morbidly obese patients undergoing bariatric surgery are discussed.

INTRODUCTION

The prevalence of obesity and severe obesity has continued to increase in the United States and around the world. According to the Centers for Disease Control and Prevention National Center for Health Statistics, the obesity prevalence in the United States was 42.4% in 2017 to 2018 with no significant differences between men and women among all adults or by age group. The prevalence of severe obesity is 9.2% and more prevalent among women and individuals over 40 years old. Obesity is associated with other comorbidities, such as hypertension, diabetes, obstructive sleep

[a] Fellow, Surgical Critical Care, Department of Anesthesiology and Critical Care, Penn Medicine, 6 Dulles, 3400 Spruce Street, Philadelphia, PA 19104, USA; [b] Anesthesiologist & Intensivist, Department of Anesthesiology, Hunter Holmes McGuire VA Medical Center, Richmond, VA, USA
* 4001 Welby Drive, Midlothian, VA 23113.
E-mail address: rileycl@gmail.com

Anesthesiology Clin 40 (2022) 119–142
https://doi.org/10.1016/j.anclin.2021.11.006
1932-2275/22/© 2021 Elsevier Inc. All rights reserved.

anesthesiology.theclinics.com

apnea (OSA), and coronary artery disease. Severe obesity further increases the risk of these obesity-related diseases and complications.[1]

Bariatric surgery continues to be the most effective and durable treatment for morbid obesity and its related comorbidities[2] compared with nonsurgical interventions. Studies on the financial impact of bariatric surgery have shown mixed results. Early studies showed decreases in health care expenditures with a return on investment within 3 to 7 years.[3] More recent data show bariatric surgery is likely cost effective (more effective but more costly) but not cost saving (more effective and less costly) when compared with medical weight loss interventions.[4,5] With the increase in obesity, the number of bariatric procedures has increased accordingly. In 2014, there were more than 575,000 surgical procedures to treat obesity worldwide, with the most common procedure being the laparoscopic sleeve gastrectomy (45.9%) followed by the laparoscopic Roux-en-Y gastric bypass (39.5%).[6] The widespread use of laparoscopic surgery and the implementation of perioperative care of the obese patient have resulted in low rates of morbidity and mortality and decreased lengths of hospital stay (LOS).[7,8] Nevertheless, efforts are still being made to further decrease postoperative complications from these elective procedures to decrease morbidity to the individual and cost to the health care system.

ENHANCED RECOVERY AFTER SURGERY IN BARIATRIC SURGERY

The implementation of the enhanced recovery after surgery (ERAS) pathways for bariatric surgery aims to incorporate evidence-based practices into the preoperative, intraoperative, and postoperative care plans with the goals to improve the quality of care, decrease complications, and shorten hospital stays. These evidence-based practices focus on modifying the metabolic response to surgical stress and accelerating functional recovery.[9] ERAS principles have been applied to multiple disciplines of surgery. General ERAS principles include counseling and education, patient optimization (weight loss, exercise, optimal management of comorbidities), and nutrition and fluid management in the preoperative period. The intraoperative period emphasizes minimally invasive surgical technique, short-acting anesthetics, optimal fluid management, normothermia, preventing postoperative nausea and vomiting (PONV), opioid-sparing analgesia, and avoiding tubes and drains. The postoperative period focuses on early mobilization, early oral fluid intake, and early removal of lines and drains while continuing to prevent PONV and use opioid-sparing analgesia.[9] Patients also are risk-stratified for postoperative care in the intensive care unit or general surgical ward based on existing comorbidities. Anesthesiologists can impact outcomes in bariatric surgery during the preoperative, intraoperative, and immediate postoperative periods, and their involvement in the application of ERAS pathways is critical.

In 2016, the ERAS Society published the first guidelines recommendations for perioperative care in bariatric surgery.[10] A summary of those recommendations is included in **Table 1**. Many of the recommendations in the guidelines are based on low levels of evidence and many recommendations were extrapolated from other surgical disciplines, such as colorectal surgery. Since the publication of ERAS Society guidelines, data from centers implementing bariatric surgery ERAS pathways have been collected and reported and suggest that ERAS is safe and capable of shortening LOS.[11,12] Postoperative LOS is used as a primary outcome in much of the ERAS literature because LOS is a surrogate measure of patient functional status recovery. Hospital discharge eligibility correlates well with the ability to resume activities of daily living, recovery of gastrointestinal functions, and adequate pain control.[11] Bariatric surgeons from 10 bariatric centers in Canada have issued national consensus

Table 1
ERAS recommendations for preoperative, intraoperative, and postoperative care in bariatric surgery

Intervention	Recommendation	Evidence	Strength
Preoperative care			
Preoperative counseling	Patient education should be provided and should include information about type of surgery, expected perioperative course, possible complications, preoperative preparation for surgery, lifestyle modifications, realistic outcome expectations, and long-term management.	Moderate	Strong
Prehabilitation	Data are limited but increasing for bariatric surgery on role of prehabilitation and exercise. Currently no recommendations but area of future research.	Low	Weak
Preoperative weight loss	Preoperative weight loss of 5%–10% of total body weight decreases postoperative complications.	High	Strong
Smoking and alcohol cessation	Recommend smoking cessation at least 4 wk before surgery. Recommend alcohol abstinence of 2 y in patients with a history of alcohol abuse.	High (smoking) Moderate (alcohol)	Strong (smoking) Strong (alcohol)
Preoperative fasting	Patients (with and without diabetes) may have clear fluids up to 2 h and solids 6 h before surgery. More data are necessary in patients with diabetes with gastroparesis.	High (nondiabetic) Moderate (diabetic) Low (gastroparesis)	Strong (nondiabetic) Weak (diabetic) Weak (gastroparesis)
Carbohydrate loading	Preoperative carbohydrate loading is associated with metabolic and clinical benefits in patients undergoing major elective abdominal surgery, but further data are required in morbidly obese patients.	Low	Strong
Premedication	Single dose glucocorticoids can be used safely to prevent PONV.	Low	Strong
Intraoperative care			
Anesthetic technique	Current data are insufficient to recommend specific anesthetic agents.	Low	Weak
Airway management	Tracheal intubation with awareness of difficulties of managing the bariatric airway.	Moderate	Strong
PONV	Multimodal approach to PONV prophylaxis should be used in all patients.	Low	Strong
Fluid management	Goal-directed fluid therapy to avoid hypotension and excessive fluid administration.	Moderate	Strong

(continued on next page)

Table 1
(continued)

Intervention	Recommendation	Evidence	Strength
Neuromuscular blockade	Deep neuromuscular blockade improves surgical performance.	Low	Weak
	Ensure full reversal of neuromuscular blockade.	Moderate	Strong
	Qualitative monitoring of neuromuscular blockade.	Moderate	Strong
Ventilation strategies	Lung-protective ventilation should be adopted for elective bariatric surgery	Moderate	Strong
Laparoscopy	Laparoscopic surgery is recommended for bariatric surgery.	High	Strong
Nasogastric tubes	Routine use not recommended.	Low	Strong
Abdominal drains	Insufficient evidence to recommend routine use.	Low	Weak
Postoperative care			
Analgesia	Multimodal systemic medications with local anesthetic infiltration are recommended.	High	Strong
Postoperative oxygen	Patients without OSA should receive supplemental oxygen.	Low	Strong
	Uncomplicated patients with OSA should receive supplemental oxygen.	High	Strong
Noninvasive positive pressure ventilation	Prophylactic routine postoperative continuous positive airway pressure is not recommended in patients without diagnosed OSA.	Moderate	Weak
	Consider continuous positive airway pressure therapy if BMI >50, severe OSA, or SpO_2 of <90 on o_2.	Low	Strong
	Patients with OSA on continuous positive airway pressure at home should use continuous positive airway pressure in postoperative period.	Moderate	Strong
	Patients with obesity hypoventilation syndrome should receive BiPAP/NIV prophylactically with intensive care unit monitoring.	Low	Strong
Thromboprophylaxis	Patients should receive mechanical and pharmacological thromboprophylaxis.	High	Strong

From Cardoso L, Rodrigues D, Gomes L, Carrilho F. Short- and long-term mortality after bariatric surgery: A systematic review and meta-analysis. *Diabetes, Obesity and Metabolism.* 2017;19(9):1223-1232. doi:10.1111/dom.12922

guidelines recommending 14 essential ERAS elements for bariatric surgery in Canada.[13] Several randomized controlled trials (RCTs) evaluating ERAS protocols in bariatric surgery have been published since the introduction of the ERAS Society guidelines that show ERAS protocol implementation in bariatric surgery reduces LOS and PONV. Anesthesiologists are increasingly participating in multidisciplinary process improvement teams and this article will review anesthetic management of the bariatric surgery patient in the context of ERAS.

PREOPERATIVE CARE PLANS

Optimal surgical outcomes begin before the patient reaches the operating room. Some interventions include patient selection, preoperative counseling and education, preoperative weight loss, prehabilitation, optimization of comorbidities, and smoking cessation.

Preoperative Counseling and Education

Any patient-centered care plan for bariatric surgery must include patient counseling that actively engages the patient to determine their preferences, needs, and values and informs them of risks and consequences of electing abdominal surgery, as well as the risks and benefits of electing not to have surgery.[14] Bariatric surgery requires patients to adhere to lifelong diet and behavior changes that may not be possible for some patients. Preoperative counseling should include information about the actual procedure to be performed, expected complications and their risks, hospital stay, postoperative recovery including expected pain, and realistic efficacy outcomes and long-term management. Different patients acquire and understand information in different ways. Patient counseling and education should be available in multiple modalities such as written, video, online, and disseminated to individuals or in group class settings. Although bariatric surgery is the most durable treatment for obesity, it does not meet the criteria for the standard of care for obesity; therefore, patients need to be involved in determining whether bariatric surgery is the weight management strategy most consistent with their preferences and values.[15] Adequate preoperative counseling and education, including anesthesia preoperative evaluation, ensures more realistic expectations about hospitalization, analgesia, mobilization, and discharge.[16]

Prehabilitation and Exercise

Despite advances in surgical technique and improvements of anesthetic care, suboptimal recovery persists for some patients. Up to 30% of patients undergoing a major abdominal surgery experience postoperative complications[17] and, even in the absence of morbid events, major abdominal surgery is associated with a 40% decrease in functional capacity.[18] Traditional interventions to improve return to baseline functional capacity have focused on the postoperative period. However, introducing new exercises and behaviors to patients concerned about interfering with postoperative recovery is challenging. A preoperative patient, however, may be more receptive to interventions that might improve recovery from surgery. Preoperative interventions may increase patient participation in their care and decrease anxiety surrounding the surgery because preoperative interventions can return a sense of control to the patient.[19]

Prehabilitation is the term applied to the concept of enhancing the functional capacity of an individual to withstand physical stress. The benefits of movement and exercise have been well-documented and include decreased sympathetic overreactivity, improved insulin sensitivity, increased antioxidant capacity, and decreased pain.[20] Physical activity has also been shown to improve functional capacity in many debilitating diseases, although the data are limited on the benefits of exercise before surgery.[19] Data on preoperative exercise before bariatric surgery are even more limited. In 2011, a systematic review of 12 studies showed preoperative exercise therapy decreased postoperative complication rates and LOS in cardiac and abdominal surgeries.[21] Outcomes after joint arthroplasty surgery were not affected by preoperative exercise routines. The studies that investigated cardiac and abdominal surgery included preoperative inspiratory muscle training and showed that the risk of developing a postoperative pulmonary complication was significantly higher in the groups who did not perform preoperative inspiratory muscle training. A case control pilot study published in 2017 investigated a 12-week pulmonary rehabilitation program in 4 morbidly obese patients with uncontrolled asthma before undergoing bariatric surgery.[22] The prehabilitation program included supervised exercise (40 minutes, 3 times per week), diet (nutritional counseling and a low-carbohydrate diet), and psychological interventions (4 group counseling sessions). The pilot study showed the feasibility of pulmonary prehabilitation in morbidly obese patients and improved asthma control in the case patients at the time of surgery compared with the control group. Owing to the study size, no difference in postoperative pulmonary complications could be shown. An RCT trial in patients undergoing colorectal resection for cancer investigated a multimodal prehabilitation program consisting of moderate-intensity exercise, nutritional counseling and protein supplementation, and anxiety reduction strategy education.[23] The study showed that more than 80% of patients who participated in the prehabilitation program returned to preoperative functional capacity by 8 weeks compared with only 40% of the control group that did not receive the prehabilitation program. A small match-paired study investigated the impact of a 30-day moderate intensity exercise program on several cardiometabolic health measures, LOS, and quality of life related to weight in patients undergoing bariatric surgery.[24] The study showed improved cardiometabolic health measures in the exercise group including decreased high-sensitivity C-reactive protein, suggesting a decrease in systemic inflammation. Cytokeratin 18, a marker of hepatic inflammation, also was decreased. Insulin sensitivity improved as measured by decreased fasting insulin levels. Adherence to preoperative diet recommendations improved in the exercise group and contributed to improved insulin sensitivity. LOS was also decreased in the exercise group, 42 hours versus 57 hours. Finally, quality of life domains for the exercise group improved significantly after the 30-day exercise intervention, including symptoms, emotions, and social interaction domains.

Systematic reviews of prehabilitation studies across multiple surgical disciplines suggest that prehabilitation confers limited clinical benefit. A 2013 review of 15 studies concluded that total body prehabilitation improved postoperative pain, LOS, and physical function, but was inconsistently improved health-related quality of life or aerobic fitness.[25] Another 2013 review that specifically evaluated studies in an attempt to quantify the effect of prehabilitation on postoperative physiology found that preoperative exercise conferred little clinical benefit.[26] Both of these reviews acknowledge the heterogeneity of prehabilitation programs, outcome measurements, and cohorts and poor methodological quality as limitations to making generalizable conclusions about the impact of prehabilitation. Although the data on prehabilitation are limited and conflicting, prehabilitation in bariatric surgery is an area for future research. The bariatric surgery patient cohort is generally younger with fewer comorbidities than cardiac, colorectal, and joint replacement patient cohorts. Future studies should focus on adequately powered RCTs specifically in bariatric surgery patient cohorts with consistent outcomes measurements and emphasis on evaluating effectiveness of intervention mode.

Preoperative Weight Loss

Preoperative weight loss is not a general requirement of the ERAS protocol because ERAS was originally developed within the colorectal surgery discipline. Bariatric patients are encouraged to achieve some reduction in their body mass before surgery (5%–10%) because studies have shown that the risk of perioperative complications is associated with the degree of obesity.[27–29] In some bariatric programs, failure to achieve a minimum mandatory preoperative weight loss results in cancellation of the surgery.[30] Preoperative weight loss decreases visceral adipose tissue and intrahepatic fat content minimizing the risk of converting to open procedure.[31,32] Preoperative weight loss has been associated with shorter operating times and LOS.[33–37] Finally, short-term postoperative weight loss is higher in patients that successfully achieve preoperative weight loss goals.[27] Interestingly, unsatisfactory preoperative weight loss among patients having bariatric surgery in accordance with ERAS principles was not associated with an increased risk of postoperative complications.[11,27] Diets used to achieve preoperative weight loss vary. Commonly, a low-calorie diet (1000–1200 kcal/d) for 5 to 7 weeks preoperatively or a very low calorie diet (500–800 kcal/d) for 2 to 3 weeks preoperatively are recommended.

Preoperative Fasting and Carbohydrate Loading

The American Society of Anesthesiologists and the European Society of Anesthesiology recommend the intake of clear fluids up to 2 hours and solids 6 hours before the induction of anesthesia in healthy and obese patients.[38,39] Recent studies suggest there are no differences in pH, gastric emptying rate, or residual gastric fluid volume after semisolid meals or liquids in either obese or lean patients.[40,41] A study of morbidly obese patients who drank 300 mL of clear fluid 2 hours before the induction of anesthesia found no difference between residual gastric volume and pH compared with patients who remained nil per os after midnight.[42,43] Another study carried out in patients with diabetes found no difference in the gastric emptying times when compared with individuals without diabetes, reinforcing the recommendation through the safety of decreased fasting times for bariatric surgery.[44] Several of the recent RCTs evaluating ERAS in bariatric surgery encouraged clear liquid intake up to 2 hours before the induction of anesthesia,[11] but a review of worldwide preoperative fasting practices in bariatric surgery ERAS protocols show that recommendations to shorten fasting times are incompletely implemented and not uniform,[45] despite evidence that low oral intake of fluids perioperatively is an independent risk factor for increased PONV and LOS.[11,46]

Iso-osmolar carbohydrate drinks taken 12 hours and 2 hours before the induction of anesthesia in major surgery have been shown to decrease the stress response to surgery, decreasing insulin resistance in the perioperative period without increasing postoperative complications.[47] Several studies have shown that preoperative carbohydrate loading can improve patient comfort after elective surgery by decreasing thirst, hunger, anxiety, and PONV.[48–51] Data on carbohydrate loading before bariatric surgery, however, are sparse. A recent small RCT looking at preoperative carbohydrate loading on bariatric surgery postoperative outcomes showed that carbohydrate drinks can be administered to bariatric surgery patients without significant risks and can decrease the occurrence and duration of PONV in patients with and without diabetes.[52] Several studies have attempted to quantify gastric volume using ultrasound examination and MRI. A small study using ultrasound examination to evaluate the gastric emptying of preoperative carbohydrate drinks found no difference in gastric volume or antral gastric cross-section between patients who fasted for 8 hours and patients who ingested oral carbohydrate drinks 2 hours before evaluation.[53] Although this study excluded patients with obesity or diabetes, another study found no difference in gastric emptying times after the ingestion of oral carbohydrate drinks in morbidly obese and nonobese patients.[54] Two studies using ultrasound examination to evaluate gastric volume after 8 hours of fasting found that patients with long-standing diabetes (>6 years) have higher residual gastric volumes than nondiabetic controls.[55,56] It is not clear, however, that this finding increases aspiration risk.

Smoking and Alcohol Cessation

Chronic tobacco smoking is associated with an increased risk of postoperative morbidity and mortality and has been linked to an increased risk of infectious complications after bariatric surgery owing to decreased tissue oxygenation.[57,58] Chronic smoking has also been associated with an increased risk of pulmonary complications and thromboembolism.[59] Cessation of smoking has been demonstrated in several controlled trials to be associated with significant reductions in postoperative complications.[60–62] The duration of smoking cessation is also important in the decrease of postoperative complications as reported in a systematic review of trials with smoking cessation duration of at least 4 weeks.[57] Although the postoperative risk reduction has not been established specifically in bariatric surgery patients, it is reasonable to assume that similar benefits would be achieved in this patient population as well.

Chronic high alcohol consumption is also associated with an increased risk of postoperative complications, especially cardiopulmonary and infectious complications.[63,64] A large retrospective study reported that the daily consumption of more than 2 alcohol equivalents per day in the 2 weeks before surgery is an independent predictor of postoperative pneumonia, sepsis, wound infection, and an increased LOS.[63] Alcohol abstinence for as little as 1 month is associated with better outcomes in colorectal surgery; therefore, the ERAS guidelines for colonic surgery recommend alcohol cessation for 4 weeks before surgery.[65] Although the evidence for the alcohol abstinence recommendation in bariatric surgery ERAS remains to be established, there are significant behavioral changes required for successful bariatric surgery and, therefore, 1 to 2 years of alcohol abstinence is recommended in patients with a prior abuse history.

INTRAOPERATIVE CARE PLANS
Premedication

Premedication is administered to decrease anxiety preoperatively and to prevent postoperative pain and PONV. Preoperative anxiety is common before surgery, and pharmacological treatment is often given to patients to decrease preoperative distress. The most common class of medication used for anxiolysis is benzodiazepines, usually midazolam. Midazolam also causes anterograde amnesia, resulting in patients not remembering much of the preoperative period. An RCT of benzodiazepines did not improve the patient experience, but were associated with longer anesthetic emergence times, especially in the elderly.[66] Dexmedetomidine, a highly selective alpha 2 adrenoceptor agonist, has broad pharmacological effects, including sedation, analgesia, anxiolysis, and inhibition of sympathetic tone. A systematic review and meta-analysis of dexmedetomidine use in the perioperative period concluded that dexmedetomidine can attenuate perioperative stress and inflammation and possibly decrease postoperative complications.[67] Melatonin is another medication that has been shown to be a potential alternative premedication. A meta-analysis of 12 RCTs found that melatonin given preoperatively decreased anxiety compared with placebo.[67] A small RCT comparing melatonin with placebo in bariatric surgery patients reported a decrease in postoperative pain and improvement in quality of recovery.[68] None of these studies compared melatonin with benzodiazepines.

Glucocorticoids have been used in elective surgery to decrease the stress response owing to its anti-inflammatory properties. Glucocorticoids have also been used to decrease PONV. The data are conflicting on the impact of glucocorticoids on postoperative outcomes. A meta-analysis of the perioperative use of corticosteroids after major abdominal surgery in 11 RCTs suggested that corticosteroids could decrease the risk of major complications.[69] In another meta-analysis, however, glucocorticoids were not associated with a decreased risk of pulmonary complications after transthoracic esophagectomy.[70] In both meta-analyses, glucocorticoid use was not associated with adverse effects compared with placebo. A recent multicenter, double-blind RCT found that dexamethasone did not significantly decrease the incidence of postoperative complications or death when compared with placebo.[71] The study also showed that, with the exception of hyperglycemia and a transient requirement for insulin, even higher doses of dexamethasone than the usual antiemetic dosing used perioperatively are well-tolerated postoperatively, consistent with an earlier Cochrane review.[71,72] The clinical relevance of mild and transient hyperglycemia reported with dexamethasone use is questionable. Data from studies including patients undergoing bariatric surgery are sparse. One retrospective analysis of patients undergoing laparoscopic gastric bypass identified a steroid bolus as a predictor of successful discharge within 24 hours, probably related to the decreased PONV.[73] A minimum dose of 2.5 to 5.0 mg dexamethasone given at the induction of anesthesia is necessary to achieve the antiemetic effect.[74,75]

Anesthetic Management

Balanced general anesthesia with endotracheal intubation is the preferred anesthetic technique for bariatric surgery. This section discusses the details of anesthetic management with particular relevance to the bariatric setting.

Airway management

The bariatric patient airway can present unique challenges. Mask ventilation has been reported to be difficult in up to 15% of patients with a higher BMI.[76,77] A higher BMI, however, has not been associated with an increased difficulty of intubation. Additionally, the usual measures to predict difficult airway in nonobese patients also predicted difficult intubation in obese patients such as the Mallampati score, Cormack–Lehane classification, and upper lip bite test.[78,79] Despite similar rates of difficult intubation between nonobese and obese patients, obese patients often present with different respiratory mechanics and impairments in ventilation and oxygenation that can affect apneic oxygenation times. Several modifications to positioning and intubation technique should be considered in obese and morbidly obese patients. The supine position is often not tolerated by a morbidly obese patient and posterior cervical adipose tissue can exaggerate flexion of the head, making a standard head support insufficient to optimize airway alignment for direct laryngoscopy. Therefore a ramped position is recommended to elevate head, neck, and shoulders with supports under the head and shoulders such that the patient's chin is higher than the chest and the patient's ear is level with the sternum.[80,81] In addition to the ramped position, the reverse Trendelenburg position can improve respiratory mechanics during preoxygenation by increasing the functional residual capacity. Several minutes of preoxygenation with an Fio_2 of 100% can increase apneic oxygenation time, thereby increasing the time available for intubation before hemoglobin oxygen desaturation occurs.[80,81]

Rapid sequence induction and the use of videolaryngoscopy can decrease the time to intubation as well.[81,82]

Mechanical ventilation

Increasing evidence exists showing the importance of lung-protective ventilation strategies during general anesthesia. Experimental studies showed that lung protective mechanical ventilation strategies such as lower tidal volume, a lower driving pressure, and a low to moderate positive end-expiratory pressure (PEEP) may protect the lung from activation of the inflammatory response and avoidance of barotrauma and volutrauma, as well as the prevention of atelectrauma from cycling opening/closing of alveoli.[83,84] The use of a low tidal volume (6–8 mL/kg predicted body weight) in obese patients was found to be associated with fewer postoperative pulmonary complications.[85,86] Additionally, a low tidal volume allows the use of pulse pressure variation and stroke volume variation measurements to determine fluid responsiveness. The optimal PEEP is a matter for debate in the obese patient; most studies that evaluated and recommended a low to moderate PEEP (<5 cm H_2O) did not include patients with a BMI of more than 35 kg/m². A higher level of PEEP and alveolar recruitment maneuvers may prevent the development of lung atelectasis and decrease atelectrauma, but may increase inflammation and impair hemodynamics. A recent large RCT that compared intraoperative high PEEP (12 cm H_2O) and recruitment maneuvers with a low PEEP (4 cm H_2O) in obese patients found no decrease in postoperative pulmonary complications with a high PEEP, despite the higher intraoperative oxygen saturation with a lower fraction of oxygen.[87] The inspiratory oxygen fraction should be set to achieve physiological oxygen saturation (92%–95%).[88,89]

Neuromuscular blockade

Most bariatric surgery is now performed laparoscopically and the pneumoperitoneum pressure required for surgical visualization will be higher in patients without neuromuscular blockade. Higher pneumoperitoneum pressures can have unfavorable cardiovascular and ventilation effects, especially in obese patients. Deep neuromuscular blockade may improve surgical conditions with lower insufflation pressures.[90,91] The primary concern for deep neuromuscular blockade is residual blockade in the recovery period, which may be of particular concern in the bariatric population. There is an association between residual blockade and pulmonary complications in the postanesthesia care unit. Some of these complications include diminished airway and pharyngeal tone, dysfunctional swallowing, and decreased aspiration defenses.[92,93] Therefore, neuromuscular blockade followed by reversal of neuromuscular blockade with binding agents (sugammadex, acetylcholine esterase inhibitors) is recommended for bariatric surgery.[94,95]

Postoperative nausea and vomiting prophylaxis

PONV decreases patient satisfaction and delays recovery. Bariatric patients often have multiple risk factors for PONV: female, less than 50 years of age, nonsmokers undergoing laparoscopic surgery. Opioid use, a history of PONV or motion sickness, and the use of volatile anesthetic also increase the risk of PONV.[96] Recent guidelines for the management of PONV recommend a multimodal approach to administering antiemetics based on patient risk factors for PONV. Decreasing opioid use and avoiding volatile anesthetics has been shown to decrease the incidence of PONV.[97] Recommended antiemetic prophylaxis medication classes include 5-hydroxytryptamine receptor antagonists, corticosteroids, butyrophenones, neurokinin-1 receptor antagonists, antihistamines, and anticholinergics.[97] A randomized trial demonstrated the superiority of a triple combination of antiemetic medication classes over a single or double combination in laparoscopic sleeve gastrectomy.[98] A meta-analysis of 3 RCTs showed a significant decrease in PONV with the use of a multimodal approach to PONV prophylaxis. PONV represents the main cause of delayed discharge and readmission after bariatric surgery.[99,100] Early PONV is usually considered to be an anesthetic complication, but may also result from postoperative ileus, a temporary disruption of gastrointestinal motility after abdominal surgery. The etiology of ileus is multifactorial and beyond the scope of this article. Briefly, factors contributing to the development of postoperative ileus include activation of the sympathetic nervous system and subsequent neurotransmitter and catecholamine release, opioid pain medications, inflammation of the intestinal wall from manipulation, and volume overload or edema of the bowel wall.[101] Postoperative ileus also delays nutritional intake and may contribute to an increased risk of adhesions. Given the role of volume overload and opioid medications in postoperative ileus, the anesthesiologist can directly impact development of postoperative ileus and PONV through judicious intraoperative fluid administration and opioid-sparing anesthetics. Therefore, PONV prophylaxis is a key component of any bariatric surgery ERAS pathway.

Analgesia

Adequate perioperative analgesia is essential to patient comfort and satisfaction, as well as decreasing the risk of postoperative complications such as pulmonary and thromboembolic complications. Inadequate analgesia in the postoperative period can delay ambulation, prolong admission, and is a common reason for readmission.[102,103] Postoperative pain is frequently underestimated and undertreated, leading to short- and long-term sequelae.[102] For these reasons, adequate perioperative analgesia is an integral element in all ERAS pathways. The ERAS goals are to manage pain, decrease overall neural and hormonal stress responses to surgery, and aid early mobilization, normal respiration, and oral nutrition.[104] All ERAS guidelines emphasize multimodal analgesia—the use of multiple mechanisms of pain control simultaneously and synergistically to improve analgesic effect while decreasing the dose of any single agent to minimize undesirable side effects. Multimodal analgesia also aims to eliminate or significantly decrease the opiate doses required in the perioperative period. Analgesia components include systemic and nonsystemic (local or regional) modalities and both are used together in a multimodal approach. Nonsteroidal antiinflammatory drugs (NSAIDs) decrease peripheral nociception and swelling associated with tissue damage and administration routes include oral, intravenous, topical, and rectal. Acetaminophen (paracetamol), thought to inhibit cyclo-oxygenase inhibitors and modulate the endogenous cannabinoid system in the central nervous system, works synergistically with NSAIDs and opioids to provide improved analgesia than NSAIDs or opioids alone.[104] Both NSAIDs and acetaminophen should be used perioperatively as a scheduled medication, with dosing based on ideal body weight.[105] N-Methyl D-aspartate (NMDA) receptor antagonists (ketamine, memantine, magnesium sulfate) modulate nociception by noncompetitive binding and allosteric inhibition of NMDA channel's excitatory glutamate receptor site. Analgesic doses of ketamine (0.1–0.3 mg/kg/h) have been showed to decrease postoperative pain and opiate requirements, both as an intravenous bolus with induction and when administered as an infusion.[106,107] At the time most ERAS Society guidelines were written, evidence on the role of the routine use of ketamine in elective surgery was limited. Therefore, most ERAS Society guidelines do not recommend routine use of ketamine for perioperative analgesia. The body of literature on a multimodal approach to perioperative pain management and perioperative opiate reduction strategies has increased in the last 5 to 10 years, including studies evaluating the safety and effectiveness of ketamine and magnesium for treating postoperative pain. The use of ketamine and magnesium in bariatric surgical patients has been shown to decrease postoperative pain scores and decrease the opioid requirement in the first 24 hours after surgery.[108–110] The use of systemic lidocaine has been shown to have clinically significant decreases in opiate requirements during and after abdominal surgery.[111] The recent bariatric surgery literature also shows improved analgesia with lidocaine intraoperatively and in the early postoperative period, decreasing opiate requirements during surgery and in the postanesthesia care unit.[112,113] The data are more conflicting in the later postoperative period and some studies do not show an opiate decrease benefit in bariatric patients postoperatively.[114]

Systemic analgesia in bariatric surgery is supplemented by the use of local anesthetic injections in the laparoscope port sites with long-acting local anesthetics such as bupivacaine or ropivacaine. There is evidence that ropivacaine and levobupivacaine are more effective than short-acting agents in bariatric surgery patients.[115] Another study comparing liposomal bupivacaine with standard bupivacaine in port site injections after bariatric surgery reported no significant difference in postoperative hospital opioid use in patients receiving liposomal bupivacaine compared with standard bupivacaine.[116] Transverseus abdominis plane blocks have been shown to be safe and effective in bariatric surgery,[117,118] but the data comparing transverseus abdominis plane blocks with local anesthetic infiltration of port sites are lacking.

Opiates continue to be used for intraoperative analgesia and postoperative pain management, but the ERAS Society recommends generally to minimize or eliminate opiate use owing to the side effects of respiratory depression, bowel ileus, nausea, constipation, and urinary retention. The bariatric patient population is especially at risk for respiratory depression from opiates and their use in this population should be minimized as much as practicable. Additionally, the use of opioids in the postoperative period has contributed to the current opioid abuse crisis; opioids remain the primary medication used to treat acute postoperative pain especially after discharge. Surgery is a critical event where many people are first exposed to opioid medications. The most commonly prescribed opioids after discharge from surgery are oxycodone and hydrocodone, the same opioids responsible for most opioid addictions and accidental opioid overdoses.[119] The multimodal management of perioperative pain is critical to minimize opioid prescription requirements after discharge to minimize addiction and accidental overdose.

Fluid management

An accurate assessment of volume status is challenging in morbidly obese patients. Total blood volume is increased in obese patients, but the overall blood volume on a volume to weight basis is decreased compared with nonobese patients (50 mL/kg compared with 75 mL/kg).[120] Preoperative rapid weight loss may lead to acute preoperative fluid and electrolyte deficiencies on the day of surgery. Obesity has been demonstrated to be a risk factor for inadvertent hypotension, which itself has been associated with organ injury, specifically acute kidney injury.[121] Noninvasive blood pressure monitoring can be difficult and inaccurate in obese patients owing to an ill-fitting blood pressure cuff. Longer intervals between noninvasive blood pressure measurements intraoperatively are associated with an increased risk of transitioning to hypotension.[122] Continuous blood pressure monitoring may be necessary in this cohort. The traditional mechanism for continuous blood pressure monitoring has been invasive arterial pressure monitoring. Noninvasive continuous blood pressure or cardiac output monitoring have been developed and validated, but most of the evidence is based on testing in lean patients.[123] Several nonrandomized studies evaluating liberal intraoperative fluid regimens (ranging from 25 to 30 mL/kg) in morbidly obese patients were associated with a lesser occurrence of rhabdomyolysis, decreased PONV, decreased incidence postoperative acute kidney injury, and shortened hospital stay.[124–128] Recently, more conservative intraoperative fluid regimens (15 mL/kg) showed no differences in postoperative rhabdomyolysis after bariatric surgery compared with liberal fluid strategies (40 mL/kg).[129] When functional parameters such as stroke volume variation were used to guide intraoperative fluid therapy, hemodynamics were maintained with lower intravenous fluid volumes in patients undergoing laparoscopic bariatric surgery, with no increases of postoperative lactate or creatinine.[130,131] In other studies, stroke volume variation monitors have been shown to be unreliable in laparoscopic procedures.[132] More recent RCTs show that a high volume of intravenous fluids are a risk factor for increased PONV and LOS.[46] Although it is difficult to draw conclusions about the optimal technique to guide fluid administration, conservative fluid administration guided by fluid responsiveness monitoring is recommended by current practice guidelines.[133]

SPECIAL POPULATIONS
Patients with Diabetes

The incidence of diabetes in the bariatric population ranges from 15% to 30% depending on the definition used. Bariatric surgery can be an effective treatment for diabetes, specifically gastric bypass, duodenal surgery, and sleeve gastrectomy. Diabetes or metabolic surgery is now considered a distinct surgical discipline from weight loss surgery, with a different primary aim to treat diabetes or metabolic disease despite obesity. The ERAS Society recommendations for glucose and lipid management are primarily for the postoperative period and are based on the 2010 Endocrine Society Clinical Practice Guideline for endocrine and nutritional management of the patient after bariatric surgery.[7,134] There is an increased amount and quality of clinical evidence available to guide clinical decision-making and that evidence has been incorporated into the current practice guidelines, a collaborative effort of 5 professional medical societies.[135] Those recommendations include perioperative intravenous insulin to achieve glycemic targets (140–180 mg/dL) in hospitalized patients. To minimize the risk of hypoglycemia in patients with type 2 diabetes perioperatively, it is recommended that all insulin secretagogues, sodium-glucose cotransporter-2 inhibitors, and thiazolidinediones should be discontinued and insulin doses adjusted (owing to low calorie intake). This practice is a change from previous recommendations. If there is no evidence of hyperglycemia, all antidiabetic medications except for metformin and incretin-based therapies should be withheld postoperatively. Endocrinology consultation is recommended for patients with type 1 diabetes or with uncontrolled type 2 diabetes.[135]

Obstructive Sleep Apnea

OSA and the related obesity hypoventilation syndrome have a prevalence in the bariatric surgical population anywhere from 35% to 94%.[136] Many of those patients are undiagnosed. Undiagnosed and untreated moderate to severe OSA is a risk factor for perioperative complications, especially postoperative pulmonary complications.[137] When OSA is diagnosed preoperatively and treated with continuous positive airway pressure, the risk of postoperative complications is decreased, regardless of OSA severity, including in patients undergoing bariatric surgery.[137,138] For these reasons, all patients undergoing bariatric surgery should be screened for OSA. The STOP-Bang questionnaire[139] for preoperative screening for OSA has a high predictive value in obese patients and is recommended in the preoperative evaluation of patients having bariatric surgery. A STOP-Bang score of 6 is both sensitive and specific for predicting severe OSA.[140] Polysomnography remains the gold standard for the diagnosis and grading of OSA, but the STOP-Bang screening tool is an easy, fast, and inexpensive tool for identifying patients at increased risk of postoperative pulmonary complications. Anesthesiologist recognition and preparation for patients with OSA are critical. Intraoperative interventions include preoxygenation with PEEP, lung protective ventilation, multimodal anesthesia with opioid avoidance or reduction, and extubation after recovery from and reversal of neuromuscular blockade.[141] Postoperative oxygen therapy alone may increase the risk of apnea or hypopnea; therefore, a combination of oxygen and continuous positive airway pressure is recommended postoperatively, especially in patients already using continuous positive airway pressure at home. Patients with a positive OSA screening and symptoms of OSA postoperatively should be monitored closely in the early postoperative period with a minimum of continuous pulse oximetry, but the routine admission of all patients with OSA to the intensive care unit postoperatively is not necessary.[138,141]

SUMMARY AND AREAS OF FUTURE RESEARCH

Since the ERAS Society issued ERAS guidelines for bariatric surgery in 2015, data have emerged on the safety and benefits of ERAS protocols applied to bariatric surgery. The data indicate that ERAS protocols in bariatric surgery are safe and do not increase perioperative morbidity. Data from several recent RCTs have also shown a decrease in hospital LOS, a decrease in PONV, earlier ambulation, and decreases pain in bariatric surgical patients when treated according to an ERAS pathway. However, some patients undergoing bariatric surgery do still experience unsatisfactory outcomes, including inadequate weight loss, postoperative pain or nausea requiring a longer hospital stay or readmission, and postoperative complications. Much of the existing literature on postoperative outcomes and complications in bariatric surgery focuses on surgical outcomes (anastomosis leak and intra-abdominal bleeding).

Data for anesthetic outcomes especially in the super morbidly obese (BMI >50) are scarce and these patients increasingly make up the bariatric and metabolic surgery population.[142] These patients are more likely to have multiple comorbidities like type 2 diabetes and OSA and are more likely to be undergoing bariatric surgery for the treatment of diabetes or another metabolic syndrome.[8] Patients selected for diabetes or metabolic surgery present with different demographic and clinical factors than patients selected for weight loss surgery and require more dedicated care and management.[143] For example, there are data to suggest that this population of bariatric surgical patients will experience a decrease in postoperative anesthetic complications (ie, pulmonary complications, thromboembolic complications, inadequate pain control) with aggressive preoperative optimization and prehabilitation.[142] Additional high-quality randomized trials are needed to better investigate prehabilitation in this population and what components of prehabilitation are effective (weight loss, exercise, functional mobility, preoperative diet, counseling, etc.). For example, emerging data show that very low carbohydrate ketogenic preoperative diets are safe and suggest that a very low carbohydrate ketogenic preoperative diet may be superior to a traditional low-calorie preoperative diet in achieving preoperative weight loss, perioperative glycemic control, a decrease in liver volume, visceral adipose tissue reduction, and even decreased LOS in patients with and without diabetes.[144–147]

The ERAS guidelines[7] for bariatric surgery (upper gastrointestinal tract surgery) were adopted from the original ERAS principles developed for colorectal surgery (lower gastrointestinal tract surgery) and relevant outcomes for bariatric surgery are different from the most relevant outcomes used to assess ERAS in colorectal surgery.[8] Relevant outcomes in ERAS for bariatric surgery include the assessment of PONV, dehydration, an inability to tolerate liquid diets, nonsedating pain control, and psychological well-being.[8] Additional adequately powered RCTs are required to investigate patient related outcomes such as PONV, postoperative pain, and fatigue as markers of return of functional status instead of LOS.[8]

Finally, the application of the ERAS recommendations for bariatric surgery is heterogenous and incomplete across the ERAS literature. ERAS pathways attempt to create many small improvements to significantly improve surgical outcomes and increase the quality of care. However, in the most recent literature evaluating ERAS pathways, only 35% to 45% of ERAS elements that were strongly recommended in the ERAS guidelines[7] were applied. Therefore, it is likely that the beneficial effects of ERAS pathways are underestimated. Additionally, strongly recommended elements that are adopted consistently are still highly variable in their application. For example, we know that immediate PONV represents the main cause of hospital readmission and increased LOS after bariatric surgery,[100,101] but PONV prophylaxis is not standardized across ERAS pathways, preventing an evaluation of the end points of ERAS in bariatric surgery. Immediate PONV is related to anesthesia, opioid use, fluid administration, and postoperative ileus. Late-onset PONV is uncommon and more often the result of surgical complications, such as dumping syndrome, anastomotic ulceration or leak, or anastomotic stricture. Standardization of bariatric surgery ERAS pathways would enhance evaluation of clinical end points and outcomes more accurately and reduce clinical heterogeneity.[8]

CLINICS CARE POINTS

- Poor oral intake is associated with PONV and patients should be counseled to continue clear fluids up until 2 hours before surgery.
- When planning airway management in bariatric patients, position patients on a ramp, perform adequate preoxygenation, and consider videolaryngoscopy for intubation.
- Use a multimodal approach to administering antiemetic medications to decrease risk of PONV.
- Use a multimodal opioid-sparing approach to analgesia to minimize respiratory depression and accelerate functional recovery from anesthesia.
- Use a conservative intraoperative fluid regimen and consider fluid responsiveness monitoring.
- Screen patients for OSA and consider the need for postoperative noninvasive ventilation and elevated level of postoperative monitoring.

DISCLOSURE

The author has nothing to disclose.

REFERENCES

1. Hales CM, Carroll MD, Fryar CD, et al. Prevalence of Obesity and Severe Obesity Among Adults: United States, 2017-2018. NCHS Data Brief 2020;(360):1–8.

2. Colquitt JL, Pickett K, Loveman E, et al. Surgery for weight loss in adults. Cochrane Database Syst Rev 2014;(8):CD003641.
3. Sampalis JS, Liberman M, Auger S, et al. The impact of weight reduction surgery on health-care costs in morbidly obese patients. Obes Surg 2004;14(7): 939–47.
4. The clinical effectiveness and cost-effectiveness of bariatric (weight loss) surgery for obesity: a systematic review and economic evaluation. Clin Governance 2010;15(1). https://doi.org/10.1108/cgij.2010.24815aae.002.
5. Padwal R, Klarenbach S, Wiebe N, et al. Bariatric surgery: a systematic review of the clinical and economic evidence. J Gen Intern Med 2011;26(10):1183–94.
6. Angrisani L, Santonicola A, Iovino P, et al. Bariatric surgery and endoluminal procedures: IFSO worldwide survey 2014. Obes Surg 2017;27(9):2279–89.
7. Cardoso L, Rodrigues D, Gomes L, et al. Short- and long-term mortality after bariatric surgery: a systematic review and meta-analysis. Diabetes Obes Metab 2017;19(9):1223–32.
8. Longitudinal Assessment of Bariatric Surgery (LABS) Consortium, Flum DR, Belle SH, King WC, et al. Perioperative safety in the longitudinal assessment of bariatric surgery. N Engl J Med 2009;361(5):445–54.
9. Ljungqvist O, Scott M, Fearon KC. Enhanced recovery after surgery: a review. JAMA Surg 2017;152(3):292–8.
10. Thorell A, MacCormick AD, Awad S, et al. Guidelines for perioperative care in bariatric surgery: Enhanced Recovery After Surgery (ERAS) Society Recommendations. World J Surg 2016;40(9):2065–83.
11. Parisi A, Desiderio J, Cirocchi R, et al. Enhanced Recovery after Surgery (ERAS): a systematic review of randomised controlled trials (RCTs) in bariatric surgery. Obes Surg 2020;30(12):5071–85.
12. Dutton J, Wadhwa A, Morton JM. ERAS protocols in bariatric surgery: a systematic review. Int Anesthesiol Clin 2020;58(3):29–33.
13. Dang JT, Szeto VG, Elnahas A, et al. Canadian consensus statement: enhanced recovery after surgery in bariatric surgery. Surg Endosc 2020;34(3):1366–75.
14. Elwyn G, Frosch D, Thomson R, et al. Shared decision making: a model for clinical practice. J Gen Intern Med 2012;27(10):1361–7.
15. Eddy DM. Designing a practice policy: standards, guidelines, and options. JAMA 1990;263(22):3077–84.
16. Elliott JA, Patel VM, Kirresh A, et al. Fast-track laparoscopic bariatric surgery: a systematic review. Updates Surg 2013;65(2):85–94.
17. Schilling PL, Dimick JB, Birkmeyer JD. Prioritizing quality improvement in general surgery. J Am Coll Surg 2008;207(5):698–704.
18. Christensen T, Kehlet H. Postoperative fatigue. World J Surg 1993;17(2):220–5.
19. Carli F, Scheede-Bergdahl C. Prehabilitation to enhance perioperative care. Anesthesiol Clin 2015;33(1):17–33.
20. Pierson LM, Herbert WG, Norton HJ, et al. Effects of combined aerobic and resistance training versus aerobic training alone in cardiac rehabilitation. J Cardiopulmonary Rehabil Prev 2001;21(2):101–10.
21. Valkenet K, van de Port IG, Dronkers JJ, et al. The effects of preoperative exercise therapy on postoperative outcome: a systematic review. Clin Rehabil 2011; 25(2):99–111.
22. Türk Y, van Huisstede A, Hiemstra PS, et al. Pre-surgical pulmonary rehabilitation in asthma patients undergoing bariatric surgery. Obes Surg 2017;27(11): 3055–60.

23. Gillis C, Li C, Lee L, et al. Prehabilitation versus rehabilitation: a randomized control trial in patients undergoing colorectal resection for cancer. Anesthesiology 2014;121(5):937–47.

24. Gilbertson NM, Eichner NZM, Khurshid M, et al. Impact of pre-operative aerobic exercise on cardiometabolic health and quality of life in patients undergoing bariatric surgery. Front Physiol 2020;11:1018.

25. Santa Mina D, Clarke H, Ritvo P, et al. Effect of total-body prehabilitation on post-operative outcomes: a systematic review and meta-analysis. Physiotherapy 2014;100(3):196–207.

26. Lemanu DP, Singh PP, MacCormick AD, et al. Effect of preoperative exercise on cardiorespiratory function and recovery after surgery: a systematic review. World J Surg 2013;37(4):711–20.

27. Stefura T, Droś J, Kacprzyk A, et al. Influence of preoperative weight loss on outcomes of bariatric surgery for patients under the enhanced recovery after surgery protocol. Obes Surg 2019;29(4):1134–41.

28. Edholm D, Kullberg J, Haenni A, et al. Preoperative 4-week low-calorie diet reduces liver volume and intrahepatic fat, and facilitates laparoscopic gastric bypass in morbidly obese. Obes Surg 2011;21(3):345–50.

29. Van Nieuwenhove Y, Dambrauskas Z, Campillo-Soto A, et al. Preoperative very low-calorie diet and operative outcome after laparoscopic gastric bypass: a randomized multicenter study. Arch Surg 2011;146(11):1300–5.

30. Nielsen LV, Nielsen MS, Schmidt JB, et al. Efficacy of a liquid low-energy formula diet in achieving preoperative target weight loss before bariatric surgery. J Nutr Sci 2016;5:e22.

31. Liu RC, Sabnis AA, Forsyth C, et al. The effects of acute preoperative weight loss on laparoscopic Roux-en-Y gastric bypass. Obes Surg 2005;15(10): 1396–402.

32. Lewis MC, Phillips ML, Slavotinek JP, et al. Change in liver size and fat content after treatment with Optifast® very low calorie diet. Obes Surg 2006;16(6): 697–701.

33. Alami RS, Morton JM, Schuster R, et al. Is there a benefit to preoperative weight loss in gastric bypass patients? A prospective randomized trial. Surg Obes Relat Dis 2007;3(2):141–5.

34. Huerta S, Dredar S, Hayden E, et al. Preoperative weight loss decreases the operative time of gastric bypass at a Veterans Administration hospital. Obes Surg 2008;18(5):508–12.

35. Giordano S, Victorzon M. The impact of preoperative weight loss before laparoscopic gastric bypass. Obes Surg 2014;24(5):669–74.

36. Cassie S, Menezes C, Birch DW, et al. Effect of preoperative weight loss in bariatric surgical patients: a systematic review. Surg Obes Relat Dis 2011;7(6): 760–7.

37. Sun Y, Liu B, Smith JK, et al. Association of preoperative body weight and weight loss with risk of death after bariatric surgery. JAMA Netw Open 2020; 3(5):e204803.

38. Practice guidelines for preoperative fasting and the use of pharmacologic agents to reduce the risk of pulmonary aspiration: application to healthy patients undergoing elective procedures: an updated report by the American Society of Anesthesiologists Task Force on Preoperative Fasting and the Use of Pharmacologic Agents to Reduce the Risk of Pulmonary Aspiration. Anesthesiology 2017; 126(3):376–93.

39. Smith I, Kranke P, Murat I, et al. Perioperative fasting in adults and children: guidelines from the European Society of Anaesthesiology. Eur J Anaesthesiol 2011;28(8):556–69.

40. Buchholz V, Berkenstadt H, Goitein D, et al. Gastric emptying is not prolonged in obese patients. Surg Obes Relat Dis 2013;9(5):714–7.

41. Seimon RV, Brennan IM, Russo A, et al. Gastric emptying, mouth-to-cecum transit, and glycemic, insulin, incretin, and energy intake responses to a mixed-nutrient liquid in lean, overweight, and obese males. Am J Physiol Endocrinol Metab 2013;304(3):E294–300.

42. Maltby JR, Pytka S, Watson NC, et al. Drinking 300 mL of clear fluid two hours before surgery has no effect on gastric fluid volume and pH in fasting and non-fasting obese patients. Can J Anesth 2004;51(2):111–5.

43. Maltby JR. Fasting from midnight – the history behind the dogma. Best Pract Res Clin Anaesthesiol 2006;20(3):363–78.

44. Gustaffson UO, Nygren J, Thorell A, et al. Pre-operative carbohydrate loading may be used in type 2 diabetes patients. Acta Anaesthesiol Scand 2008; 52(7):946–51.

45. Rossoni C, Oliveira Magro D, Santos ZC, et al. Enhanced Recovery After Surgery (ERAS) protocol in bariatric and metabolic surgery (BMS)—analysis of practices in nutritional aspects from five continents. Obes Surg 2020;30(11): 4510–8.

46. Major P, Wysocki M, Torbicz G, et al. Risk factors for prolonged length of hospital stay and readmissions after laparoscopic sleeve gastrectomy and laparoscopic Roux-en-Y gastric bypass. Obes Surg 2018;28(2):323–32.

47. Colles SL, Dixon JB, Marks P, et al. Preoperative weight loss with a very-low-energy diet: quantitation of changes in liver and abdominal fat by serial imaging. Am J Clin Nutr 2006;84(2):304–11.

48. Hausel J, Nygren J, Thorell A, et al. Randomized clinical trial of the effects of oral preoperative carbohydrates on postoperative nausea and vomiting after laparoscopic cholecystectomy. Br J Surg 2005;92(4):415–21.

49. Nygren J, Thorell A, Jacobsson H, et al. Preoperative gastric emptying effects of anxiety and oral carbohydrate administration. Ann Surg 1995;222(6):728–34.

50. Hausel J, Nygren J, Lagerkranser M, et al. A carbohydrate-rich drink reduces preoperative discomfort in elective surgery patients. Anesth Analg 2001;93(5): 1344–50.

51. Cheng P-L, Loh E-W, Chen J-T, et al. Effects of preoperative oral carbohydrate on postoperative discomfort in patients undergoing elective surgery: a meta-analysis of randomized controlled trials. Langenbecks Arch Surg 2021;406(4): 993–1005.

52. Suh S, Hetzel E, Alter-Troilo K, et al. The influence of preoperative carbohydrate loading on postoperative outcomes in bariatric surgery patients: a randomized, controlled trial. Surg Obes Relat Dis 2021;17(8):1480–8.

53. Cho E-A, Huh J, Lee SH, et al. Gastric ultrasound assessing gastric emptying of preoperative carbohydrate drinks: a randomized controlled noninferiority study. Anesth Analg 2021;133(3):690–7.

54. Shiraishi T, Kurosaki D, Nakamura M, et al. Gastric fluid volume change after oral rehydration solution intake in morbidly obese and normal controls: a magnetic resonance imaging-based analysis. Anesth Analg 2017;124(4):1174–8.

55. Sabry R, Hasanin A, Refaat S, et al. Evaluation of gastric residual volume in fasting diabetic patients using gastric ultrasound. Acta Anaesthesiol Scand 2019; 63(5):615–9.

56. Garg H, Podder S, Bala I, et al. Comparison of fasting gastric volume using ultrasound in diabetic and non-diabetic patients in elective surgery: an observational study. Indian J Anaesth 2020;64(5):391–6.

57. Mills E, Eyawo O, Lockhart I, et al. Smoking cessation reduces postoperative complications: a systematic review and meta-analysis. Am J Med 2011; 124(2):144–54.e8.

58. Sorensen LT, Karlsmark T, Gottrup F. Abstinence from smoking reduces incisional wound infection: a randomized controlled trial. Ann Surg 2003;238(1):1–5.

59. Gourgiotis S, Aloizos S, Gakis C, et al. Platypnea-orthodeoxia due to fat embolism. Int J Surg Case Rep 2011;2(6):147–9.

60. Levin L, Herzberg R, Dolev E, et al. Smoking and complications of onlay bone grafts and sinus lift operations. Int J Oral Maxillofac Implants 2004;19(3): 369–73.

61. Myles PS, Leslie K, Angliss M, et al. Effectiveness of bupropion as an aid to stopping smoking before elective surgery: a randomised controlled trial. Anaesthesia 2004;59(11):1053–8.

62. Warner DO, Patten CA, Ames SC, et al. Effect of nicotine replacement therapy on stress and smoking behavior in surgical patients. Anesthesiology 2005; 102(6):1138–46.

63. Nath B, Li Y, Carroll JE, et al. Alcohol exposure as a risk factor for adverse outcomes in elective surgery. J Gastrointest Surg 2010;14(11):1732–41.

64. Tønnesen H, Kehlet H. Preoperative alcoholism and postoperative morbidity. Br J Surg 1999;86(7):869–74.

65. Tønnesen H, Rosenberg J, Nielsen HJ, et al. Effect of preoperative abstinence on poor postoperative outcome in alcohol misusers: randomised controlled trial. BMJ 1999;318(7194):1311.

66. Maurice-Szamburski A, Auquier P, Viarre-Oreal V, et al. Effect of sedative premedication on patient experience after general anesthesia: a randomized clinical trial. JAMA 2015;313(9):916–25.

67. Wang K, Wu M, Xu J, et al. Effects of dexmedetomidine on perioperative stress, inflammation, and immune function: systematic review and meta-analysis. Br J Anaesth 2019;123(6):777–94.

68. Ivry M, Goitein D, Welly W, et al. Melatonin premedication improves quality of recovery following bariatric surgery – a double blind placebo controlled prospective study. Surg Obes Relat Dis 2017;13(3):502–6.

69. Dexamethasone in Hospitalized Patients with Covid-19. N Engl J Med 2021; 384(8):693–704.

70. Weijs TJ, Dieleman JM, Ruurda JP, et al. The effect of perioperative administration of glucocorticoids on pulmonary complications after transthoracic oesophagectomy: a systematic review and meta-analysis. Eur J Anaesthesiol 2014; 31(12):685–94.

71. Asehnoune K, Le Moal C, Lebuffe G, et al. Effect of dexamethasone on complications or all cause mortality after major non-cardiac surgery: multicentre, double blind, randomised controlled trial. BMJ 2021;373. https://doi.org/10.1136/bmj.n1162.

72. Polderman JAW, Farhang-Razi V, Van Dieren S, et al. Adverse side effects of dexamethasone in surgical patients. Cochrane Database Syst Rev 2018;11. https://doi.org/10.1002/14651858.CD011940.pub3.

73. McCarty TM, Arnold DT, Lamont JP, et al. Optimizing outcomes in bariatric surgery: outpatient laparoscopic gastric bypass. Ann Surg 2005;242(4):494–501.

74. Wang J-J, Ho S-T, Lee S-C, et al. The use of dexamethasone for preventing post-operative nausea and vomiting in females undergoing thyroidectomy: a dose-ranging study. Anesth Analg 2000;91(6):1404–7.

75. Wang J-J, Ho S-T, Wong C-S, et al. Dexamethasone prophylaxis of nausea and vomiting after epidural morphine for post-Cesarean analgesia. Can J Anaesth 2001;48(2):185.

76. Cattano D, Killoran PV, Iannucci D, et al. Anticipation of the difficult airway: pre-operative airway assessment, an educational and quality improvement tool. Br J Anaesth 2013;111(2):276–85.

77. Leoni A, Arlati S, Ghisi D, et al. Difficult mask ventilation in obese patients: anal-ysis of predictive factors. Minerva Anestesiol 2014;80(2):149–57.

78. Dohrn N, Sommer T, Bisgaard J, et al. Difficult tracheal intubation in obese gastric bypass patients. Obes Surg 2016;26(11):2640–7.

79. Aceto P, Perilli V, Modesti C, et al. Airway management in obese patients. Surg Obes Relat Dis 2013;9(5):809–15.

80. Soleimanpour H, Safari S, Sanaie S, et al. Anesthetic considerations in patients undergoing bariatric surgery: a review article. Anesth Pain Med 2017;7(4): e57568.

81. Bazurro S, Ball L, Pelosi P. Perioperative management of obese patient. Curr Opin Crit Care 2018;24(6):560–7.

82. Lewis SR, Butler AR, Parker J, et al. Videolaryngoscopy versus direct laryngos-copy for adult patients requiring tracheal intubation. Cochrane Database Syst Rev 2016;11. https://doi.org/10.1002/14651858.CD011136.pub2.

83. Schultz MJ, Gama de Abreu M, Pelosi P. Mechanical ventilation strategies for the surgical patient. Curr Opin Crit Care 2015;21(4):351–7.

84. Maia L de A, Samary CS, Oliveira MV, et al. Impact of different ventilation stra-tegies on driving pressure, mechanical power, and biological markers during open abdominal surgery in rats. Anesth Analg 2017;125(4):1364–74.

85. Schultz MJ, Neto AS, Pelosi P, et al. Should the lungs be rested or open during anaesthesia to prevent postoperative complications? Lancet Respir Med 2018; 6(3):163–5.

86. Güldner A, Kiss T, Serpa Neto A, et al. Intraoperative protective mechanical ventilation for prevention of postoperative pulmonary complications: a compre-hensive review of the role of tidal volume, positive end-expiratory pressure, and lung recruitment maneuvers. Anesthesiology 2015;123(3):692–713.

87. Writing Committee for the PROBESE Collaborative Group of the PROtective VEntilation Network (PROVEnet) for the Clinical Trial Network of the European Society of Anaesthesiology. Effect of intraoperative high positive end-expiratory pressure (PEEP) with recruitment maneuvers vs low peep on postop-erative pulmonary complications in obese patients: a randomized clinical trial. JAMA 2019;321(23):2292–305.

88. Ball L, Lumb AB, Pelosi P. Intraoperative fraction of inspired oxygen: bringing back the focus on patient outcome. Br J Anaesth 2017;119(1):16–8.

89. Robba C, Ball L, Pelosi P. Between hypoxia or hyperoxia: not perfect but more physiologic. J Thorac Dis 2018;10(Suppl 17):S2052–4.

90. Staehr-Rye AK, Rasmussen LS, Rosenberg J, et al. Surgical space conditions during low-pressure laparoscopic cholecystectomy with deep versus moderate neuromuscular blockade: a randomized clinical study. Anesth Analg 2014; 119(5):1084–92.

91. Martini CH, Boon M, Bevers RF, et al. Evaluation of surgical conditions during laparoscopic surgery in patients with moderate vs deep neuromuscular block. Br J Anaesth 2014;112(3):498–505.

92. Sauer M, Stahn A, Soltesz S, et al. The influence of residual neuromuscular block on the incidence of critical respiratory events. A randomised, prospective, placebo-controlled trial. Eur J Anaesthesiol 2011;28(12):842–8.

93. Murphy GS, Szokol JW, Marymont JH, et al. Intraoperative Acceleromyographic Monitoring Reduces the Risk of Residual Meeting Abstracts and Adverse Respiratory Events in the Postanesthesia Care Unit. Anesthesiology 2008;109(3): 389–98.

94. Suzuki T, Masaki G, Ogawa S. Neostigmine-induced reversal of vecuronium in normal weight, overweight and obese female patients. Br J Anaesth 2006; 97(2):160–3.

95. Jones RK, Caldwell JE, Brull SJ, et al. Reversal of profound rocuronium-induced blockade with sugammadex: a randomized comparison with neostigmine. Anesthesiology 2008;109(5):816–24.

96. Apfel CC, Heidrich FM, Jukar-Rao S, et al. Evidence-based analysis of risk factors for postoperative nausea and vomiting. Br J Anaesth 2012;109(5):742–53.

97. Gan TJ, Belani KG, Bergese S, et al. Fourth consensus guidelines for the management of postoperative nausea and vomiting. Anesth Analg 2020;131(2): 411–48.

98. Benevides ML, Oliveira Sde S, Aguilar-Nascimento JE. Combination of haloperidol, dexamethasone, and ondansetron reduces nausea and pain intensity and morphine consumption after laparoscopic sleeve gastrectomy. Braz J Anesthesiol 2013;63(5):404–9.

99. Aman MW, Stem M, Schweitzer MA, et al. Early hospital readmission after bariatric surgery. Surg Endosc 2016;30(6):2231–8.

100. Berger ER, Huffman KM, Fraker T, et al. Prevalence and risk factors for bariatric surgery readmissions: findings from 130,007 admissions in the metabolic and bariatric surgery accreditation and quality improvement program. Ann Surg 2018;267(1):122–31.

101. Kreis ME. Postoperative nausea and vomiting. Auton Neurosci Basic Clin 2006; 129(1):86–91.

102. Lynch M. Pain as the fifth vital sign. J Intravenous Nurs 2001;24(2):85–94.

103. Breivik H, Stubhaug A. Management of acute postoperative pain: still a long way to go! Pain 2008;137(2):233–4.

104. Beverly A, Kaye AD, Ljungqvist O, et al. Essential elements of multimodal analgesia in enhanced recovery after surgery (ERAS) guidelines. Anesthesiol Clin 2017;35(2):e115–43.

105. Maund E, McDaid C, Rice S, et al. Paracetamol and selective and non-selective non-steroidal anti-inflammatory drugs for the reduction in morphine-related side-effects after major surgery: a systematic review. Br J Anaesth 2011;106(3): 292–7.

106. Jalili M, Bahreini M, Doosti-Irani A, et al. Ketamine-propofol combination (ketofol) vs propofol for procedural sedation and analgesia: systematic review and meta-analysis. Am J Emerg Med 2016;34(3):558–69.

107. Siddiqui KM, Khan FA. Effect of preinduction low-dose ketamine bolus on intra operative and immediate postoperative analgesia requirement in day care surgery: a randomized controlled trial. Saudi J Anaesth 2015;9(4):422–7.

108. Jabbour H, Jabbour K, Abi Lutfallah A, et al. Magnesium and ketamine reduce early morphine consumption after open bariatric surgery: a prospective randomized double-blind study. Obes Surg 2020;30(4):1452–8.
109. Kasputytė G, Karbonskienė A, Macas A, et al. Role of ketamine in multimodal analgesia protocol for bariatric surgery. Medicina (Kaunas) 2020;56(3):96.
110. Mehta SD, Smyth D, Vasilopoulos T, et al. Ketamine infusion reduces narcotic requirements following gastric bypass surgery: a randomized controlled trial. Surg Obes Relat Dis 2021;17(4):737–43.
111. Marret E, Rolin M, Beaussier M, et al. Meta-analysis of intravenous lidocaine and postoperative recovery after abdominal surgery. Br J Surg 2008;95(11):1331–8.
112. De Oliveira GS, Duncan K, Fitzgerald P, et al. Systemic lidocaine to improve quality of recovery after laparoscopic bariatric surgery: a randomized double-blinded placebo-controlled trial. Obes Surg 2014;24(2):212–8.
113. Sakata RK, de Lima RC, Valadão JA, et al. Randomized, double-blind study of the effect of intraoperative intravenous lidocaine on the opioid consumption and criteria for hospital discharge after bariatric surgery. Obes Surg 2020;30(4):1189–93.
114. Plass F, Nicolle C, Zamparini M, et al. Effect of intra-operative intravenous lidocaine on opioid consumption after bariatric surgery: a prospective, randomised, blinded, placebo-controlled study. Anaesthesia 2021;76(2):189–98.
115. Hilvering B, Draaisma WA, van der Bilt JDW, et al. Randomized clinical trial of combined preincisional infiltration and intraperitoneal instillation of levobupivacaine for postoperative pain after laparoscopic cholecystectomy. Br J Surg 2011;98(6):784–9.
116. Ma P, Lloyd A, McGrath M, et al. Efficacy of liposomal bupivacaine versus bupivacaine in port site injections on postoperative pain within enhanced recovery after bariatric surgery program: a randomized clinical trial. Surg Obes Relat Dis 2019;15(9):1554–62.
117. Wassef M, Lee DY, Levine JL, et al. Feasibility and analgesic efficacy of the transversus abdominis plane block after single-port laparoscopy in patients having bariatric surgery. J Pain Res 2013;6:837–41.
118. Földi M, Soós A, Hegyi P, et al. Transversus abdominis plane block appears to be effective and safe as a part of multimodal analgesia in bariatric surgery: a meta-analysis and systematic review of randomized controlled trials. Obes Surg 2021;31(2):531–43.
119. Hah JM, Bateman BT, Ratliff J, et al. Chronic opioid use after surgery: implications for perioperative management in the face of the opioid epidemic. Anesth Analg 2017;125(5):1733–40.
120. Sharma SK, McCauley J, Cottam D, et al. Acute changes in renal function after laparoscopic gastric surgery for morbid obesity. Surg Obes Relat Dis 2006;2(3):389–92.
121. Wesselink EM, Kappen TH, Torn HM, et al. Intraoperative hypotension and the risk of postoperative adverse outcomes: a systematic review. Br J Anaesth 2018;121(4):706–21.
122. Eley VA, Christensen R, Guy L, et al. Perioperative blood pressure monitoring in patients with obesity. Anesth Analg 2019;128(3):484–91.
123. Boly CA, Schraverus P, van Raalten F, et al. Pulse-contour derived cardiac output measurements in morbid obesity: influence of actual, ideal and adjusted bodyweight. J Clin Monit Comput 2018;32(3):423–8.
124. de Menezes Ettinger JEMT, dos Santos Filho PV, Azaro E, et al. Prevention of rhabdomyolysis in bariatric surgery. Obes Surg 2005;15(6):874–9.

125. Domi R, Laho H. Anesthetic challenges in the obese patient. J Anesth 2012; 26(5):758–65.
126. Schuster R, Alami RS, Curet MJ, et al. Intra-operative fluid volume influences postoperative nausea and vomiting after laparoscopic gastric bypass surgery. Obes Surg 2006;16(7):848–51.
127. Ogunnaike BO, Jones SB, Jones DB, et al. Anesthetic considerations for bariatric surgery. Anesth Analg 2002;95(6):1793–805.
128. Nossaman VE, Richardson WS, Wooldridge JB, et al. Role of intraoperative fluids on hospital length of stay in laparoscopic bariatric surgery: a retrospective study in 224 consecutive patients. Surg Endosc 2015;29(10):2960–9.
129. Wool DB, Lemmens HJM, Brodsky JB, et al. Intraoperative fluid replacement and postoperative creatine phosphokinase levels in laparoscopic bariatric patients. Obes Surg 2010;20(6):698–701.
130. Matot I, Paskaleva R, Eid L, et al. Effect of the volume of fluids administered on intraoperative oliguria in laparoscopic bariatric surgery: a randomized controlled trial. Arch Surg 2012;147(3):228–34.
131. Jain AK, Dutta A. Stroke volume variation as a guide to fluid administration in morbidly obese patients undergoing laparoscopic bariatric surgery. Obes Surg 2010;20(6):709–15.
132. DeBarros M, Causey MW, Chesley P, et al. Reliability of continuous non-invasive assessment of hemoglobin and fluid responsiveness: impact of obesity and abdominal insufflation pressures. Obes Surg 2015;25(7):1142–8.
133. Haren AP, Nair S, Pace MC, et al. Intraoperative monitoring of the obese patient undergoing surgery: a narrative review. Adv Ther 2021;38(7):3622–51.
134. Heber D, Greenway FL, Kaplan LM, et al. Endocrine and nutritional management of the post-bariatric surgery patient: an Endocrine Society Clinical Practice Guideline. J Clin Endocrinol Metab 2010;95(11):4823–43.
135. Mechanick JI, Apovian C, Brethauer S, et al. Clinical practice guidelines for the perioperative nutrition, metabolic, and nonsurgical support of patients undergoing bariatric procedures – 2019 update: cosponsored by American Association of Clinical Endocrinologists/American College of Endocrinology, The Obesity Society, American Society For Metabolic & Bariatric Surgery, Obesity Medicine Association, and American Society of Anesthesiologists. Endocr Pract 2019; 25:1–75.
136. de Raaff CAL, Gorter-Stam MAW, de Vries N, et al. Perioperative management of obstructive sleep apnea in bariatric surgery: a consensus guideline. Surg Obes Relat Dis 2017;13(7):1095–109.
137. Weingarten TN, Kor DJ, Gali B, et al. Predicting postoperative pulmonary complications in high-risk populations. Curr Opin Anaesthesiol 2013;26(2):116–25.
138. Goucham AB, Coblijn UK, Hart-Sweet HB, et al. Routine postoperative monitoring after bariatric surgery in morbidly obese patients with severe obstructive sleep apnea: ICU admission is not Necessary. Obes Surg 2016;26(4):737–42.
139. Chung F, Abdullah HR, Liao P. STOP-bang questionnaire: a practical approach to screen for obstructive sleep apnea. CHEST 2016;149(3):631–8.
140. Chung F, Yang Y, Liao P. Predictive Performance of the STOP-Bang score for identifying obstructive sleep apnea in obese patients. Obes Surg 2013; 23(12):2050–7.
141. de Raaff CAL, de Vries N, van Wagensveld BA. Obstructive sleep apnea and bariatric surgical guidelines: summary and update. Curr Opin Anesthesiol 2018;31(1).

142. Sinha A, Jayaraman L, Punhani D, et al. Enhanced recovery after bariatric surgery in the severely obese, morbidly obese, super-morbidly obese and super-super morbidly obese using evidence-based clinical pathways: a comparative study. Obes Surg 2017;27(3):560–8.
143. Rubino F, Shukla A, Pomp A, et al. Bariatric, metabolic, and diabetes surgery: what's in a name? Ann Surg 2014;259(1):117–22.
144. Albanese A, Prevedello L, Markovich M, et al. Pre-operative very low calorie ketogenic diet (VLCKD) vs. very low calorie diet (VLCD): surgical impact. Obes Surg 2019;29(1):292–6.
145. Pilone V, Tramontano S, Renzulli M, et al. Metabolic effects, safety, and acceptability of very low-calorie ketogenic dietetic scheme on candidates for bariatric surgery. Surg Obes Relat Dis 2018;14(7):1013–9.
146. Leonetti F, Campanile FC, Coccia F, et al. Very low-carbohydrate ketogenic diet before bariatric surgery: prospective evaluation of a sequential diet. Obes Surg 2015;25(1):64–71.
147. Schulman AR, Thompson CC. Complications of bariatric surgery: what you can expect to see in your GI practice. Am J Gastroenterol 2017;112(11):1640–55.

Enhanced Recovery After Cardiac Surgery

Mike Charlesworth, MSci, MBChB, PGCert, FRCA, MSc, FFICM[a],[*],
Andrew Klein, MBBS, FRCA, FFICM[b]

KEYWORDS

- Cardiac surgery • Enhanced recovery • Peri-operative • Pathways

KEY POINTS

- The aims of "Fast track" cardiac anesthesia including shortening time to tracheal extubation and to hospital discharge in selected patients.
- The evidence is weak and recommendations are mostly based on observational, non-randomized data and expert opinion.
- The majority of outcomes studied include: time to tracheal extubation, hospital/ICU length of stay, procedure-related financial costs, and the type/amount of opioids used in the peri-operative period.
- There should be a shift in focus to generating higher quality evidence supporting the use of enhanced recovery protocols in cardiac surgical patients and finding ways to tailor enhanced recovery principles to all cardiac surgical patients.
- Research should focus on the quality of care for individual patients and the delivery of health care to the public.

INTRODUCTION

The aims of enhanced recovery after cardiac surgery (ERACS) are similar to those of any enhanced recovery program—to at once improve patient outcomes and optimize the delivery of health care to all patients. That said, cardiac surgery is different. It involves, almost exclusively: major surgery; the need for postoperative critical care and mechanical ventilation; periods of hemodynamic instability; cardiopulmonary bypass; bleeding and the frequent need for allogeneic transfusion of blood components; and a baseline mortality risk higher than for most other types of surgery. Our aim is to provide an evidence-based synthesis of pre, intra, and postoperative strategies that might constitute an enhanced recovery program for cardiac surgical patients, but also to comment on barriers to implementation as well as future directions.

[a] Department of Cardiothoracic Anaesthesia, Critical Care and ECMO, Wythenshawe Hospital, Manchester University NHS Foundation Trust, Southmoor Road, Manchester, M23 9LT, UK;
[b] Department of Cardiothoracic Anaesthesia and Critical Care, Royal Papworth Hospital NHS Foundation Trust, Papworth Road, Trumpington, Cambridge CB2 0AY, UK
* Corresponding author.
E-mail address: mike.charlesworth@doctors.org.uk

Anesthesiology Clin 40 (2022) 143–155
https://doi.org/10.1016/j.anclin.2021.11.007
anesthesiology.theclinics.com
1932-2275/22/© 2021 Elsevier Inc. All rights reserved.

EVIDENCE

Enhanced recovery after surgery has arguably come later for cardiac surgery as compared with other surgical specialties. There has nevertheless been much interest in developing ways to provide it and there are many areas whereby urgent research is required. The evidence to support such programs is limited to retrospective observations and a small number of prospective/randomized studies (**Table 1**). The majority of outcomes studied include: time to tracheal extubation, length of ICU/hospital stay, incidence of postoperative complications, procedure-related financial costs, opioid use, and mortality. Although such studies generally demonstrate favorable outcomes, the outcomes studied may not always be clinically relevant (eg, time to tracheal extubation), and the influence of confounding and bias cannot be excluded.

GUIDELINES

The most recent guidelines for ERACS come from the Enhanced Recovery after Surgery Society and split goals of care into pre-, intra-, and postoperative domains.[12] This is the first consensus review of evidence-based enhanced recovery after cardiac surgical practices, which given that it was published in 2019, shows the relative infancy of enhanced recovery as applied to cardiac surgery. The most important aspects of this guidance are summarised and provided herein (**Fig. 1**).

GOALS
Preoperative

Prehabilitation

Prehabilitation, which is arguably an area of practice and study in its own right, should now be a standard of care for all patients undergoing major elective surgery, with components including: education; exercise; nutritional optimization; psychological support; smoking and hazardous substance cessation and support; optimization of anemia, diabetes mellitus, and other comorbidities; comprehensive frailty and geriatric assessment; and oral hygiene.[13] Initiatives such as 'surgery school' are key, as these consultant-led sessions with support from the whole multidisciplinary team provide educational sessions on how patients can address their modifiable risk factors. The literature in regard to prehabilitation before cardiac surgery is sparse and trials are urgently required.

Clear fluid intake

Encouraging clear fluid intake should be an important component of all ERAS programs. Current European[14] and American[15] guidelines promote the intake of clear fluids up to 2 h before elective surgery and this should also be the case for cardiac surgical patients.[12]

Preoperative carbohydrate loading

A clear carbohydrate drink 2 h before surgery is a very low-risk and low-cost intervention that may yield a range of benefits. As there is minimal supportive data only, it was only a weak recommendation in recent guidance.[12]

Anticoagulation

For elective cardiac surgical patients, management of oral anticoagulants is relatively straightforward.[16] The period of cessation for warfarin is usually 5 days and it would be unusual to "bridge" this period with low molecular weight or unfractionated heparin. For direct oral anticoagulants (DOACs), the cessation period is dependent on renal function. In patient with no renal impairment, the minimum cessation period should

Table 1
A sample of studies comparing fast-track care and enhanced recovery following cardiac surgery against conventional management

	Methods	Number of Patients	Main Conclusions
Engelman et al,[1] 1994	Retrospective observational study	280 fast-track vs 282 conventional	Shorter time to tracheal extubation and ICU length of stay, as well as lower incidence of mediastinal or sternal infections in the fast-track group.
Dunstan et al,[2] 1997	Retrospective observational study	303 fast-track vs 312 conventional	Significantly shorter ICU and hospital length of stay as well as lower procedure-related financial costs for the fast-track group.
Fernandes et al,[3] 2004	Retrospective observational study	107 fast-track vs 68 conventional	Shorter length of hospital stay and lower procedure-related financial costs for the fast-track group.
Yanatori et al,[4] 2007	Retrospective observational study	54 fast-track vs 40 conventional	Shorter length of hospital stay and lower procedure-related financial costs for the fast-track group.
Ender et al,[5] 2008	Retrospective observational study	421 fast-track vs 421 conventional	Shorter time to tracheal extubation and ICU length of stay, as well as lower incidence of mediastinal or sternal infections and lower mortality in the fast-track group.
Salhiyyah et al,[6] 2011	Prospective observational study	84 fast-track vs 52 conventional	Shorter time to tracheal extubation and ICU/hospital length of stay, as well as lower procedure-related financial costs for the fast-track group.
Hardman et al,[7] 2015	Retrospective observational study	37 enhanced recovery vs 37 conventional	Shorter hospital length of stay in the enhanced recovery group.
Fleming et al,[8] 2016	Prospective observational study with historical controls	52 enhanced recovery vs 53 conventional	Fewer postoperative complications, shorter duration of opioids, lower pain scores, and less nausea in the enhanced recovery group.

(continued on next page)

	Methods	Number of Patients	Main Conclusions
Table 1 ***(continued)***			
Li et al,[9] 2018	Randomized controlled trial	104 enhanced recovery vs 105 conventional	Less duration of mechanical ventilation, shorter ICU length of stay, lower financial costs, and lower pain scores in the enhanced recovery group.
Markham et al,[10] 2019	Retrospective observational study	25 enhanced recovery vs 25 conventional	More tracheal extubations in theater, shorter tracheal intubation time, less intraoperative fentanyl, and postoperative morphine in the enhanced recovery group.
Williams et al,[11] 2019	Prospective observational study	443 enhanced recovery vs 489 conventional	Less ICU/hospital length of stay, less opioid use, and fewer gastrointestinal complications in the enhanced recovery group.

Note that most of the studies use retrospective observations and historical controls.

be 2 days for dabigatran, apixaban, and edoxaban. Rivaroxaban requires a longer cessation period of 3 days and longer periods are required in patients with varying degrees of renal impairment.[17] Specific reversal agents are of limited use in cardiac surgical patients due to a lack of evidence in this cohort and concerns about the subsequent use of heparin for cardiopulmonary bypass. However, prothrombin complex concentrate seems a reasonable "tried and tested" antidote to DOAC-associated peri-operative bleeding.[18] In terms of enhanced recovery, the decision to restart a DOAC after surgery is usually taken following removal of chest drainage tubes and epicardial pacing wires as well as the occasional requirement for subsequent procedures, such as permanent pacemaker implantation.

Intraoperative

Anti-fibrinolysis
A discussion of the use of tranexamic acid versus aprotinin[19] or the principles of patient blood management[20] lies outside the scope of this article, but there is reasonable evidence for tranexamic acid to be given intraoperatively to reduce blood loss by its antifibrinolytic action at a maximum dose of 100 mg kg^{-1}.[12,21,22]

Glycemic control
Glycemic control arguably extends from the preoperative period all the way through to discharge from hospital and beyond. Most of the recommendations for cardiac surgical patients suggest that moderate glycemic control (6.7–10.0 mmmol.l^{-1}) is an

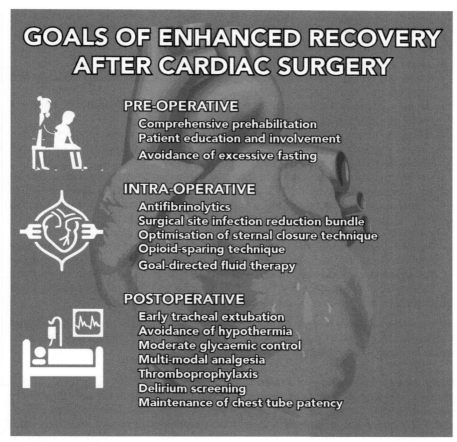

Fig. 1. The proposed goals of an enhanced recovery after the cardiac surgery program.

appropriate goal.[23] A preoperative hemoglobin A_{1C} level of less than 6.5% should be aimed for, but there is evidence of sparse screening of patients and optimization of glycemic control in the preoperative period, with calls for clearer guidance.[24] The recent ERAS society guidelines nevertheless recommends hemoglobin A_{1C} screening preoperatively to assist with risk stratification.[12] Intra- and postoperatively, glycemic control is best achieved with an intravenous infusion of short-acting insulin, with plasma glucose targets to ensure hypoglycemia is avoided. Only following discharge to the ward should be switching back to oral agents be considered, which should be done gradually and with input from specialist diabetes mellitus teams.

Goal-directed fluid therapy

The recent ERAS society recommendations for cardiac surgery recommend the use of goal-directed fluid therapy, but it is not clear exactly what this is or which algorithm should be used.[12] One definition of goal-directed fluid therapy in cardiac surgical patients is the use of hemodynamic parameters, beyond standard ones such as heart rate and blood pressure, to maximize oxygen delivery.[25] For patients undergoing non-cardiac surgery, a recent Cochrane review found low-quality evidence for goal-directed fluid therapy and was not able to conclude with certainty that it is superior to restrictive fluid therapy.[26]

The data for goal-directed fluid therapy in cardiac surgery are even more sparse and it is perhaps better to think of goal-directed therapy in cardiac surgery as individualized hemodynamic care for high-risk patients. One approach is to:

- define a target population of high-risk patients
- define the timing of the intervention, which should ideally be started early and continue throughout the peri-operative period
- define the type of intervention, which should be an appropriate combination of fluids, inotropes, and vasopressors
- define the target variables, which may include heart rate, mean arterial pressure, central venous pressure, pulmonary artery occlusion pressure, stroke volume variation, cardiac output, stroke volume, and their indices
- define the target values for these variables. A reasonable starting point would be targeting stroke volume variation first (<10%), mean arterial pressure next (<20% baseline), and then cardiac index (>2.2 L.min^{-1}.m^{-2}) last. Continuous cardiac output monitoring with a Swann Ganz catheter in combination with transoesophageal echocardiography remains the gold standard and much information about the performance of the right heart can also be gained which allows for specific interventions, such as inhaled nitric oxide or an intravenous phosphodiesterase inhibitor. However, the peri-operative course is dependent on multiple factors which are patient- and procedure-specific and any one algorithm or range of targets may fail to account for this complexity sufficiently.

The variables introduced by cardiopulmonary bypass must also be considered, and modern techniques such as retrograde autologous priming encouraged. There remains an urgent need for randomized trials in this area.

Opioid sparing anesthesia and analgesia techniques

Although opioid-sparing techniques are recommended widely in enhanced recovery protocols, applications to cardiac surgery have limited evidence and clinical experience. For many years, parenteral opioids have been the mainstay of anesthesia and analgesia strategies in the intra- and postoperative period. Induction of anesthesia is usually with, among other agents, high dose opioids, with an intravenous opioid infusion started thereafter and continued until oral intake is possible following tracheal extubation on the ICU.[19] Although "opioid-free anesthesia" as a concept has been challenged,[27] strategies to use opiates sparingly may include:

- the use of total intravenous anesthesia with shorter acting opiates such as remifentanil replacing the need for longer acting agents such as fentanyl or alfentanil[28]
- The use of regional anesthesia techniques such as, whereby practicable, paravertebral blockade[29] or ultrasound-guided fascial plane blocks of the chest wall, such as the erector spinae plane block which may also be used postoperatively with an appropriately sited catheter[30]
- The avoidance of modified release preparations in the postoperative period[31]
- The avoidance of the use of unidimensional pain scores alone to guide prescribing and titration of postoperative opioids[31]
- The use of the preoperative period to prepare patients psychologically for appropriate expectations of peri-operative analgesia targets.

Although the recent consensus recommendations suggest the peri-operative use of acetaminophen, tramadol, dexmedetomidine, and pregabalin,[12] the evidence is sparse and determining the ideal enhanced recovery regimen for cardiac surgical patients remains a fertile area for further research, with much work to be done and implemented into clinical practice.

Avoidance of hypothermia

The need and means to prevent peri-operative hypothermia for noncardiac surgery has a reasonable evidence base.[32] Cardiac surgery is arguably somewhat more problematic, more so when there becomes a need for cardiopulmonary bypass, cooling, and even deep hypothermic circulatory arrest with neuroprotection. It is of no less relevance, however, as hypothermia has known associations with bleeding, infection, prolonged critical stay, and death.[33] The recent ERAS society guidelines refer to the need to avoid persistent hypothermia, which is arguable of more relevance in the postoperative period.[12] Strategies include the use of forced-air warming blankets; raising the ambient room temperature; and the use of fluid warmers for intravenous fluid administration. Important also is the need to avoid hyperthermia during the rewarming phase of cardiopulmonary bypass.

Postoperative

Early tracheal extubation

Before enhanced recovery came "fast-track" cardiac anesthesia, with the primary outcome being that of early tracheal extubation. However, a recent Cochrane review found no difference in postoperative outcomes for those receiving "fast track" and conventional management.[34] It is nevertheless reasonable that efforts should be made to ensure patients tracheas are extubated as soon as feasible following surgery, and within 6 h of arrival on the critical care unit.[12] The patient must be stable from a hemodynamic and respiratory perspective before emergence, neurologic assessment, and tracheal extubation.

Early detection and management of acute kidney injury

Acute kidney injury, depending on the definition used, is common following cardiac surgery with an incidence of ~30% in all cases.[35] The need for postoperative renal replacement therapy is currently ~2–3%, yet the associated mortality in this group is high, ~50%.[35] Although recent guidelines suggest early identification of acute kidney injury with the use of plasma biomarkers,[12] there remains much work to be done on validating the use of such tests and implementing preventative strategies.

Chest drain management

Placement of chest drains are normal practice following cardiac surgery, and the recent ERAS society guidelines recommend ensuring patency without breaking the sterile field to avoid retained blood and associated complications, such as cardiac tamponade.[12,36] Complications related to bleeding more generally, which may result in resternotomy, are associated with adverse outcomes.[37] More important in our opinion than ensuring chest tube patency is the need to have in place agreed criteria for chest drain removal following surgery, as chest drains may cause pain and delay mobilization and recovery.

Thromboprophylaxis

As with most patients undergoing major surgery, a full preoperative venous thromboembolism assessment must be undertaken in the pre, intra, and postoperative periods. It is usual for cardiac surgical patients to receive mechanical thromboprophylaxis immediately following surgery, unless there are contraindications. On postoperative day 1, if there are no bleeding concerns, pharmacologic prophylaxis should be initiated and continued until discharge.[12]

Delirium screening

There is reasonable evidence that delirium is associated with poor postoperative outcomes for patients undergoing noncardiac and cardiac surgery.[38,39] To manage delirium, it has to be detected systematically by using screening methods, such as the confusion assessment method (CAM),[40] at regular intervals. The recent guideline suggests this should be done once per nursing shift.[12] Once identified, the underlying cause can be sought and managed. Management strategies should first be nonpharmacological, with reality reorientation methods and reassurance of far greater use than pharmacologic agents such as haloperidol. Pharmacologic agents of use include mirtazapine, olanzapine and increasingly, dexmedetomidine. Each institution should develop its own guidance and pathways for the management of delirium after cardiac surgery in collaboration with the whole multidisciplinary team.

Surgical Techniques

Minimally invasive surgery

Some centers undertake minimal access surgery, which encompasses a variety of procedures, including: port access mitral valve surgery; minimal access aortic valve surgery; tricuspid valve repair/replacement; ASD and PFO closure; AF ablation; and resection of atrial myxomas. Purported benefits include: reduced need for median sternotomy; reduced pain; shorter hospital stay; better cosmesis; and earlier mobilization, all of which are in line with the aims of enhanced recovery. That said, the use of minimally invasive surgical techniques is yet to appear in enhanced recovery guidelines due to the lack of evidence of superiority in terms of clinically relevant outcomes.[41]

Rigid sternal fixation

Deep sternal wound infections are a common cause of postoperative morbidity and are associated with: obesity, diabetes, coronary artery disease, low ejection fraction, chronic steroid therapy, chronic infections, end-stage renal disease, smoking, and advanced age. However, they are also associated with surgical factors such as: inadequate skin preparation, use of bone wax, emergency sternotomy, bilateral harvesting of the internal mammary artery, blood product transfusion, prolonged bypass, sternal rewiring, and postoperative bleeding. In those with risk factors, there is emerging evidence that rigid sternal fixation with plating, as opposed to wire cerclage, might be associated with reduced incidence of sternal wound complications.[42,43] In the United Kingdom, however, chest closure with sternal wires remains the most common approach due to the need in some patients for resternotomy following cardiac surgery,[37] which is more difficult to undertake with rigid sternal fixation.

Controversies

There are many areas of controversy in the field of ERACS. These include:

- The lack of patient representation in formulating the recently published enhanced recovery recommendations.[12]
- The definition of ERACS as compared with conventional management, especially given that many of the principles of enhanced recovery may have now become standard practice.
- The lack of consensus on what outcomes are clinically important when studying ERACS.
- How to account for intraoperative complications associated with cardiac surgery and their impact on outcomes in patients who are otherwise suitable for enhanced recovery.

- How enhanced recovery protocols and pathways can be implemented in complex organizations providing cardiac surgery.
- The lack of evidence on which guidelines are based, which many might suggest is simply new dogma replacing the old.

Recommendations

In addition to the clinical recommendations provided in recent guidelines,[12] there are several patient-centered recommendations we feel should receive focus that has perhaps been overlooked. We hope this can guide future iterations of ERACS guidelines. These are that:

- ERACS should be for all patients regardless of surgical risk profile, comorbidities, or operation type.
- Patients should be admitted to the hospital on the day of surgery, having been assessed thoroughly as an outpatient by all teams including the anesthetist.
- Patients should be educated about the goals of enhanced recovery in the preoperative period and be involved fully in their care and progress throughout the perioperative period.
- Patients should complete a daily progress record documenting items such as: the period sat out in a chair; number of times attempted to march on the spot; distance walked; oral intake; pain score; nausea score; and lines/monitoring/drains/dressings removed or discontinued each day until discharge from hospital.
- There should be a shift from the outcomes studied to the documentation of morbidity using a postoperative morbidity survey[44] and/or quality of recovery score[45] together with a metric of a successful recovery to return home such as counting the number of days alive and at home up to 30 days after surgery.[46,47]

FUTURE DIRECTIONS

It has been argued that the ERACS guidelines[12] are just an important first step on the road to implementation of the enhanced recovery philosophy into cardiac surgical peri-operative pathways.[48] Further research should now focus on the implementation of these strategies in all cardiac surgical patients, and determining the barriers to their use. A large multicentre randomized trial of enhanced recovery versus conventional management would not be without significant challenge, but such a study would be easy to justify scientifically. There must also be more focus placed on the patient experience through the use of appropriate patient-related outcome and patient-reported experience measures.[49] Finally, there must be efforts made to understand practice variations between individuals, clinicians, centers, departments, and countries, because only when we understand how to define what "conventional" management is will we be able to work out how enhanced recovery may be implemented.

SUMMARY

ERACS is relatively new as compared with established pathways in general and orthopedic surgery, but the aims are broadly the same. It has evolved from "fast track" cardiac surgery and now envelopes the whole peri-operative process, from listing for surgery through to discharge from the hospital. Early mobilization and restoration of normal function as soon as possible after surgery are important aims for cardiac surgical patients and although we now have a set of guidelines to work with, centers need to work together to ensure optimal implementation and data collection. Rather than simply encompassing a list of interventions or strategies for carefully selected patients, it should instead signify a different way of improving the quality of care for all patients undergoing cardiac surgery.

CLINICS CARE POINTS

- There is reasonable evidence to support:
  - antifibrinolytics in the intraoperative period
  - moderate glycemic control throughout the perioperative period
  - bundles to reduce the incidence of surgical site infections
  - goal-directed hemodynamic therapy
  - smoking, alcohol, and hazardous substance cessation in the preoperative period
  - opioid-sparing anesthesia and analgesia techniques
  - avoidance of postoperative hypothermia
  - maintenance of chest tube patency
  - screening for postoperative delirium

- It may be of benefit to:
  - have mechanisms to detect kidney injury associated with surgery
  - engage patients in prehabilitation pathways before surgery
  - use an intravenous infusion of insulin in all patients postoperatively
  - aim for tracheal extubation within 4 hours of the end of surgery in most patients, but with an appreciation that some patients require individualized targets
  - ensure appropriate chemical or mechanical thromboprophylaxis is in place postoperatively and until discharge from hospital
  - continue consumption of clear fluids until 2 hours before general anesthesia
  - encourage preoperative carbohydrate drinks before surgery

---

DISCLOSURE

A. Klein or his institution has received unrestricted educational grant funding, honoraria or travel assistance from Nordic Pharma, Fisher and Paykel, Pharmacosmos, Vifor Pharma, HemoSonics, and Hemonetics and Masimo. No other competing interests were declared.

REFERENCES

1. Engelman RM, Rousou JA, Flack JE, et al. Fast-track recovery of the coronary bypass patient. Ann Thorac Surg 1994;58(6):1742–6.
2. Dunstan JL, Riddle MM. Rapid recovery management: the effects on the patient who has undergone heart surgery. Heart Lung 1997;26(4):289–98.
3. Fernandes AM da S, Mansur AJ, Canêo LF, et al. The reduction in hospital stay and costs in the care of patients with congenital heart diseases undergoing fast-track cardiac surgery. Arq Bras Cardiol 2004;83(1):27–34, 18-26.
4. Yanatori M, Tomita S, Miura Y, et al. Feasibility of the fast-track recovery program after cardiac surgery in Japan. Gen Thorac Cardiovasc Surg 2007;55(11):445–9.
5. Ender J, Borger MA, Scholz M, et al. Cardiac surgery fast-track treatment in a postanesthetic care unit: six-month results of the Leipzig fast-track concept. Anesthesiology 2008;109(1):61–6.
6. Salhiyyah K, Elsobky S, Raja S, et al. A clinical and economic evaluation of fast-track recovery after cardiac surgery. Heart Surg Forum 2011;14(6):E330–4.
7. Hardman G, Bose A, Saunders H, et al. Enhanced recovery in Cardiac surgery. J Cardiothorac Surg 2015;10(Suppl 1):A75.

8. Fleming IO, Garratt C, Guha R, et al. Aggregation of Marginal Gains in Cardiac Surgery: Feasibility of a Perioperative Care Bundle for Enhanced Recovery in Cardiac Surgical Patients. J Cardiothorac Vasc Anesth 2016;30(3):665–70.

9. Li M, Zhang J, Gan TJ, et al. Enhanced recovery after surgery pathway for patients undergoing cardiac surgery: a randomized clinical trial. Eur J Cardiothorac Surg 2018;54(3):491–7.

10. Markham T, Wegner R, Hernandez N, et al. Assessment of a multimodal analgesia protocol to allow the implementation of enhanced recovery after cardiac surgery: Retrospective analysis of patient outcomes. J Clin Anesth 2019;54: 76–80.

11. Williams JB, McConnell G, Allender JE, et al. One-year results from the first US-based enhanced recovery after cardiac surgery (ERAS Cardiac) program. J Thorac Cardiovasc Surg 2019;157(5):1881–8.

12. Engelman DT, Ben Ali W, Williams JB, et al. Guidelines for Perioperative Care in Cardiac Surgery: Enhanced Recovery After Surgery Society Recommendations. JAMA Surg 2019;154(8):755–66.

13. McCann M, Stamp N, Ngui A, et al. Cardiac Prehabilitation. J Cardiothorac Vasc Anesth 2019;33(8):2255–65.

14. Smith I, Kranke P, Murat I, et al. Perioperative fasting in adults and children: guidelines from the European Society of Anaesthesiology. Eur J Anaesthesiol 2011;28(8):556–69.

15. Practice Guidelines for Preoperative Fasting and the Use of Pharmacologic Agents to Reduce the Risk of Pulmonary Aspiration: Application to Healthy Patients Undergoing Elective Procedures: An Updated Report by the American Society of Anesthesiologists Task Force on Preoperative Fasting and the Use of Pharmacologic Agents to Reduce the Risk of Pulmonary Aspiration. Anesthesiology 2017;126(3):376–93.

16. Charlesworth M, Arya R. Direct oral anticoagulants: peri-operative considerations and controversies. Anaesthesia 2018;73(12):1460–3.

17. Erdoes G, Arroyabe BMLD, Bolliger D, et al. International consensus statement on the peri-operative management of direct oral anticoagulants in cardiac surgery. Anaesthesia 2018;73(12):1535–45.

18. Charlesworth M, Hayes T, Erdoes G. Reversal Agents for the Management of Direct Oral Anticoagulant-Related Bleeding in Cardiac Surgical Patients: The Emperor's New Clothes? J Cardiothorac Vasc Anesth 2021;35(8):2480–2.

19. Charlesworth M, Martinovsky P. The principles of cardiac anaesthesia. Anaesth Intensive Care Med 2018;19(7):335–8.

20. Spahn DR, Muñoz M, Klein AA, et al. Patient Blood Management: Effectiveness and Future Potential. Anesthesiology 2020;133(1):212–22.

21. Tengborn L, Blombäck M, Berntorp E. Tranexamic acid–an old drug still going strong and making a revival. Thromb Res 2015;135(2):231–42.

22. Myles PS, Smith JA, Forbes A, et al. Tranexamic Acid in Patients Undergoing Coronary-Artery Surgery. N Engl J Med 2017;376(2):136–48.

23. Reddy P, Duggar B, Butterworth J. Blood glucose management in the patient undergoing cardiac surgery: A review. World J Cardiol 2014;6(11):1209–17.

24. Navaratnarajah M, Rea R, Evans R, et al. Effect of glycaemic control on complications following cardiac surgery: literature review. J Cardiothorac Surg 2018; 13(1):10.

25. Fergerson BD, Manecke GR. Goal-Directed Therapy in Cardiac Surgery: Are We There Yet? J Cardiothorac Vasc Anesth 2013;27(6):1075–8.

26. Wrzosek A, Jakowicka-Wordliczek J, Zajaczkowska R, et al. Perioperative restrictive versus goal-directed fluid therapy for adults undergoing major non-cardiac surgery. Cochrane Database Syst Rev 2019;12. https://doi.org/10.1002/14651858.CD012767.pub2.

27. Elkassabany NM, Mariano ER. Opioid-free anaesthesia – what would Inigo Montoya say? Anaesthesia 2019;74(5):560–3.

28. Beverstock J, Park T, Alston RP, et al. A Comparison of Volatile Anesthesia and Total Intravenous Anesthesia (TIVA) Effects on Outcome From Cardiac Surgery: A Systematic Review and Meta-Analysis. J Cardiothorac Vasc Anesth 2020. https://doi.org/10.1053/j.jvca.2020.10.036.

29. Caruso TJ, Lawrence K, Tsui BCH. Regional anesthesia for cardiac surgery. Curr Opin Anesthesiol 2019;32(5):674–82.

30. Chin KJ, Versyck B, Pawa A. Ultrasound-guided fascial plane blocks of the chest wall: a state-of-the-art review. Anaesthesia 2021;76(S1):110–26.

31. Levy N, Quinlan J, El-Boghdadly K, et al. An international multidisciplinary consensus statement on the prevention of opioid-related harm in adult surgical patients. Anaesthesia 2021;76(4):520–36. https://doi.org/10.1111/anae.15262.

32. Torossian A, Bräuer A, Höcker J, et al. Preventing Inadvertent Perioperative Hypothermia. Dtsch Arztebl Int 2015;112(10):166–72.

33. Karalapillai D, Story D, Hart GK, et al. Postoperative hypothermia and patient outcomes after major elective non-cardiac surgery. Anaesthesia 2013;68(6):605–11.

34. Wong W-T, Lai VK, Chee YE, et al. Fast-track cardiac care for adult cardiac surgical patients. Cochrane Database Syst Rev 2016;9. https://doi.org/10.1002/14651858.CD003587.pub3.

35. Hu J, Chen R, Liu S, et al. Global Incidence and Outcomes of Adult Patients With Acute Kidney Injury After Cardiac Surgery: A Systematic Review and Meta-Analysis. J Cardiothorac Vasc Anesth 2016;30(1):82–9.

36. Baribeau Y, Westbrook B, Baribeau Y, et al. Active clearance of chest tubes is associated with reduced postoperative complications and costs after cardiac surgery: a propensity matched analysis. J Cardiothorac Surg 2019;14(1):192.

37. Agarwal S, Choi SW, Fletcher SN, et al. The incidence and effect of resternotomy following cardiac surgery on morbidity and mortality: a 1-year national audit on behalf of the Association of Cardiothoracic Anaesthesia and Critical Care. Anaesthesia 2021;76(1):19–26.

38. Brown CHIV, Probert J, Healy R, et al. Cognitive Decline after Delirium in Patients Undergoing Cardiac Surgery. Anesthesiology 2018;129(3):406–16.

39. Gleason LJ, Schmitt EM, Kosar CM, et al. Effect of Delirium and Other Major Complications After Elective Surgery in Older Adults. JAMA Surg 2015;150(12):1134–40.

40. Ely EW, Inouye SK, Bernard GR, et al. Delirium in mechanically ventilated patients: validity and reliability of the confusion assessment method for the intensive care unit (CAM-ICU). JAMA 2001;286(21):2703–10.

41. Cheng DCH, Martin J, Lal A, et al. Minimally Invasive versus Conventional Open Mitral Valve Surgery a Meta-Analysis and Systematic Review. Innovations (Phila) 2011;6(2):84–103.

42. Allen KB, Thourani VH, Naka Y, et al. Randomized, multicenter trial comparing sternotomy closure with rigid plate fixation to wire cerclage. J Thorac Cardiovasc Surg 2017;153(4):888–96.e1.

43. Allen KB, Thourani VH, Naka Y, et al. Rigid Plate Fixation Versus Wire Cerclage: Patient-Reported and Economic Outcomes From a Randomized Trial. Ann Thorac Surg 2018;105(5):1344–50.

44. Bennett-Guerrero E, Welsby I, Dunn TJ, et al. The use of a postoperative morbidity survey to evaluate patients with prolonged hospitalization after routine, moderate-risk, elective surgery. Anesth Analg 1999;89(2):514–9.

45. Myles PS. Measuring quality of recovery in perioperative clinical trials. Curr Opin Anaesthesiol 2018;31(4):396–401.

46. Myles PS, Shulman MA, Heritier S, et al. Validation of days at home as an outcome measure after surgery: a prospective cohort study in Australia. BMJ Open 2017;7(8):e015828.

47. Myles PS. More than just morbidity and mortality – quality of recovery and long-term functional recovery after surgery. Anaesthesia 2020;75(S1):e143–50.

48. Gregory AJ, Grant MC, Manning MW, et al. Enhanced Recovery After Cardiac Surgery (ERAS Cardiac) Recommendations: An Important First Step—But There Is Much Work to Be Done. J Cardiothorac Vasc Anesth 2020;34(1):39–47.

49. Shah A, Bailey CR. Outcomes following surgery: are we measuring what really matters? Anaesthesia 2019;74(6):696–9.

Updates in Enhanced Recovery Pathways for Gynecologic Surgery

Andres Zorrilla-Vaca, MD[a], Javier D. Lasala, MD[b],
Gabriel E. Mena, MD[b],*

KEYWORDS

- Enhanced recovery after surgery • Fast track • ERAS • Anesthesia • Analgesia
- Gynecologic surgery

KEY POINTS

- Substantial advances in surgical and anesthetic techniques have contributed to improvements in enhanced recovery after surgery (ERAS) protocols over the last decade.
- ERAS protocols have gained widespread acceptance in gynecologic surgery by tailoring the complexity of women's health and institutional demands.
- Evidence is now supporting the implementation of ERAS protocols in gynecologic surgery to ensure faster recovery with lower complications rates.
- Multimodal analgesia, prehabilitation, and perioperative nutritional supplementation are becoming important components of ERAS programs in gynecologic surgery, which comprise physical, immune-nutrition, and psychological interventions.
- Implementation of ERAS pathways in gynecologic oncologic surgery has been associated with an improvement in patient satisfaction and patient-reported outcomes.

INTRODUCTION

Gynecologic surgery encompasses over a quarter of inpatient surgical procedures for US women, and current projections estimate an increase of the US female population by nearly 50% in 2050.[1] In parallel to this growing population and as a response to its complexity, enhanced recovery pathways (ERPs) for gynecologic surgeries emerged and have been evolving over the past few years with the main goal of ensuring faster functional recovery that lead to early hospital discharges and lower postoperative complication rates.[2] These pathways consist of a bundle of multidisciplinary

a Department of Anesthesiology, Brigham and Women's Hospital, 75 Francis Street, Boston, MA 02115, USA; b Department of Anesthesiology and Perioperative Medicine, The University of Texas MD Anderson Cancer Center, 1515 Holcombe Boulevard, Unit 409 13th floor, Houston, TX 77030, USA
* Corresponding author.
E-mail address: gmena@mdanderson.org

Anesthesiology Clin 40 (2022) 157–174
https://doi.org/10.1016/j.anclin.2021.11.008
1932-2275/22/© 2021 Elsevier Inc. All rights reserved.

interventions, evidence-based perioperative management, and patient-centered strategies, including a systematic approach to patient care, which for gynecology, it is based on a set of measures categorized as preoperative (counseling, multimodal prehabilitation), intraoperative (goal-directed fluid therapy ([GDFT] optimization, minimally invasive surgical techniques, adequate pain control, and minimal use of surgical drains), and postoperative (quick resumption of a general diet, opioid-sparing analgesia, limited fluid therapy, and early mobilization).[3]

Over the last decade, US hospitals have embraced ERPs in many specialties. They have increasingly been used in multiple institutions worldwide, becoming the standard of care for patient optimization.[4] Although they were initially introduced in colorectal surgery programs, they have gained widespread acceptance in many more surgical subspecialties, leading to favorable patient outcomes, including early bowel recovery, decreased length of stay, lower rates of surgical site infections (SSI), and lower rates of readmission. In 2014, an international group of experts in areas related to gynecology summoned and developed the first enhanced recovery after surgery (ERAS) guidelines for Gynecology/Oncology in 2018 based on the ERAS colonic surgery and rectal/pelvis guidelines as templates.[5] Currently, several gynecologic and anesthesiology societies advocate for the introduction of ERPs into their practice,[5,6] especially given the vulnerable women's population undergoing gynecologic procedures, as well as the substantial clinical benefits in patient-reported outcomes (PROs) and cost savings to the health care system demonstrating better results after implementation.[7–10]

According to the last updated ERAS guideline published in 2019, there are several new considerations behind each practice in ERAS protocols.[11] More items have now been included, and others have escalated their quality of evidence, making them impactful when applied and promoted in the perioperative care setting. This article discusses the most updated evidence regarding ERAS programs for gynecologic surgery in light of the new considerations endorsed by the ERAS societies.[11–13] The best evidence is categorized based on the type of gynecologic surgery (malignancy vs benign) and aimed at 8 specific aspects of the ERAS protocols: prehabilitation, nutritional strategies, bowel management, GDFT, anesthetic technique, surgical approach, multimodal perioperative analgesia, and postoperative nausea and vomiting prophylaxis.

ENHANCED RECOVERY AFTER SURGERY PRINCIPLES

Perioperative care demands the implementation of evidence-based practices with clinically significant impact. ERAS protocols for the gynecologic surgical population have addressed this critical point by conceiving the synergistic effects of multiple interventions along the major phases of the hospital journey (preoperative, intraoperative, and postoperative) with the main goal of mitigating the physiologic stress of surgery and optimizing patient outcomes across the phases of recovery (**Fig. 1**).[14] Over the last 2 decades, the ERAS societies have actively been engaged to merge the best clinical practices and consolidate consensus for the establishment of standardized protocols.[15] They have taken into consideration some key principles of ERAS programs, which include the following: (1) the reduction of the stress response associated with surgery (eg, inflammatory and metabolic responses), (2) early recovery of baseline functional capacity, (3) adequate pain control by implementing multimodal analgesia, (4) cost savings to the health care system, and (5) active engagement of the patients in their perioperative care and recovery.[15] Those principles are typically used for the introduction of new practices in the protocols as well

Phases of recovery

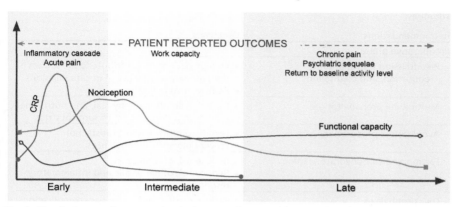

Fig. 1. The 3 phases of recovery (early, intermediate, and late) and its characteristic markers. CRP, C-reactive protein. (Source: Authors Own Work.)

as to build up the 3 main pillars on which ERAS lies, which include evidence-based perioperative care processes, multidisciplinary teamwork, and continuous audit. In **Table 1**, the updated ERAS practices for gynecologic surgery are summarized. Furthermore, all these principles delineate the rationale of ERAS programs, which is to reduce prolonged hospital stay while prioritizing patient outcomes and cost savings, which have been clearly shown in recent cohorts reporting a decrease in 15% of hospital charges per patient mostly attributed to less laboratory, pharmacy, and room charges.[8]

Although an important ERAS objective is to help integrate evidence-based knowledge into practice, align perioperative care, and minimize practice variations making them feasible and easily applicable,[16] it is also important to tailor the ERAS approach to each institution and workflow.[17] Several institutions have adopted different approaches, understanding that ERAS is a concept, which includes several components that are implemented in various ways but applying its principles. Despite the highly heterogeneous ERAS protocols between institutions, several randomized controlled trials (RCTs) have surfaced over the past few years reporting the successful implementation of this multimodal approach in the perioperative care of the gynecologic surgical patients.

A particular issue in gynecologic surgical patients is the comorbidity indices in this population as well as the high risk for developing chronic postoperative pain, which may significantly impact functional recovery and mental health in the long term.[18] All these reasons have promoted the increased interest implementing ERAS protocols in gynecologic surgeries in several institutions, becoming feasible programs with growing evidence supporting the benefits in terms of faster recovery, lower complications, lower readmission rates, and reduction of hospital costs.[14]

ORGANIZATION FOR ENHANCED RECOVERY AFTER SURGERY IMPLEMENTATION IN GYNECOLOGY

It is noteworthy to prioritize the ERAS pathway organization, which plays an important role in developing these programs and translating them into an actual protocol for gynecologic surgeries.[19] There is a vast amount of evidence that demonstrates the

Table 1
Description of the enhanced recovery after surgery recommendations in gynecologic surgeries

Recommendations	Outcomes
Preoperative phase	
Preadmission information, education, and counseling	• Engage patients to contribute to the success of the pathway and be active in care decisions • Reduce anxiety levels
Multimodal prehabilitation	• Optimize emotional, physical, and nutritional aspects to reduce impact of surgical stress
Avoid bowel preparation	• Less discomfort, patient satisfaction • Prevent electrolyte imbalances
Fasting and carbohydrate loading	• Reduce risk of aspiration • Reduce risk of metabolic and inflammatory response
DVT prophylaxis	• Reduce cardiac and pulmonary complications
SSI reduction bundles	• Reduce rates of SSI
Intraoperative phase	
Minimally invasive surgical techniques	• Reduce surgical stress • Improve pain scores, less ileus and blood loss, shorter length of stay
Fluid management/GDFT	• Reduce cardiac and pulmonary complications • Maintain adequate tissue perfusion and oxygen delivery.
Opioid-sparing analgesia	• Diminish opioid-induced side effects (ie, postoperative nausea and vomiting, ileus, pruritus)
Antiemetic prophylaxis	• Shorter PACU length of stay
Postoperative phase	
Multimodal analgesia	• Lower pain scores postoperatively Shorter length of stay • Diminish opioid-induced side effects Better patient satisfaction
Early ambulation	• Reduce cardiac and pulmonary complications • Return to baseline functional capacity
Early feeding	• Faster recovery of bowel function (less ileus) • Shorter length of stay
Discharge pathways	• Follow-up and patient satisfaction
ERAS audit & reporting	• Continuous improvements and pathway optimization

Abbreviations: DVT, deep venous thrombosis; PACU, postanesthesia care unit.

importance of changing initiatives in a climate of engagement, powerful guiding coalition, and continued quality improvement.[19] A more complete series of recommendations was recently published by Nelson and colleagues,[19] including ERAS order sets and instructions for a successful protocol implementation. A summary of recommendations stratified by the timing of implementation and Deming model (plan-do-study-act cycle)[20] is listed in **Table 2**.[20] The Deming model has been the traditional breakthrough strategy for ERAS implementation in gynecologic surgery with the use of standard cycles for planning and executing improvements,[20] but newer models, such as the innovative stepped strategy, which comprise 4 levels of intensity support (digital tool

Table 2
Recommendations to implement enhanced recovery after surgery programs in gynecologic surgery stratified by timing of implementation and the Deming model[20]

Recommendations	Objective	Deming Model
Before implementing	Standardize management in a	PLAN
Generate climate of change	multidisciplinary team	
Assemble the team		
Empower broad-based action		
During implementation	Consolidate the momentum and	DO
Implement teamwork and	discuss weaknesses within the	
communication	team	
Continuous ongoing education		
and training		
Embrace short-term wins		
Consolidate and build on change		
Identify defects through sense-		
making		
Frequent updates on the successes/		CHECK
challenges		
Developing a plan for testing the		
effectiveness		
After implementation	Analyze and reconfigure the	
Audit & monitor outcomes	program based on collected	
Use patient feedback in	data and patient feedback	
developing care pathways		
Anchor ERPs changes into the		
organization		
Use process measures to track		
quality		
Follow-up with multidisciplinary		
team		
Implement solutions to barriers		ACT
Generate appropriate		
modifications		

promoting awareness, interactive educational sessions, regional opinion leader, tailored and labor-intensive activities), are being evaluated in an ongoing Dutch trial with the aim of further improving cost-effectiveness of ERAS protocols during their implementation.[21]

At the beginning of ERAS implementation, it is mandatory that the patient's interdisciplinary team has a patient-centered vision with a clear understanding of this stepwise process.[22] All the practices before introduction of ERAS programs should be established in an appropriate environment that promotes the culture of leadership, dissemination, and participation.[22] As for gynecologic surgeries, it is suggested that institutions examine their own infrastructure and create an organizational culture that emphasizes quality and safety.

Other key elements for a successful program are as follows: (1) strong commitment for ownership and continued excellence from all participants; (2) coordination of care support and continuous monitoring of compliance (at least 80%), which has been shown to correlate with the level of positive impact on patient outcomes[23,24]; and (3) patient feedback and continuous monitoring of PROs. There are some tools that have been shown to significantly increase the level of compliance in gynecology, such as the ERAS Interactive Audit System, which increased compliance from 56%

to 77%[25]; another method is by integrating electronic health records (RedCap) and scheduling systems that have been shown to improve safety, compliance, and efficacy.[26] Although there is no consensus regarding the minimum number of ERAS items associated with improved outcomes, some data suggest that avoidance of salt-water overload, early mobilization, early oral nutrition, and early removal of the Foley catheter have been shown to lead to less postoperative complications in the gynecology surgical population.[23]

Another special consideration besides clinical endpoints is the inclusion of patient feedback or PROs throughout the enhanced recovery process. This helps analyze and strengthen some key elements of the ERAS program.

GYNECOLOGIC ONCOLOGY SURGERY

Oncologic population accounts for a significant health and economic burden worldwide. ERPs in Gynecologic/Oncology share several similarities with protocols in colorectal cancer, but only a few modifications have been introduced to the protocols based on the neurohormonal differences in the women's population as well as pharmacokinetic/dynamic considerations. Until 2017, almost all the evidence in ERAS Gynecologic/Oncologic surgery was based on a broad range of nonrandomized studies at high risk of bias.[27] Since that time, a great number of randomized data have been published allowing to strongly support ERPs in this arena. **Table 3** shows an updated list of all the RCTs in ERAS for gynecologic surgery. According to this updated evidence, the most impactful ERAS aspects in gynecology/oncologic surgery are presented in the following sections. Most of the recommendations are also applicable for ERAS in benign gynecologic surgeries.

Counseling and Education

Patient self-engagement and control of their own recovery are imperative in ERAS programs. Some strategies include easy access to appropriate educational material preoperatively, good communication and understanding of the procedural risks, expectations as well as the commitments of health care providers and patients. A recent trial in patients undergoing hysterectomy suggested that the use of audiovisual/multimedia, as a preoperative counseling strategy, is effective to improve patient comprehension while reducing physician time.[37] Other communication interventions, such as extended discussions and test/feedback techniques, have also been shown to facilitate the feasibility and acceptability of the interventions to clinicians and patients.[38]

As for gynecologic oncologic surgeries, a thorough description regarding the impact of cancer treatment on future fertility is necessary because both fertility counseling and fertility-sparing surgery have been associated with decreased distress in reproductive-aged women with gynecologic cancers.[39,40] Therefore, early referral to reproductive specialists before initiation of chemo/radiation is crucial to success in the field of female fertility preservation and consequently patient satisfaction.

Multimodal Prehabilitation

This ERAS aspect was recently included in the updated guidelines for Gynecology/Oncologic surgery with low level of evidence and weak recommendation given the prematurity of the research in this area.[11] However, several investigators have noted this as a revolutionary item, especially in oncologic surgery, as more attention is now being directed toward longer preoperative periods.[41] Furthermore, oncologic patients typically have nutritional deficits, psychological impairments, and physical

Table 3
Updated best quality of evidence (randomized controlled trials) summarized in randomized controlled trials of enhanced recovery after surgery in gynecologic surgeries

Trial	Number of Patients	Diagnosis	Special Interventions	Compliance	Outcomes Improved
Burgos et al,[28] 2016	24	Ovarian cancer	Not reported	Not reported	Lower postoperative complications (wound infections, ileus, pleural effusion) Lower readmissions (16% vs 33%) Cost-effectiveness (saving 1700 euros per patient)
Lashkul et al,[29] 2017	39	Laparoscopic hysterectomy	Early multimodal rehabilitation & restrictive fluid management (5 mL/kg/h)	Not reported	Lower length of hospital stay (5 vs 7 d) Lower intraoperative blood loss (282 vs 547 mL)
Dickson et al,[30] 2017	112	Oncology	Preoperative counseling, clear liquids until 2 h before surgery, routine mechanical bowel preparation was discouraged, TAP block using liposomal bupivacaine, acetaminophen, ibuprofen, early ambulation within 2 h	87%	Lower opioid consumption at day 2 postoperative
Antypin et al,[31] 2013	48	Hysterectomy	Not reported	Not reported	Lower proinflammatory C-reactive protein levels up to 7 d postoperative
Bourazani et al,[32] 2019	61	Oncology	Not reported	Not reported	Lower length of hospital stay (3 vs 5 d) Lower pain scores
Ferrari et al,[33] 2019	138	Endometrial or ovarian cancer	Not reported	Not reported	Lower length of hospital stay (3.5 d difference)
Sánchez-Iglesias et al,[34] 2019	99	Advanced ovarian cancer	Not reported	>90%	Lower length of hospital stay (7 vs 9 d) Lower readmissions Cost-effectiveness (saving 13,330 euros per patient)

(continued on next page)

Table 3
(continued)

Trial	Number of Patients	Diagnosis	Special Interventions	Compliance	Outcomes Improved
Johnson et al,[35] 2019	50	Hysterectomy	Early mobilization, early transition to oral pain medications, oral feeding, chewing gum	88%	Better patient satisfaction Lower length of hospital stay
Yi et al,[36] 2020	118	Oncology	Special formulated whey protein-carbohydrate loading 3 h prior surgery, early oral feedings, opioid-sparing analgesia, fluid therapy based on total body fluid losses	96%	Decrease in readmission (6% vs 16%) Less length of bowel function return Less nausea/vomiting Better handgrip strength in recovery

*All studies considered standard.

deconditioning, all of which are associated with poor postoperative outcomes.[42] In response to these problems, multimodal prehabilitation emerged as a multidisciplinary process of improving physical, emotional, and nutritional status before surgery. A recent systematic review of this area in Gynecology/Oncologic surgery comprised little evidence and created a framework for future studies.[43] Despite the promising results and increasing interest in this area, the last guidelines emphasized standardizing this ERAS item (eg, recognize the selective group of patients with most benefits and definition of minimum duration of prehabilitation) and considering other items, such as weight loss.

Nutritional Considerations

Oncologic patients typically have high nutritional demands because of the elevated metabolic rate and permanent inflammatory status. Supplementation with polyunsaturated fatty acids, arginine, glutamine, antioxidants, and nucleotides has been an emerging area showing promising results in terms of inflammation and postoperative healing.[44] Interestingly, both arginine and high-protein feeds have been shown to have clinically significant effects on a reduction of overall infections and shorter hospital stay. Although apparently no effects on mortality have been observed from nutritional supplementation, there are still ongoing studies assessing the role of vitamin A and arginine.[45] However, further well-designed evidence is needed in order to draw definitive recommendations.

On the other hand, it is highly recommended to follow the fasting standards by the American Society of Anesthesiology and avoid prolonged periods of fasting.[11] Therefore, patients should be encouraged to eat a light meal up until 6 hours and clear fluids until 2 hours before surgery.[46] Preoperative carbohydrate loading is also strongly suggested as a way to reduce insulin resistance, but there is low evidence on improving clinical outcomes with this measure.[11] In addition, there is a call to abandon the routine use of preoperative bowel preparation because recent literature has shown no benefits in both minimally invasive surgery and open gynecologic procedures, whereas, oppositely, it can potentially cause fluid and electrolyte imbalance. In cases of concomitant colonic resection, it is suggested to use oral antibiotics alone preferably or in combination with bowel preparation.

High-protein oral feedings within the first 24 hours after surgery should be the main component of postoperative nutrition. Although early postoperative feeding is the most frequently implemented nutritional practice and best-supported strategy in ERAS programs,[47] other recommended interventions, such as drinking coffee and chewing gum, have also robust evidence showing to be effective in shortening length of stay, hastening bowel recovery, preventing ileus, and decreasing the risk of nausea/vomiting.[35,48,49] All these strategies were recently recommended in the last guidelines with high quality of evidence and for being simple, inexpensive, and feasible.[11]

Preoperative Metabolic Screening

In the United States, approximately 17% of gynecologic/oncologic surgical patients are hyperglycemic preoperatively, being at higher risk of developing SSI. According to recent studies, hyperglycemic patients have significantly higher reductions in SSI (approximately 33%–50%) if they are controlled with intensive approaches.[50,51] Nevertheless, glucose management must avoid hypoglycemic events, as both extremes have been associated with mortality. Recent guidelines from the ERAS Society and the American College of Obstetricians and Gynecologists concur that the intraoperative glucose levels should be maintained bellow 180 to 200 mg/dL.

Surgical Approach

Minimally invasive surgical techniques are highly recommended for appropriate patients when feasible.[11] Laparoscopic surgery has been associated with reduced operative morbidity, shorter hospital length of stay, lower postoperative pain, less bowel complications (ileus), and in-hospital cost savings when compared with open procedures.[52] High-quality evidence summarized in meta-analyses supports the preference for laparoscopic techniques within ERAS protocols with similar survival rates compared with open surgical techniques.[53] Other surgical techniques that might alleviate the postoperative inflammatory stress is robotic assistance, which has also shown superior results when compared with the open approach but still comparable with laparoscopic procedures in terms of postoperative complications.[54]

Fluid Management/Goal-Directed Fluid Therapy

Fluid optimization is an essential component of ERAS. It is well known that a liberal fluid therapy approach leads to overload conditions, which can worsen the lung compliance, compromise tissue perfusion, and increase the risk of postoperative complications, such as ileus, which is particularly common in intraabdominal and gynecologic surgeries. On the other hand, a very restrictive approach is also associated with harmful effects secondary to insufficient perfusion to highly dependent organs, such as the kidney or brain. Therefore, euvolemia and optimization of fluid therapy are major ERAS components to positively impact patient outcomes. Goal-directed reductions of intravenous fluids and the zero-balance approach are 2 strategies frequently used to guide fluid administration intraoperatively and have become fundamental concepts central to ERAS. More recent literature has opted for patient risk-based algorithms where there is a tendency to limit the use of GDFT to patients with high-complexity procedures and those with multiple comorbidities.[55] For high-risk surgical patients, goal-directed therapy (GDT), a simple technique to manipulate hemodynamics with the use of fluids and inotropes to improve tissue perfusion and oxygenation, has been associated with improvements in short- and long-term outcomes.[56,57] Although the previous studies observing the effect of GDT delivered in the intensive care unit were conducted in the perioperative period, in 2005, Pearse and colleagues[57] showed that even GDT in the immediate postoperative period only led to improved postoperative outcomes and a lower in-hospital length of stay. As such, GDT may have the potential to improve the quality of care while avoiding excessive expenditures. Despite these favorable results, the widespread implementation of GDT has not been accomplished. Some of the main obstacles are limited resource availability, additional costs related to acquisition and maintenance of new devices, a reluctance of health professionals toward change,[58] and an academic debate about the clinical and cost-effectiveness of the technique.

A meta-analysis comparing GDFT versus conventional therapy within ERAS programs showed no major differences using either technique.[59] Although there is still conflicting evidence and mixed opinions, ERAS societies have suggested for gynecologic surgeries to use a risk-based algorithmic fluid replacement approach in which "zero balance" is used for low-risk patients or low-risk surgeries, whereas GDFT is used in high-risk patients with multiple cocomorbidities or expected increased blood loss.[11]

Emerging literature has associated ERAS implementation with increased rates of postoperative acute kidney injury (AKI).[60] The plausible causes behind this phenomenon can be the indiscriminate use of nonsteroidal anti-inflammatory drugs, epidural-associated hypotensive events, and highly restrictive fluid approaches in some protocols. Another reason to consider is the fact that approximately 20% to 30% of patients with gynecologic cancer arrive to surgery with altered renal function secondary to obstructive uropathy.[61] Keeping this point in mind, it is recommended to individualize patient care and develop institutional risk-stratification systems to identify the group of patients at higher risk of AKI.

Anesthetic Technique

Multiple factors might influence the best anesthetic choice in gynecologic surgery. ERAS guidelines recommend the use of short-acting anesthetics, either inhalational agents (ie, sevoflurane or desflurane) or continuous controlled infusions of intravenous pharmacologic agents (propofol, lidocaine, ketamine) to allow a faster neurocognitive recovery and minimal adverse effects (nausea, vomiting).[11] Recent evidence suggests that total intravenous anesthesia could potentially provide better pain control and less opioid consumption when compared with inhalational anesthesia, but still further validation is needed to prove this finding within ERAS programs.[62] In addition to these recommendations, a high-impact antiemetic prophylactic regimen with at least 2 drugs is also recommended. Although faster emergence can also be obtained by using nitrous oxide, it is reasonable to avoid this gas because of the increased risk of nausea and vomiting, especially in the surgical gynecologic population.

Intraoperative infusion of opioid-sparing agents and regional anesthetic techniques are major components of ERAS in gynecologic surgery. Neuraxial anesthesia is frequently used in gynecologic surgery,[63] as this technique has less systemic effects and better postoperative recovery compared with general anesthesia. In addition, moderate quality of evidence suggests the potential benefits of epidural and spinal anesthesia strategies, when compared with general anesthesia, including less risk of venous thromboembolism, blood loss, pneumonia, respiratory depression, arrhythmias, and renal failure.[64] Moreover, there is evidence showing the use of intrathecal fentanyl as an adjuvant that prolongs analgesia and reduces the risk of shivering, nausea, and vomiting.[65] Despite these benefits, it is also suggested to be selective in the use of epidurals and to outweigh its risks given some concerns of delaying mobilization, the need of more opioids if epidural anesthesia is not effective, and even the risk of iatrogenic hypervolemia or inotropic overuse because of the higher risk of hypotension.[66]

Certainly, some intravenous analgesics are preferred depending on particular scenarios, such as chronic opioid dependence (eg, methadone, hydromorphone), elderly patients at high risk of delirium (dexmedetomidine), concomitant neuropathic pain (gabapentinoids and ketamine), or cases at risk of opioid-induced hyperalgesia (magnesium sulfate).[67] The later section "Multimodal Analgesia" provides more details.

In addition to the conventional anesthetic management, ventilation should use the necessary protective lung measures with lower tidal volumes (5–7 mL/kg), positive end-expiratory pressure (6–8 cm H_2O), and alveolar recruitment maneuvers (increasing airway pressure up to 30–40 cmH_2O for 20–30 seconds). The use of the bispectral index to guide anesthetic depth is also recommended with limited quality of evidence, as well as monitoring of neuromuscular block depth and ensuring complete reversal with strong evidence. Other major outcomes, such as survival or cancer recurrence, have been associated with avoidance of inhalational anesthesia based on observational data; however, a recent large multicenter trial published by Sessler and colleagues[68] found no differences between the 2 anesthetic modalities.

Multimodal Analgesia

Postoperative pain causes significant economic and disability burden with nearly half of the patients experiencing severe pain after gynecologic procedures,[69] of which mostly accounts for oncologic patients.[70] Pain control using multiple modalities has been considered the cornerstone of ERAS protocols in gynecology.[63] Multimodal analgesia means the synergistic combination of multiple pharmacologic analgesics aiming for a superior control of pain. The main reason behind its effectiveness is the blockade of different pain pathways (ie, ascending or descending) at multiple targets along the nervous system (both central and peripheral), which allows better pain control and potentially reduces the risk of central sensitization.[18] This technique has become popular in many other areas besides acute postoperative pain, such as in chronic and neuropathic pain. Several pain medications have been proposed (see **Table 3**), and varied combinations are frequently administered in ERAS programs with the main goal of avoiding opioid consumption (opioid sparing) and consequently preventing opioid-induced side effects.

A recent evidence-based review by Grant and colleagues[71] summarized a consensus of experts about best practices in perioperative care for ERPs in gynecologic surgeries. With regards to multimodal analgesia, it is suggested to use neuraxial techniques (epidural or spinal), preemptive pain medications (acetaminophen, gabapentin), intraoperative incisional infiltration or intraperitoneal instillation of local anesthetic, and postoperative peripheral nerve blocks. An increasingly evolving analgesic modality in gynecologic surgery is regional blocks, especially transversus abdominis plane (TAP) block with inconsistent results,[72] quadratus lumborum block with superior analgesia,[73] or sacral plexus blocks, which are mainly used for pelvic surgery.[63]

On average, physicians prescribe 4 times the necessary amount of opioids after gynecologic surgery. Undoubtedly this has led to a dramatic increase in excesses opioids with deleterious health consequences, such as opioid misuse, diversion, abuse, suicide, readmission, and reoperation.[74] Recent efforts have been made to predict the risk of postoperative opioid use and individualize patients' opioid prescriptions, which may help to lessen the contribution to the opioid epidemic in the United States.[75,76] A recent cohort study showed that ERAS in gynecologic surgery is feasible and safe to reduce postoperative opioid prescribing, particularly in the subset of older Caucasian patients.[76] In recent years of the era of pro-ERAS, there has been an increased interest for the development of ultrarestrictive opioid regimens, which possesses favorable evidence[77] but still needs further research. Future updates on ERAS guidelines will need to address these insights (preoperative opioid management and ultrarestrictive opioid regimens).

BENIGN GYNECOLOGIC SURGERY

Hysterectomy is the most frequent procedure indicated for benign gynecologic entities. ERAS protocols for hysterectomies have similar structure, principles, and items to the protocols in Gynecology/Oncologic surgery, but existing evidence has yielded controversial results regarding its cost-effectiveness and reduction of complications. Several cohort studies in hysterectomy have shown benefit only in length of stay, but no difference in complications or readmissions.[24,78] As for the surgical technique, although there is a tendency to prefer the vaginal approach over laparoscopy for hysterectomies, recent evidence suggests that either of those approaches will result in similar outcomes with the exception of lower costs and rates of vaginal dehiscence when using the vaginal approach.[79] Similarly, ERAS guidelines have been applied in many other elective procedures, such as urogynecologic surgeries, pelvic floor reconstruction surgeries,[80] and ambulatory minor surgeries with conflicting results in terms of cost-effectiveness and complications.[81]

PITFALLS OF IMPLEMENTING ENHANCED RECOVERY AFTER SURGERY IN GYNECOLOGIC SURGERY

Although ERAS guidelines pretend to standardize the most impactful practices in order to improve patient outcomes, there is still a wide interinstitutional variability, which may limit the external validation of the ERAS practices, as well as contribute to the increase in the heterogeneity of ERAS effectiveness across the studies. Recent survey studies have shown that the adherence to ERAS elements in gynecologic surgeries remains highly variable even within the members of ERAS societies.[82] This clearly reflects the need for further studies looking at the barriers for ERAS implementation. Some investigators have proposed introducing an ERAS nurse specialist in order to assist with protocol compliance and goal attainment.[83] Other barriers of compliance include the health care disparities, poor communication between the teams, and lack of a culture to adopt goals.

FUTURE INCLUSIONS IN ENHANCED RECOVERY AFTER SURGERY IN GYNECOLOGICAL SURGERY

Upcoming insights for ERAS in gynecologic surgery will be focused on its effectiveness in high risk of gynecologic surgeries, such as pelvic exenteration and hyperthermic intraperitoneal chemotherapy, which possess tremendous morbidity and complication rates. The minimization of complications in these surgeries remains challenging, and the few published cohort studies have not appreciated significant benefits in this population.[84] Further clarification regarding new analgesic regimens, better antiemetic prophylaxis, and introduction of new preventive measures against postoperative ileus is needed to hasten the recovery for these major procedures. Future insights on prehabilitation, multimodal analgesia, and GDFT would also be at the center of expert discussions, especially some unclear considerations, such as the optimal time to initiate prehabilitation, who will most likely obtain benefit from prehabilitation, and how to use a selective fluid therapy strategy depending on surgical and patient risks.

Furthermore, it is noteworthy to mention that an important weakness of ERAS research in gynecology, as evidenced in this review, is the lack of compliance reporting of ERAS interventions in most of the trials conducted to the date (only 4 out of 9 RCTs reported compliance rates based on **Table 3**). As mentioned previously, this is a critical component not only to enhance the benefits of ERAS protocols but also to be able to critically appraise the literature on ERAS in gynecologic surgery and to drive further recommendations in the future.

SUMMARY

Recent advances on the quality of the evidence, surgical techniques, and perioperative care have included or modified some practices within recovery pathways. Newly updated ERAS guidelines for gynecologic surgeries comprise a more complete bundle of multidisciplinary interventions aimed to provide faster recovery while minimizing complications and health care costs. Further research efforts should focus on the unclear effects of ERAS on patient satisfaction, optimal prehabilitation, methods to improve compliance, and restrictive opioid management.

DISCLOSURE

The authors have no conflicts of interests.

REFERENCES

1. Oliphant SS, Jones KA, Wang L, et al. Trends over time with commonly performed obstetric and gynecologic inpatient procedures. Obstet Gynecol 2010;116: 926–31.

2. Miralpeix E, Nick AM, Meyer LA, et al. A call for new standard of care in perioperative gynecologic oncology practice: impact of enhanced recovery after surgery (ERAS) programs. Gynecol Oncol 2016;141:371–8.

3. Ljungqvist O, Scott M, Fearon KC. Enhanced recovery after surgery: a review. JAMA Surg 2017;152:292–8.

4. Altman AD, Helpman L, McGee J, et al. Enhanced recovery after surgery: implementing a new standard of surgical care. CMAJ 2019;191:E469–75.

5. Nelson G, Kalogera E, Dowdy SC. Enhanced recovery pathways in gynecologic oncology. Gynecol Oncol 2014;135:586–94.

6. Committee on Gynecologic P. ACOG committee opinion no. 750: perioperative pathways: enhanced recovery after surgery. Obstet Gynecol 2018;132:e120–30.

7. Pache B, Joliat GR, Hubner M, et al. Cost-analysis of enhanced recovery after surgery (ERAS) program in gynecologic surgery. Gynecol Oncol 2019;154: 388–93.

8. Harrison RF, Li Y, Guzman A, et al. Impact of implementation of an enhanced recovery program in gynecologic surgery on healthcare costs. Am J Obstet Gynecol 2020;222:66.e1–9.

9. Meyer LA, Lasala J, Iniesta MD, et al. Effect of an enhanced recovery after surgery program on opioid use and patient-reported outcomes. Obstet Gynecol 2018;132:281–90.

10. Marcus RK, Lillemoe HA, Rice DC, et al. Determining the safety and efficacy of enhanced recovery protocols in major oncologic surgery: an institutional NSQIP analysis. Ann Surg Oncol 2019;26:782–90.

11. Nelson G, Bakkum-Gamez J, Kalogera E, et al. Guidelines for perioperative care in gynecologic/oncology: Enhanced Recovery after Surgery (ERAS) Society recommendations—2019 update. Int J Gynecol Cancer 2019;29:651–68.

12. Nelson G, Altman AD, Nick A, et al. Guidelines for pre- and intra-operative care in gynecologic/oncology surgery: Enhanced Recovery after Surgery (ERAS(R)) Society recommendations–part I. Gynecol Oncol 2016;140:313–22.

13. Nelson G, Altman AD, Nick A, et al. Guidelines for postoperative care in gynecologic/oncology surgery: Enhanced Recovery after Surgery (ERAS(R)) Society recommendations–part II. Gynecol Oncol 2016;140:323–32.

14. Bauchat JR, Habib AS. Evidence-based anesthesia for major gynecologic surgery. Anesthesiol Clin 2015;33:173–207.

15. Elias KM, Stone AB, McGinigle K, et al. The reporting on ERAS compliance, outcomes, and elements research (recover) checklist: a joint statement by the ERAS((R)) and ERAS((R)) USA societies. World J Surg 2019;43:1–8.

16. Altman AD, Nelson GS. Society of Gynecologic Oncology of Canada Annual General Meeting CPD, Communities of Practice Education C. The Canadian Gynaecologic Oncology Perioperative Management survey: baseline practice prior to implementation of Enhanced Recovery After Surgery (ERAS) Society guidelines. J Obstet Gynaecol Can 2016;38:1105–9.e2.

17. Modesitt SC, Sarosiek BM, Trowbridge ER, et al. Enhanced recovery implementation in major gynecologic surgeries: effect of care standardization. Obstet Gynecol 2016;128:457–66.

18. Jarrell J, Robert M, Giamberardino MA, et al. Pain, psychosocial tests, pain sensitization and laparoscopic pelvic surgery. Scand J Pain 2018;18:49–57.

19. Nelson G, Dowdy SC, Lasala J, et al. Enhanced recovery after surgery (ERAS(R)) in gynecologic oncology - practical considerations for program development. Gynecol Oncol 2017;147:617–20.

20. Simon NV, Heaps KP, Chodroff CH. Improving the processes of care and outcomes in obstetrics/gynecology. Jt Comm J Qual Improv 1997;23:485–97.

21. de Groot JJ, Maessen JM, Slangen BF, et al. A stepped strategy that aims at the nationwide implementation of the enhanced recovery after surgery programme in major gynaecological surgery: study protocol of a cluster randomised controlled trial. Implement Sci 2015;10:106.

22. de Groot JJ, van Es LE, Maessen JM, et al. Diffusion of enhanced recovery principles in gynecologic oncology surgery: is active implementation still necessary? Gynecol Oncol 2014;134:570–5.

23. Iniesta MD, Lasala J, Mena G, et al. Impact of compliance with an enhanced recovery after surgery pathway on patient outcomes in open gynecologic surgery. Int J Gynecol Cancer 2019;29:1417–24.

24. Wijk L, Udumyan R, Pache B, et al. International validation of Enhanced Recovery After Surgery Society guidelines on enhanced recovery for gynecologic surgery. Am J Obstet Gynecol 2019;221:237.e1–11.

25. Bisch SP, Wells T, Gramlich L, et al. Enhanced recovery after surgery (ERAS) in gynecologic oncology: system-wide implementation and audit leads to improved value and patient outcomes. Gynecol Oncol 2018;151:117–23.

26. Gan TJTJ, Miller TE, Scott MJ, et al. Enhanced recovery for major abdominopelvic surgery. West Islip (NY): NY Professional Communications; 2016.

27. de Groot JJ, Ament SM, Maessen JM, et al. Enhanced recovery pathways in abdominal gynecologic surgery: a systematic review and meta-analysis. Acta Obstet Gynecol Scand 2016;95:382–95.

28. Burgos R, Sanchez-Iglesias JL, Cardenas G, et al. Mon-p240: enhanced recovery after surgery protocol (ERAS) for advanced gynecological cancer. Preliminary results. Clin Nutr 2016;35:S241.

29. Lashkul OS, Gavrylyuk VP, Pavelko NO. Fast track surgery - multimodal strategy of postoperative period management in gynecological patients. The role of anesthesiologists. Clin Anesthesiology Intensive Care 2017;1:21–8.

30. Dickson EL, Stockwell E, Geller MA, et al. Enhanced recovery program and length of stay after laparotomy on a gynecologic oncology service: a randomized controlled trial. Obstet Gynecol 2017;129:355–62.

31. Antypin E, Uvarov D, Antypina N, et al. Effect of enhanced recovery after surgery (ERAS) on secretion of pro-inflammatory cytokines and C-reactive protein after hysterectomy. Eur J Anesthesiology 2013;30:13.

32. Bourazani M, Karopoulou E, Fyrfiris N. Ep1096 Implementing enhanced recovery after surgery (ERAS) pathways in major gynecologic oncology operations in Greece (the pre-eliminary results of our department). Int J Gynecol Cancer 2019;29:A573–4.

33. Ferrari F, Forte S, Sbalzer N. Validation of an ERAS protocol in gynecological surgery: interim analysis of an Italian randomized controlled trial. Int J Gynecol Cancer 2019;29:A40.

34. Sánchez-Iglesias J, Carbonell Socias M, Pérez Benavente A, et al. Enhanced recovery after surgery in advanced ovarian cancer: a prospective randomized trial. Int J Gynecol Cancer 2019;29:A33.

35. Johnson K, Razo S, Smith J, et al. Optimize patient outcomes among females undergoing gynecological surgery: a randomized controlled trial. Appl Nurs Res 2019;45:39–44.

36. Yi HC, Ibrahim Z, Abu Zaid Z, et al. Impact of enhanced recovery after surgery with preoperative whey protein-infused carbohydrate loading and postoperative

early oral feeding among surgical gynecologic cancer patients: an open-labelled randomized controlled trial. Nutrients 2020;12(1):264.

37. Pallett AC, Nguyen BT, Klein NM, et al. A randomized controlled trial to determine whether a video presentation improves informed consent for hysterectomy. Am J Obstet Gynecol 2018;219:277.e1–7.

38. Schenker Y, Fernandez A, Sudore R, et al. Interventions to improve patient comprehension in informed consent for medical and surgical procedures: a systematic review. Med Decis Making 2011;31:151–73.

39. Chan JL, Letourneau J, Salem W, et al. Regret around fertility choices is decreased with pre-treatment counseling in gynecologic cancer patients. J Cancer Surviv 2017;11:58–63.

40. Dolmans MM. Recent advances in fertility preservation and counseling for female cancer patients. Expert Rev Anticancer Ther 2018;18:115–20.

41. Kalogera E, Dowdy S. Prehabilitation: enhancing the enhanced recovery after surgery pathway. Int J Gynecol Cancer 2019;29:1233–4.

42. McLennan E, Oliphant R, Moug SJ. Limited preoperative physical capacity continues to be associated with poor postoperative outcomes within a colorectal ERAS programme. Ann R Coll Surg Engl 2019;101:261–7.

43. Miralpeix E, Mancebo G, Gayete S, et al. Role and impact of multimodal prehabilitation for gynecologic oncology patients in an enhanced recovery after surgery (ERAS) program. Int J Gynecol Cancer 2019;29:1235–43.

44. Bisch S, Nelson G, Altman A. Impact of nutrition on enhanced recovery after surgery (ERAS) in gynecologic oncology. Nutrients 2019;11(5):1088.

45. Sanusi RS. Outcome of combined neoadjuvant chemotherapy and vitamin a in advanced cervical carcinoma: a randomized double-blind clinical trial. Asian Pac J Cancer Prev 2019;20:2213–8.

46. Practice guidelines for preoperative fasting and the use of pharmacologic agents to reduce the risk of pulmonary aspiration: application to healthy patients undergoing elective procedures: an updated report by the American Society of Anesthesiologists Task Force on preoperative fasting and the use of pharmacologic agents to reduce the risk of pulmonary aspiration. Anesthesiology 2017;126:376–93.

47. Lindemann K, Kok PS, Stockler M, et al. Enhanced recovery after surgery for advanced ovarian cancer: a systematic review of interventions trialed. Int J Gynecol Cancer 2017;27:1274–82.

48. Xu C, Peng J, Liu S, et al. Effect of chewing gum on gastrointestinal function after gynecological surgery: a systematic literature review and meta-analysis. J Obstet Gynaecol Res 2018;44:936–43.

49. Terzioglu F, Simsek S, Karaca K, et al. Multimodal interventions (chewing gum, early oral hydration and early mobilisation) on the intestinal motility following abdominal gynaecologic surgery. J Clin Nurs 2013;22:1917–25.

50. Hopkins L, Brown-Broderick J, Hearn J, et al. Implementation of a referral to discharge glycemic control initiative for reduction of surgical site infections in gynecologic oncology patients. Gynecol Oncol 2017;146:228–33.

51. Al-Niaimi AN, Ahmed M, Burish N, et al. Intensive postoperative glucose control reduces the surgical site infection rates in gynecologic oncology patients. Gynecol Oncol 2015;136:71–6.

52. Galaal K, Donkers H, Bryant A, et al. Laparoscopy versus laparotomy for the management of early stage endometrial cancer. Cochrane Database Syst Rev 2018;10:CD006655.

53. Wang YZ, Deng L, Xu HC, et al. Laparoscopy versus laparotomy for the management of early stage cervical cancer. BMC Cancer 2015;15:928.
54. Lawrie TA, Liu H, Lu D, et al. Robot-assisted surgery in gynaecology. Cochrane Database Syst Rev 2019;4:CD011422.
55. Miller TE, Roche AM, Mythen M. Fluid management and goal-directed therapy as an adjunct to enhanced recovery after surgery (ERAS). Can J Anaesth 2015;62: 158–68.
56. Michard F. The burden of high-risk surgery and the potential benefit of goal-directed strategies. Crit Care 2011;15:447.
57. Pearse R, Dawson D, Fawcett J, et al. Early goal-directed therapy after major surgery reduces complications and duration of hospital stay. A randomised, controlled trial [ISRCTN38797445]. Crit Care 2005;9:R687–93.
58. Bennett D, Chaloner E, Mythen M. Modernising care for Patients Undergoing Major Surgery: Improving Patient Outcomes and Increasing Clinical Efficiency. A Report by the Improving Surgical Outcomes Group. 2005.
59. Rollins KE, Lobo DN. Intraoperative goal-directed fluid therapy in elective major abdominal surgery: a meta-analysis of randomized controlled trials. Ann Surg 2016;263:465–76.
60. Koerner CP, Lopez-Aguiar AG, Zaidi M, et al. Caution: increased acute kidney injury in enhanced recovery after surgery (ERAS) protocols. Am Surg 2019;85: 156–61.
61. Patel K, Foster NR, Kumar A, et al. Hydronephrosis in patients with cervical cancer: an assessment of morbidity and survival. Support Care Cancer 2015;23: 1303–9.
62. Lin WL, Lee MS, Wong CS, et al. Effects of intraoperative propofol-based total intravenous anesthesia on postoperative pain in spine surgery: comparison with desflurane anesthesia - a randomised trial. Medicine (Baltimore) 2019;98: e15074.
63. Munro A, Sjaus A, George RB. Anesthesia and analgesia for gynecological surgery. Curr Opin Anaesthesiol 2018;31:274–9.
64. Popping DM, Elia N, Van Aken HK, et al. Impact of epidural analgesia on mortality and morbidity after surgery: systematic review and meta-analysis of randomized controlled trials. Ann Surg 2014;259:1056–67.
65. Uppal V, Retter S, Casey M, et al. Efficacy of intrathecal fentanyl for cesarean delivery: a systematic review and meta-analysis of randomized controlled trials with trial sequential analysis. Anesth Analg 2020;130:111–25.
66. Huepenbecker SP, Cusworth SE, Kuroki LM, et al. Continuous epidural infusion in gynecologic oncology patients undergoing exploratory laparotomy: the new standard for decreased postoperative pain and opioid use. Gynecol Oncol 2019;153: 356–61.
67. Lee C, Song YK, Jeong HM, et al. The effects of magnesium sulfate infiltration on perioperative opioid consumption and opioid-induced hyperalgesia in patients undergoing robot-assisted laparoscopic prostatectomy with remifentanil-based anesthesia. Korean J Anesthesiol 2011;61:244–50.
68. Sessler DI, Pei L, Huang Y, et al. Recurrence of breast cancer after regional or general anaesthesia: a randomised controlled trial. Lancet 2019;394:1807–15.
69. Henschke N, Kamper SJ, Maher CG. The epidemiology and economic consequences of pain. Mayo Clin Proc 2015;90:139–47.
70. Cata JP, Lasala J, Bugada D. Best practice in the administration of analgesia in postoncological surgery. Pain Manag 2015;5:273–84.

71. Grant MC, Gibbons MM, Ko CY, et al. Evidence review conducted for the AHRQ Safety Program for improving surgical care and recovery: focus on anesthesiology for gynecologic surgery. Reg Anesth Pain Med 2019. https://doi.org/10.1136/rapm-2018-100071.

72. Bacal V, Rana U, McIsaac DI, et al. Transversus abdominis plane block for post hysterectomy pain: a systematic review and meta-analysis. J Minim Invasive Gynecol 2019;26:40–52.

73. Yousef NK. Quadratus lumborum block versus transversus abdominis plane block in patients undergoing total abdominal hysterectomy: a randomized prospective controlled trial. Anesth Essays Res 2018;12:742–7.

74. Soffin EM, Lee BH, Kumar KK, et al. The prescription opioid crisis: role of the anaesthesiologist in reducing opioid use and misuse. Br J Anaesth 2019;122:e198–208.

75. Johnson CM, Makai GEH. A systematic review of perioperative opioid management for minimally invasive hysterectomy. J Minim Invasive Gynecol 2019;26:233–43.

76. Hillman RT, Sanchez-Migallon A, Meyer LA, et al. Patient characteristics and opioid use prior to discharge after open gynecologic surgery in an enhanced recovery after surgery (ERAS) program. Gynecol Oncol 2019;153:604–9.

77. Mark J, Argentieri DM, Gutierrez CA, et al. Ultrarestrictive opioid prescription protocol for pain management after gynecologic and abdominal surgery. JAMA Netw Open 2018;1:e185452.

78. Yoong W, Sivashanmugarajan V, Relph S, et al. Can enhanced recovery pathways improve outcomes of vaginal hysterectomy? Cohort control study. J Minim Invasive Gynecol 2014;21:83–9.

79. Sandberg EM, Twijnstra ARH, Driessen SRC, et al. Total laparoscopic hysterectomy versus vaginal hysterectomy: a systematic review and meta-analysis. J Minim Invasive Gynecol 2017;24:206–17.e2.

80. Gong R, Hu Q, Liu D, et al. Enhanced recovery after surgery versus traditional care in total pelvic floor reconstruction surgery with transvaginal mesh. Int J Gynaecol Obstet 2020;148:107–12.

81. Carter-Brooks CM, Du AL, Ruppert KM, et al. Implementation of a urogynecology-specific enhanced recovery after surgery (ERAS) pathway. Am J Obstet Gynecol 2018;219:495.e1–10.

82. Ore AS, Shear MA, Liu FW, et al. Adoption of enhanced recovery after laparotomy in gynecologic oncology. Int J Gynecol Cancer 2020;30:122–7.

83. Kahokehr A, Sammour T, Zargar-Shoshtari K, et al. Implementation of ERAS and how to overcome the barriers. Int J Surg 2009;7:16–9.

84. Funder JA, Tolstrup R, Jepsen BN, et al. Postoperative paralytic ileus remains a problem following surgery for advanced pelvic cancers. J Surg Res 2017;218:167–73.

Anaesthesia for Major Urological Surgery

Jaishel Patel, MBChB, BSc, FRCA*, Christopher N. Jones, MBBS(LOND), FRCA, MD(Res)

KEYWORDS

- Enhanced recovery • Shared decision making • Perioperative anesthesia
- Robotic surgery • Laparoscopic • Prostatectomy • Cystectomy
- Analgesia for major surgery

KEY POINTS

- Anesthesia for major urology surgery has changed with the advent of laparoscopic and robot-assisted surgical techniques.
- Enhanced recovery pathways are now established in complex major urologic surgery and are reducing lengths of stay and postoperative complications.
- The success of enhanced recovery pathways in urologic surgery depends on preoperative assessment, preparation, and compliance with all the perioperative elements.
- Attention to detail and fastidious preparation are the keys to successful anesthesia and outcomes in robotic surgery.

PATIENT POPULATION

Bladder Cancer

Bladder cancer is the eighth most common cancer in the United Kingdom (UK). There is a male preponderance with a ratio of approximately 3:1. Most cases are diagnosed in people aged more than 75. 1 in 3 cases of bladder cancer are due to smoking.[1] Treatment options for muscle-invasive bladder cancer include cystectomy with urinary diversion, with the formation of an ileal conduit or neobladder, systemic chemotherapy, and radiotherapy. Individualized patient treatment plans are formulated according to disease progression, risk of recurrence, and patient clinical status.[2]

Renal Cell Carcinoma

The vast majority ($\sim$90%) of solid renal masses are renal cell carcinomas (RCC); the remainder comprising mainly of transitional cell carcinoma or Wilms' tumor (in

Royal Surrey NHS Foundation Trust, Royal Surrey County Hospital, Egerton Road, Guildford, Surrey, GU2 7XX, UK
* Corresponding author.
E-mail address: jaishelpatel@nhs.net

Anesthesiology Clin 40 (2022) 175–197
https://doi.org/10.1016/j.anclin.2021.11.009
1932-2275/22/© 2021 Elsevier Inc. All rights reserved.

anesthesiology.theclinics.com

children). RCC accounts for between 1% and 3% of all visceral malignancies. It is twice as common in men when compared with women and most commonly presents in the seventh decade of life. The main environmental risk factor is cigarette smoking, contributing to one-third of all cases. Other important risk factors include obesity, hypertension, asbestos exposure, and acquired polycystic kidney disease. Surgical management of RCC includes radical or partial nephrectomy with nephron-sparing surgery reserved for those with metastatic disease.[3]

PROSTATE CANCER

Prostate cancer is predominantly a disease of older men (aged 65–79 years) and is the most common cancer in men in the UK. In the UK, about 1 in 8 men will be diagnosed with prostate cancer in their lifetime.[4,5] Options for the management of prostate cancer include conservative surveillance, radiotherapy, hormone therapy, or radical prostatectomy. Radical prostatectomy is usually recommended for patients whereby disease is confined to the prostate and life expectancy is over 10 years.[6]

PREASSESSMENT

Patients undergoing major urologic procedures are elderly patients with significant other systemic comorbidities. There is clear evidence that older and frail patients run a higher risk for complications following major abdominal surgery (British Geriatrics Society).

Patients with cancer pose additional challenges for the peri-operative team. Assessment and optimization of these high-risk patients are achieved via specialized high-risk clinics. These provide the opportunity for shared decision-making with a strong multidisciplinary team input, whereby the risks and benefits of the proposed surgery can be comprehended fully by the patient within the context of their own lives. Risk assessment facilitates meaningful informed patient consent and shared decision-making, empowering patients to make decisions in partnership with clinicians.[7]

Perioperative morbidity and mortality are significant health issues as they impact on patients' short- and long-term survival and resource utilization within health services.[8] Accurate risk stratification helps identify those at increased risk of adverse perioperative events who may benefit from targeted interventions. These include preoperative optimization, intraoperative goal-directed fluid therapy, postoperative respiratory support, and admission to critical care.[8] It allows for preoperative patient optimization and modification of the surgical pathway as required.

Comorbidities such as COPD, ischemic heart disease, hypertension, diabetes, and anemia can be addressed in clinic allowing clinicians to optimize medications and formulate anticoagulation bridging plans. A retrospective cohort analysis found that unresolved most of these comorbidities were identified risk factors for complications after cystectomy.[9]

Essential blood tests, ECGs and imaging, and correspondence can be requested at this stage to enable the risk of the stratification process.

Cardiopulmonary exercise testing (CPET) is an individualized assessment of a patient's cardiorespiratory function and provides objective functional data (anaerobic threshold (AT), peak oxygen consumption (peak V_{O_2}), and ventilatory equivalents

(VE/VECO2) that have specifically been shown to be independent predictors of mortality, morbidity, and length of hospital stay.[10,11]

Several risk stratification tools exist, though it is not established which scoring system or model is the best predictor of risk for major urology surgery. Current commonly used scores include P-POSSUM, Surgical Outcomes Risk Tool (SORT), and the Surgical Risk Calculator Score (ACS NSQIP).[12–14] Clinical judgment alone is not a reliable predictor of an adverse outcome.[8] The combination of a good patient history and an objective measure of functional capacity helps to risk stratify.

Prehabilitation

Prehabilitation refers to the multimodal process of improving a patient's functional status before surgery to enhance their body's ability to cope with a stressful event and therefore improve their postoperative outcome.[15]

Key aspects of prehabilitation focus on:

1. Preoperative exercise.
2. *Nutritional optimization*: Up to 33% of urology patients undergoing surgery are at nutritional risk.[16] For Open cystectomy surgery, preoperative malnutrition independently increases the mortality rate.[17]
3. *Psychological counseling*: This has been shown to reduced anxiety in abdominal surgery. Multi-disciplinary team (MDT) counseling has been a component of ERAS implementation by Pang and colleagues,[18] involving the surgeon, cancer nurse specialist, and stoma therapist in the preoperative patient education.
4. *Lifestyle modification*: Smoking, obesity and excessive alcohol have all shown to have a negative impact on postoperative outcomes. Smoking cessation for 4 to 8 weeks before surgery has been shown to significantly reduce pulmonary and wound complications.[19] Just 4 weeks of alcohol abstinence has been shown to decrease morbidity and shorten patient hospital stay.[20]

A narrative review looking at the current evidence based on prehabilitation concluded that there are no randomized controlled trials (RCTs) that have evaluated the effect of smoking or alcohol cessation interventions on complications or health relayed quality of life (HRQoL) in radical cystectomy. Patient education interventions focusing on stoma care significantly improve self-efficacy regarding independent change of stoma-appliance up to 1-year postoperatively.[21]

Published data to date indicate that a group of preoperative multi-professional interventions including physical exercises, supportive nutritional care, and stoma education can postoperatively improve early mobilization, self-efficacy, and health-related quality of life (HRQoL). However, this has not yet translated into reducing the length of stay or complications.[22]

ENHANCED RECOVERY AFTER SURGERY IN MAJOR SURGERY

Enhanced recovery after surgery (ERAS) protocols are a combination of multimodal evidence-based strategies, applied to conventional perioperative techniques, to reduce postoperative morbidity and achieve early recovery. ERAS pathways aim to standardize the variations in practice while delivering high quality to care patients from the point of diagnosis to discharge (**Fig. 1**).

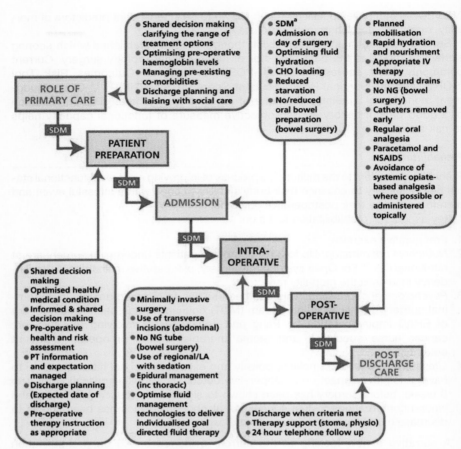

Fig. 1. ER for gastrointestinal surgery (Department of Health). [a] SDM, shared decision-making. (Information from the NHS website is licensed under the Open Government License v3.0.)

ERAS protocols were initially designed for colorectal surgeries and have now been widely adapted and implemented by many different surgical subspecialties throughout the UK.[23] ERAS programs within urology are predominantly adapted from colorectal protocols[24].

These protocols have been shown to reduce the surgical stress response to surgery, improve postoperative recovery and reduce LOS.[25] Postsurgical complications following colorectal surgery have been reduced by up to 50%, and hospital stay by 2.5 days.[26]

There are 4 key areas to any ERAS protocol:

1. Appropriate preoperative assessment, patient identification, and preparation before admission.
2. Reducing physical stress of the operation—through a series of modifications to surgical and anesthetic intraoperative care.
3. A structured approach to immediate postoperative care, including pain relief and nutrition.
4. Early mobilization (**Fig. 2**).

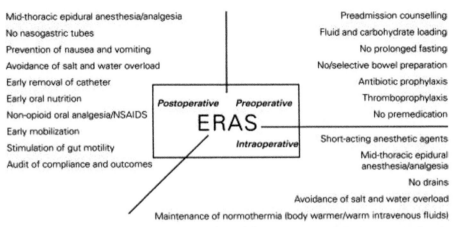

Mid-thoracic epidural anesthesia/analgesia
No nasogastric tubes
Prevention of nausea and vomiting
Avoidance of salt and water overload
Early removal of catheter
Early oral nutrition
Non-opioid oral analgesia/NSAIDS
Early mobilization
Stimulation of gut motility
Audit of compliance and outcomes

Postoperative   Preoperative

ERAS

Intraoperative

Preadmission counselling
Fluid and carbohydrate loading
No prolonged fasting
No/selective bowel preparation
Antibiotic prophylaxis
Thromboprophylaxis
No premedication

Short-acting anesthetic agents
Mid-thoracic epidural anesthesia/analgesia
No drains
Avoidance of salt and water overload
Maintenance of normothermia (body warmer/warm intravenous fluids)

Fig. 2. Key aspects of ERAS protocols. (*Adapted from* Donat et al. Early nasogastric tube removal combined with metoclopramide after radical cystectomy and urinary diversion. J Urol 1999;162:1599–602.(63).)

ENHANCED RECOVERY AFTER SURGERY IN UROLOGY
Minimally Invasive Surgery

Minimally invasive surgery using laparoscopic and robotic techniques are widely used across a variety of surgical specialties (head and neck, thoracic, upper gi, colorectal, hepato-biliary, gynecology, and urology). These advances allow for major complex surgery to take place with a convincing reduction in postoperative surgical and nonsurgical complications, reduced blood loss, improved recovery rates, improved cosmesis, and reduced length of stay in comparison with open surgery.[27–29] Outcomes in the elderly have been shown to be better after robotic surgery in comparison with open surgery, with reduced surgical and medical complications, improved length of stay, and quicker discharge home.[30]

Open radical cystectomy with pelvic lymph node dissection has remained the gold standard for muscle-invasive bladder carcinoma.[31]

This operation presents a significant surgical challenge. The proinflammatory cascade to surgical insult results in a high postoperative oxygen demand and significant fluid shifts.

Despite the standardization of the surgical technique, improved anesthesia and perioperative care protocols, morbidity after open radical cystectomy with bilateral pelvic lymph node dissection and urinary diversion or bladder reconstruction was noted to be up to 30% to 64%.[32]

However, most centers in the UK now use a minimally invasive (MIS, minimally invasive surgery) approach to cystectomy surgery as it is associated with a reduced inflammatory response, reduced risk of postoperative ileus, complications, and length of stay (LOS).[33] MIS encompasses laparoscopic and robotic-assisted surgical techniques.

A recent meta-analysis concluded that MIS approaches were associated with fewer 30-day overall complication and had a trend toward fewer 90-day overall complications. When stratified by type of MIS approaches, robotic-assisted radical cystectomy (RARC) only had a trend toward *fewer* 30- day and 90-day overall complications but laparoscopic radical cystectomy (LRC) was *significantly* associated with fewer risk of 30-day and 90-day overall complications. Although MIS approaches had a longer operative time, they had a significantly shorter time to flatus, time to diet, and LOS.[34]

MIS approaches had better perioperative outcomes, less overall complications, and similar pathologic and oncological outcomes compared with ORC (Open radical cystectomy). When stratified by type of MIS techniques (RARC and LRC), the results were similar.[34]

MIS techniques are associated with reduced narcotic requirements and thus earlier return to bowel function, reduced complications, and reduced LOS.[35,36]

A USA-based multi-centre RCT entitled RAZOR concluded noninferiority between ORC and RARC, having explored data from 350 patients.[37]

PROSTATECTOMY

Radical prostatectomy (RP) is a first-line treatment of patients with low and intermediate-risk localized prostate cancer.[38,39] Open radical prostatectomy is accompanied by extensive operative trauma, a high risk of intraoperative hemorrhage, high rate of operative mortality, pneumonia, DVT, and anastomotic leakage as a result of prolonged postoperative bed rest.[40]

The development of laparoscopic technology has greatly reduced postoperative complications and minimally invasive radical prostatectomies (RPs) are widely applied. Techniques include laparoscopic radical prostatectomy (LRP) and robot-assisted laparoscopic radical prostatectomy (RALP). RALP has become the mainstay invasive treatment of localized prostate cancer.

A retrospective study carried out by Lin and colleagues showed that the times from LRP to first water intake, ambulation, defecation, pelvic drainage-tube removal, and length of hospital stay (LOS) were all significantly shorter. Hospitalization costs and the incidence of postoperative complications were significantly lower in the ERAS group compared with the control group. No deaths or reoperations occurred in either group and there were no readmissions in the ERAS group, within 90 days after surgery. They conclude that ERAS protocols may effectively accelerate patient rehabilitation and reduce LOS and hospitalization costs in patients undergoing LRP.[40]

Recent studies have highlighted the advantages of minimally invasive surgery with many centers opting to carry out day case or up to 48 hour stays post robotic prostatectomies. Abaza and colleagues, 2018 published a single-center study of 500 men showed that same-day discharge following robot-assisted laparoscopic prostatectomy can be safely routinely offered with no increase in readmissions or emergency visits. They highlight a significant cost saving.[41]

A retrospective observational study of 32 patients concluded that radical prostatectomy can be performed routinely in an outpatient setting with no increase in morbidity or decrease in functional and oncological results, with a high patient-family satisfaction rate.[42]

NEPHRECTOMY

RCC commonly presents in patients aged greater than 70 years and most patients undergoing nephrectomy are elderly with comorbidities.

Nephrectomy is the standard treatment of RCC. Partial or radical nephrectomy may be performed according to the tumor characteristics. The European Association of Urology guidelines recommend that patients with mass less than 4 cm may undergo partial nephrectomy.[43]

The surgical approach is individualized and determined by surgeon preference and by disease stage. Radical nephrectomy is considered for patients with cancer with stage I, II, and III diseases. However, those patients with metastatic disease, at risk of developing severe renal impairment, and those with bilateral tumors are likely to be considered for nephron-sparing surgery. Open radical nephrectomy surgery has the same incumbent risks as other major open surgeries the physiologic effects of the surgical stress response, pain, bleeding, and postop complications.

Laparoscopic partial nephrectomy (LPN) and robotic-assisted partial nephrectomy (RaPN) are becoming the standard of care.[44]

A meta-analysis carried out by Tsai and colleagues reviewing 60,000 patients showed that compared with OPN (open nephrectomy), RaPN (robotic-assisted partial nephrectomy) is associated with decreased blood loss, blood transfusion and complication rates, longer operative time, shorter hospital stay, lower readmission rate, and minor eGFR change.[45]

ANESTHETIC CONSIDERATIONS FOR OPEN SURGERY
Preassessment and Preoperative Considerations

Even though most centers are using a minimally invasive approach, conversion to open surgery is still a possibility. There are a proportion of patients who will not be able to undergo these approaches as their disease is inaccessible or they have cardio-respiratory issues which will not allow them to withstand the physiologic demands of a pneumoperitoneum, steep Trendelenburg, or length of surgery.

Typically, these patients tend to be elderly, frail, and have the additional physiologic burdens of cancer, which poses its own set of challenges for the peri-operative anesthetist.

Most factors should have been assessed as part of the preoperative work up of these patients but specific issues to consider are highlighted below with a particular focus on open radical cystectomy.

Carbohydrate loading

While there is no study evaluating carbohydrate loading in cystectomy patients, it has been shown that preoperative loading decreases thirst, reduces insulin resistance, and helps maintain lean body mass and muscle strength in colorectal surgery. It involves the use of clear carbohydrate drinks the day before surgery and up to 2 hours before. In addition to the metabolic effects, it facilitates accelerated recovery through the early return of bowel function and shorter hospital stay.[46]

Carbohydrate drinks are specially formulated for rapid gastric transit with low osmolality. Current consensus from the Association of Anaesthetists of Great Britain and Ireland (AAGBI) is that 2 hours fasting for liquids and 6 hours for solids is correct practice.[47] However, emerging evidence suggests that the liberal consumption of clear fluids before the induction of scheduled day-case anesthesia reduced the rates of postoperative nausea and vomiting.[48]

Bowel preparation

There is no evidence supporting the routine use of bowel preparation in radical cystectomy patients[49].

Preoperative

On the day consultation with the patient should include discussion of the common general anesthesia anesthetic risks (postoperative nausea and vomiting, dental damage, sore throat, presence of endotracheal tube, and positive pressure ventilation).

Further discussion should include analgesia modalities (regional, wound catheter infusions, or patient-controlled analgesia and explanation of the specific benefits and risks pertinent to these.

This encounter is also an opportunity to encourage the patient about postoperative engagement with physiotherapy and early mobilization and engagement with dieticians.

All patients should be consented to large bore intravenous access, invasive lines (central venous catheter and arterial), potential neuropraxias related to positioning, presence of NGT (nasogastric tubes) catheter, and consent for potential transfusion of blood products and requirements for postoperative critical care admission.

Renal impairment: After a radical nephrectomy, one-third of patients will be left with significantly reduced renal reserve, that is, a glomerular filtration rate (GFR) of less than 45 mL/min (CKD stage 3B)

NSAIDS should be avoided and other renally excreted drugs should be dosed appropriately to reflect the reduction glomerular filtration.

Induction

The WHO checklist is a mandated practice for most centers to ensure the surgical safety of patients. A team brief, and "sign in" of the patient should be completed before any procedure takes place.

Mode of anesthesia either using volatile agents or TIVA (total intravenous anesthesia) will be dictated by anesthetist preference, experience, and patient characteristics (avoidance of postoperative nausea and vomiting).

A retrospective analysis by Wigmore and colleagues demonstrated an association between the type of anesthetic delivered and survival. A meta-analysis suggested that propofol-TIVA use may be associated with improved recurrence-free survival and overall survival in patients having major cancer surgery. To date, there has been no RCT evidence to suggest that either TIVA or volatile anesthesia has any impact on cancer recurrence rates.[50]

Intraoperative

Blood loss: The average blood loss during cystectomy is reported to range from 0.56 to 3 L.[48,51]

Assessment of transfusion requirements, optimization of anemia, and intraoperative cell salvage should be considered.[52]

Pain Relief

The etiology of acute postoperative pain is multifactorial and complex. Surgical procedures cause injury to tissues. This triggers a cascade of responses in the pain matrix, from the sensitization of peripheral and central pain pathways to feelings of fear, anxiety, and frustration. Pain post-open urology surgery can be attributed to wound incisional pain, pelvic organ nociception, and urinary catheter discomfort.

For analgesia to be adequate and effective the size and site of the incision should be taken into consideration. The approach for both radical open cystectomy and prostatectomy is lower midline (sub-umbilical). For nephrectomy, 3 incision sites are commonly used, Flank (T9–T1),1 Thoraco-abdominal (T7–T12) Trans-abdominal (T6–T10).

Multimodal (paracetamol, NSAIDs) opioid-sparing analgesia is recommended to reduced postoperative ileus and enhance bowel recovery.[53]

Thoracic epidural analgesia (TEA) has been the mainstay of analgesia for open abdominal and pelvic surgeries. It provides superior pain relief, counteracts the stress response to surgery, and a reduction in postoperative cardiopulmonary complications. The optimum vertebral level not clear but between T9 and T11 have been used in RC with the suggested duration of up to 48 to 72 hours postcystectomy.[54]

For nephrectomies epidural analgesia to level T6 maybe required depending on the incision approach used (see above).

A systematic review and meta-analysis reviewing analgesia after open abdominal surgery in the setting of enhanced recovery surgery found no advantage for the use of epidurals over any other form of analgesic regimen in terms of overall complication rate, systemic complication rate, and length of hospital stay. The analysis acknowledged that greater pain scores were achieved by epidurals over the alternative techniques (PCA, wound catheter infusions) when providing pain relief. However, in the context of enhanced recovery protocols whereby complications and LOS are key outcomes, merely looking at pain scores and opiate consumption does not provide all the information that is required by the clinician to make a sound choice. The results of this review revealed inferior analgesic capabilities of the alternative methods compared with epidurals, but this did not translate into prolonged LOS or higher morbidity rates. This review showed a faster time to the return of bowel functioning with epidurals; however, no difference in ileus rates was observed. Current evidence comparing analgesic techniques within an ERAS protocol is limited.[55]

Alternatives to epidurals (difficulty siting, contraindicated or unsuccessful insertion) with varying reports of analgesia adequacy include catheters placed in the preperitoneal space (rectus sheath) and transverse abdominis plane (TAP) blocks. These may also help reduce postop reduced morphine consumption.[56]

Temperature regulation: Maintenance of normothermia to prevent postop complications is recommended ERAS guidance. The use of warming blankets, fluid warming devices, and active warmers is warranted.[57]

Goal-directed fluid therapy

Fluid excess or hypovolemia can provoke splanchnic hypoperfusion, which can then result in ileus, increased morbidity, and LOS.[58]

Fluid management in cystectomy patients remains a challenge with patients who are mostly ASA III/IV and accurate measure of urine output are unreliable. Individualized goal-directed fluid management led by experienced anesthetists is recommended to ensure adequate tissue perfusion.[59]

Postoperative

ERAS principles guide the recovery process. The postoperative plan should be discussed and documented by the theater team as part of the "sign out" process.

Anesthesia

- Prescriptions should include multimodal oral analgesics both regular and as required (paracetamol, NSAIDS if not contraindicated, PCA, epidurals wound infiltration catheters) to enable sparing of opioids and improving bowel recovery.[60]
- Multimodal anti-emetic prophylaxis should be considered for patients with a high risk of PONV, alongside anesthetic planning to minimizing PONV risks such as the avoidance of inhalational agents and minimization of opioids.
- Following open cystectomies, patients are nursed in the critical care environment to allow close monitoring.

Surgical

- Drains and tubes: The need for NGT and catheters should be reviewed, and a plan should be documented for drain reviews on the ward or critical care.
- Ileus Prevention: Prevention of postoperative ileus using mu receptor antagonists such as alvimopam has been used in some centers for open cystectomy. They

have a limited ability to cross the blood–brain barrier so do not antagonize the analgesic effects of opioids but reduce the peripheral effects such as ileus.

- Chewing gum has also demonstrated earlier first defecation, but with no effect on LOS or comorbidity.[61]
- Early mobilization may help reduce chest complications, encourage blood flow (reducing venous thrombosis risk), and help reduce the risk of insulin resistance and muscle loss associated with prolonged bed rest.
- Nutrition: Normal diet, as opposed to parental nutrition, should be encouraged and reestablished as soon as possible as no evidence supports the routine prolonged fasting after cystectomy.[59]
- Thromboprophylaxis: The incidence of clinically significant deep vein thrombosis (DVT) after cystectomy is estimated at 5%.[62] For all major pelvic surgeries, thromboprophylaxis with LMWH (low-molecular-weight Heparin) or unfractionated heparin should be considered in addition to compressive stockings or intermittent pneumatic compression devices to further reduced the risk.[63] The European Association of Urologists (EAU Thromboprophylaxis, March 2017) recommends commencing thromboprophylaxis the morning after surgery and the optimal duration of pharmacologic prophylaxis is approximately 4-weeks postsurgery.[27]

ANESTHETIC CONSIDERATION FOR MINIMALLY INVASIVE SURGERY

The development of minimally invasive techniques using robotic and laparoscopic techniques has allowed patients to undergo complex and high-risk surgery, limiting the harmful consequences and physiologic sequelae of open surgery.

Robots are designed to allow the surgeon to control their instruments from a distance with a higher degree of precision and with better visualization of tissues than is possible with standard laparoscopic techniques. The most used system is the da Vinci TM surgical robot (Intuitive Surgical, USA).

The surgeon operates from a nonsterile, seated control unit that separates from the robot. The patient is first placed in the lithotomy position and the operating arms are positioned between, the legs of the patient, and then a pneumoperitoneum is created. The patient is changed to the steep Trendelenburg position. This positioning allows for an intraabdominal workspace as well as the retraction of the bowel from the surgical field by the way of gravity.

Four operating arms attached to the intra-abdominal ports extend over the patient. These ports remain in place for the duration of the procedure and the instruments, inserted via the ports, are manipulated by the surgeon in the control unit (**Fig. 3**).

The systemic and hemodynamic changes for this type of surgery are highlighted later in discussion.

Specific Differences from the Traditional Laparoscopic Approach

- Emergency access to the patient: a plan to disengage instruments, remove the trocars and unlock the robot, before leveling the patient, must be decided, communicated, and rehearsed by any airway emergency or cardiac arrest scenarios
- Muscle relaxation: Maintenance of neuromuscular block and avoidance of patient movement while trocars are fixed is mandatory to avoid potential vascular or visceral injury

Specific Consideration with Robot-Assisted Surgery

Duration of surgery: Long.

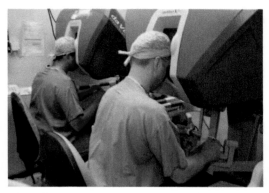

Fig. 3. Robotic Console unit.

- RALP (robotic-assisted laparoscopic prostatectomy): 2 to 3 hours, maybe more
- RARC (robotic-assisted radical cystectomy) 8 to 10 hours on average
- RAPN (robotic-assisted laparoscopic partial nephrectomy) 3 to 4 hours

Prolonged lithotomy position can predispose to the following nerve injuries and consequences. Risk factors for injury include diabetes, thin body habitus, and improper placement or inadequate padding of the robot's immobile arms on the patient's lower extremities.

- Common peroneal nerve injury (0.3% of patients experiencing a sensory deficit and one in 4500 patients, a motor deficit)
- Femoral nerve (1 in 50,000 chance of a persistent motor deficit)
- Obturator nerve (0.5% injury rate)
- Sciatic nerve (0.3%−2% risk of sensory injury and motor involvement in 1 in 25,000 cases)
- Pressure areas, compartment syndrome, and rhabdomyolysis have all been reported in the literature

Prolonged Trendelenburg Position

- Once the robot has been docked the patient cannot be removed or repositioned from the steep Trendelenburg position without undocking the robot first
- Raised Intracranial pressure leading to cerebral edema; this is due to a reduction in cerebral venous return due to high intraabdominal pressures and head-down position.
- Facial and laryngeal edema causing respiratory distress on extubation
- Raised intraocular pressure and orbital edema
- Reduction in pulmonary compliance and functional residual capacity resulting in high ventilatory pressures and atelectasis (**Fig. 4, Table 1**)

A pneumoperitoneum is required to create a surgical operating space. Carbon dioxide is insufflated into the abdomen using a veress needle. Carbon dioxide is inert and will not support combustion if diathermy is used. It also has a significantly increased blood solubility than nitrogen or oxygen, minimizing the risk of a significant venous embolus should inadvertent intravascular insufflation occur.

There are 3 major areas to consider when managing patients with a pneumoperitoneum:

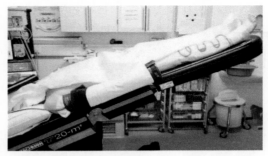

Fig. 4. Steep Trendelenburg position.

(1) Increase in intraabdominal pressure (IAP)
(2) Patient's position (flat, reverse Trendelenburg, and Trendelenburg)
(3) Biochemical changes resulting from CO2 absorption

Systemically the following issues can occur:

Cardiovascular.
A complex series of CV changes ensue due to the compression of major arteries and organs and the varying degree of the IAP and.

- Low IAP (10 mm Hg) increases venous return and cardiac output (CO).
- Moderate IAP changes (10–20 mm Hg) reduce CO and increased systemic vascular resistance (SVR). The effect on Mean arterial pressure (MAP) mirrors the product of CO and SVR and is often variable.
- High IAP (>20 mm Hg) decreases MAP as CO is reduced markedly.
- Compression of the inferior vena cava (IVC) leads to a reduction in preload and CO.
- Rising SVR resulting from compression of the major arteries and catecholamine release (epinephrine and norepinephrine) leads to tachycardia and increases in systolic and diastolic BP.

Table 1 Pneumoperitoneum		
System	**Increased**	**Decreased**
Neurologic	Intracranial pressure	
	Intraocular pressure	
	Cerebral blood flow	
	Risk of neuropraxia	
Endocrine	Catecholamine release	
	Renin-angiotensin system activation	
Cardiovascular	Systemic vascular resistance	Splanchnic blood flow
	Mean arterial pressure	Venous return
	Oxygen consumption	Cardiac output
	Risk of venous air emboli	
	Risk of visceral/vascular injury	
Respiratory	Ventilation-perfusion mismatch	Functional residual capacity
	Peak airway pressure	Vital capacity
	Hypercarbia	Compliance
	Risk of tracheal tube displacement	
	Risk of surgical emphysema	
	Risk of facial/airway edema	
Gastrointestinal	Regurgitation	
Renal		Glomerular filtration rate
		Urine output

- This consequential increase in myocardial workload may lead to ventricular failure especially if preexisting ventricular function is poor.
- Vascular compression reduces visceral perfusion and causes venous pooling, predisposing to deep venous thrombosis (DVT).

Respiratory

- Functional residual capacity (FRC) is reduced by supine position and being under general anesthesia
- Increased IAP contributes to this leading reduced lung volumes due to the splinting of the diaphragm.
- The associated atelectasis and ventilation-perfusion mismatch results in hypoxia, hypercarbia, and respiratory acidosis. Minute ventilation must be adjusted to combat this.
- The high ventilatory pressures required once in steep head down position also increase the injury of barotrauma and pneumothoraces.

Renal and gastrointestinal

- IAP increased the renal vascular resistance resulting in reduced renal blood flow, and glomerular filtration rate. This is compounded by the reduction in cardiac output and can lead to a low urine output. Activation of RAS (renin–angiotensin system) and the consequential neuroendocrine response further adds to the physiologic insult
- IAP reduced splanchnic bloods flow can result in ischemic organ injury and regurgitation of gastric contents

Physiologic effects of gas absorption

- Carbon dioxide is readily absorbed from the peritoneum, and it has direct and indirect (from increasing catecholamine release) effects on the CV system.
- The resulting tachycardia, increased myocardial contractility, and reduction in diastolic filling can lead to poo myocardial oxygen supply and ischemia.

Effects of gas insufflation

- Nodal arrhythmias, bradycardia, and asystole can occur from the vagal response to rapid peritoneal stretch
- Subcutaneous emphysema, pneumothorax, and pneumomediastinum may occur due to poor needle positioning
- Venous gas embolisms from the injection of gas into blood vessels
- Trauma from trocars lacerating vessels or organs. The small bowel is the structure most frequently damaged (25%), followed by the iliac artery (19%), colon (12%), and iliac veins.[64]

Preoperative Visit

Following a standard assessment, high-risk patients should be identified. Urinary tract infections should be treated preoperatively, and a urine dipstick should be performed on admission. Preassessing patients undergoing robotic surgery requires careful consideration of cardiac and respiratory function as these are key determinants as to whether a patient will be able to cope with the physiologic demands imposed by abdominal insufflation and steep Trendelenburg position.

Discussion with patient
General and common to all the surgeries.

- Consent for general anesthesia and common risks: ETT, Sore throat, dental damage, PONV (postoperative nausea and vomiting), regional anesthesia or PCA explanation, (see later in discussion), facial and orbital edema, insertion of NGT, and catheter
- Insertion of CVC, arterial cannulation, and minimum of 2 peripheral venous catheters
- Opportunity to encourage postop early mobilization
- Carbohydrate loading preop before surgery resulting in patient arriving euvolemic to theater
- Ensure routine blood (FBC, UE, and clotting) are up to date and that valid group and save screens are available in case of inadvertent injury.

INTRAOPERATIVE

- Maintenance of anesthesia with volatile anesthesia or TIVA. Remifentanil intraoperatively helps to obtund the physiologic responses to surgery.
- High PEEP, low tidal volumes, and allowance of permissive hypercapnia as a ventilation strategy
- Use of peripheral nerve stimulator to ensure adequate paralysis
- Consider the use of depth of anesthesia monitoring-most centers use BIS or Entropy
- Fluid warmers and forced air warmers to chest
- Preincision surgical antibiotics as per local guidance.
- IV dexamethasone to help with inflammation and swelling.
- Tranexamic acid 1g for bleeding prevention
- Preinsufflation use of anti-muscarinic (glycopyrrolate or atropine) or drawn up and accessible in case of brady-arrythmia
- Fluid therapy should be limited during the procedure or while ureters are clamped and GDFT using noninvasive cardiac output monitoring should be used to guide fluids and vasopressors.
- Assess adequacy of perfusion with arterial blood gas sampling, monitoring for hyperkalaemia is important, particularly when the ureters have been clamped surgically before urinary diversion (either through an ileal conduit or formation of a neobladder)
- Calf compression devices and thromboembolic stockings should be encouraged to be worn before arriving at the theater (**Table 1**).
- Set up considerations and strategies to avoid common issues highlighted in **Table 2**. Meticulous attention to pressure areas is required and most centers use bolsters under the shoulder and under the knees as well as gel pads under the ankles to help minimize injuries.
- Nephrectomy surgery may involve positioning the patient in the lateral position and breaking the table.

Analgesia

- There are multiple sources of postoperative pain: port site pain, incisional pain, shoulder tip pain, and visceral pain. Pain is also experienced following peritoneal stretch and distension secondary to carbon dioxide insufflation. Rapid insufflation of the peritoneum with carbon dioxide causes tearing of blood vessels, traumatic traction of nerves, and release of inflammatory mediators. Residual gas postprocedure causes shoulder tip pain, back pain, and upper abdominal pain by diaphragmatic stretching and phrenic nerve irritation. The major aim in

Table 2
Summary of the common problems with minimally invasive surgery and solutions

Position	Risk	Consequences	Solution
All	Patient Sliding	Direct trauma visceral injury from indwelling instruments	Nonslip padding/eggshell straps foot /should
	Pressure injuries	Neuropraxia/neuropathy Pressure sores	Avoiding excess stretch (eg, use of level arm boards). Gel padding/eggshell Padding to plastic IV connectors and monitoring devices (eg, arterial catheter connectors) Padded angle bar below patients chin to protect head from instruments
			Insert all lines/monitoring before docking the robot
			Insert on one side (usually opposite to robot assistant)
	Access to intravenous catheters and monitoring devices	Difficult to access once underway (especially robotic surgery)	Arms wrapped at sides- ensure no kinking of lines
			Arterial transducer fixed at the level of shoulder
Trendelenburg	Tracheal tube movement	Bronchial intubation	Secure tracheal tube effectively Check tube length after positioning, including auscultation
	Edema	Cerebral edema	Limit volumes of IV fluids. Avoid tracheal tube ties(tape)
		Conjunctival edema/chemosis	Periodic leveling of patient Consider "leak test" before extubation
		Airway edema	Use of PEEP
	Pulmonary	Atelectasis	Use a tracheal tube with sufficient balloon pressure
	Gastric content spillage	Pulmonary aspiration Oral ulceration Conjunctival chemical burns around the eyes	Insert and drain nasogastric tube (NGT Use extrapadding and lubrication ointment around the eyes Periodic monitoring of face

(continued on next page)

Table 2
(continued)

Position	Risk	Consequences	Solution
	Compartment syndrome (especially lithotomy syndrome)	(Bilateral) calf compartment syndrome Gluteal compartment syndrome	Adequate padding Avoid the use of compression stockings Use heel/ankle supports Periodic "leveling out"/moving patients legs perioperatively Monitor foot pulses
	Upper extremity neuropathy	C5-7 distribution	Caution with the use of beanbag head and neck/joint positioning (eg, avoiding abduction >90and head contralateral extension) Use padded shoulder bolsters (especially over acromioclavicular joint) Use sufficient padding of supports
	Lower extremity neuropathy (especially in lithotomy position)	Lateral femoral cutaneous nerve Common peroneal nerve Obturator nerve Sciatic nerve	
	Reduced venous return	Hypotension on leveling the patient	Preload with IV fluids and consider the use of vasopressors before leveling
Reverse Trendelenburg	Reduced venous return	Hypotension	Preload/Vasopressor use

Table 3
An example of ERAS pathway for Cystectomy at the Authors' center at the Royal Surrey County Hospital, Guildford, UK

Day	Clinic	-1	PRE-OP	0 / INTRA-OP	POST-OP	1	2	3	4	5 / AIM DISCHARGE
Date	/ /	/ /	/ /			/ /	/ /	/ /	/ /	/ /
Exercise	Normal exercise				Sit up in bed. Deep breathing + coughing every hour (when awake)	7 AM Sit into chair; March on spot Walk 2 x 20m	7 AM Mobilize to chair; Walk 3 x 20m	Sit out in own clothes Mobilizing independently; Walk 3 x 40m	Walk 4 x 60m	Mobilize independently at least 4x/day
Nutrition	CHO preload info NB. Not for diabetic pts unless on VRII	Phosphate enema 8 PM; CHO preload 9 PM; Clear fluids from 12 AM	CHO preload 6 AM	Induction antibiotics: 1.5 g cefuroxime (redose at 4 h or after 1.5 L blood loss) + 120 mg gentamicin; Spinal diamorphine; Paracetamol; GDFT once ureters unclamped; Hypothermia management; AKI Bundle: TXA 1g Avoid nephrotoxic drugs; Keep SBP within 10% baseline; Limit starvation time; Post op prescription: Fortisip compact 125 mL TDS; Chewing gum 15 min; TDS LMWH 1st night – check with surgeons	Free fluids. Fortisip compact. Offer evening meal.	7.30 AM Breakfast in chair; Discontinue IVs; Encourage oral fluids; 3 meals/d	Eating and drinking (little & often)	Monitor for paralytic ileus (abdominal discomfort/ distension, nausea, vomiting, excessive belching, lack of flatus) – if signs present, contact surgeon; Full diet as tolerated (little & often); Dietician referral if not on oral diet		
Analgesia		Continue regular meds			Paracetamol 1g QDS PO/IV Tramadol 50100 mg QDS PRN Oramorph 10 mg 2°-3° PRN	Regular oral analgesia		Pain team if required Optimise analgesia (including consider NSAID)		Oral analgesia Prepare discharge medication prescription
Tubes & Drains	If IC: See stoma nurse If NB: Shown self-catheterization		Stoma nurse to		No nasogastric tube. Drains on free drainage.	If IC: Review stoma regularly (should be pink, warm & healthy); monitor stoma UO; commence stoma care plan. If NB: Record UO from urethral catheter; 6hrly 50 mL saline catheter flushes. Urologists to consider urethral/ pelvic drain removal	ICU staff to change	All remaining drains/lines reviewed & removed if able. Or plan for removal as outpatient.		Stoma nurse assist pt independence with stoma care (if IC)/self-catheterization & catheter flushing (if NB) Wound care teaching
		Admitted to ESU				Encourage completion				Prepare to go home Follow-up arranged

(continued on next page)

Table 3
(continued)

Day	Clinic	−1	0	1	2	3	4	5
Education Planning & Patient	ERAS explained to pt Receive ERAS Booklet Given patient diary Predicted LOS 5 d		mark stoma site	of patient diary *Voice any questions at any time to your team* Engage with stoma care to aid discharge (if IC) Learn self-catheterization and later flushing of catheter (if NB) Learn how to do LMWH injections (if require extended DVT prophylaxis)	stoma bag	Begin discharge planning		

Abbreviations: AKI, acute kidney injury; CHO, carbohydrate; GDFT, goal-directed fluid therapy; IC, ileal conduit; LOS, Length of stay, UO, urine output; NB, neobladder; pt, patient; TXA, tranexamic acid; VRII, variable rate insulin infusion.

providing perioperative analgesia for patients undergoing MIS abdominal and pelvic surgery is to use multimodal opioid-sparing drugs.

- Spinal anesthesia has been widely and successfully used to manage intraop and immediate postoperative pain for both laparoscopic and robotic surgeries with the aim of converting to multimodal oral analgesia. It has also been helpful in the prevention of bladder spasm.
- Local anesthetic (0.5% Heavy Bupivacaine or plain 0.25% levobupivacaine and intrathecal diamorphine is a popular choice to reduce the need for systemic opioid. Doses range from 250 mcg to as high as 1 mg, depending on the type and duration of surgery, the associated comorbidities, and the location of postoperative care. Preservative-free (PF) morphine has also been used successfully in robotic prostatectomies; however, its use is limited by intense pruritis experienced by patients in the postoperative setting and by the limited availability of PF morphine.[65]
- Although laparoscopic nephrectomy has proven reduced analgesic requirements, patients will still require regular strong opioids, usually a PCA (Patient Controlled Analgesia) pump as well as regular simple analgesics such as paracetamol. The use of drugs that rely on renal metabolism and excretion should be used cautiously in those with preoperative evidence of poor renal reserve and complete avoidance of nonsteroidal anti-inflammatory drugs is recommended.
- Local anesthetic techniques, such as transversus abdominis plane block, may decrease opioid consumption, especially when the block is sited before surgery.[65]

End of surgery

- Administer antiemetics: Ondansetron 4 mg IV
- Once the robot has been disengaged, flatten the patient out, and perform recruitment maneuvers.
- Suction and remove unnecessary NGT
- Reverse any residual neuromuscular blockade
- Sit up, assess, and facial edema or subcutaneous emphysema
- Perform cuff leak to check for laryngeal edema before extubating

Postoperative

Common considerations

- Multi-modal analgesia (Caution with NSAIDs) and Buscopan for bladder spasm (prostatectomy)
- Multimodal antiemetics
- Low-molecular-weight heparin for VTE prophylaxis
- Suspension of intravenous fluids and resumption of oral hydration and nutrition once patient alert and not being sick
- Prostatectomies and nephrectomies are usually discharged from recovery to a ward that is set up to look after these patients
- Uncomplicated RALP maybe considered for 23 hour stays and early discharge on day one postop. Most patients eat and drink within a couple of hours from wakeup and minimal oral analgesia (paracetamol ± ibuprofen) is sufficient analgesia.

Specific for cystectomy

- Cystectomy patients will require critical care in the immediate postoperative setting (adequacy of monitoring, fluid requirement assessments, and close monitoring for ileus)

- Triaging patient postoperative destination according to preop CPET results.[66]

Degree of Cardiac Failure	At Peak ml.min^{-1}kg^{-1}	Vo$_2$ ml.min^{-1}kg^{-1}	Triage
Mild to none	>14	>20	Ward
Mild to moderate	11–14	16–20	Ward
Moderate to severe	8–11	10–16	HDU/ICU
Severe	5–8	6–10	ICU

- Consider prescription of chewing gum, 15 mins, three times a day. Chewing gum has also demonstrated earlier first defecation, but with no effect on LOS or comorbidity.[61]
- Early engagement with stoma care nurses and teaching the patient how to care for their stoma.

CYSTECTOMY AND ILEAL CONDUIT/NEOBLADDER ERAS.

Recommended Suggestions. Modify as required based on clinical judgement (**Table 3**)

REFERENCES

1. Cancer Research UK. Available at: www.cancerresearchuk.org. Accessed November, 2020.
2. Crabb SJ, Douglas James. The latest treatment options for bladder cancer. Br Med Bull 2018;128(Issue 1):85–95.
3. Chapman E, Pichel AC. Anaesthesia for Nephrectomy. BJA Education 2016; 16(3):98–101.
4. NHS England. Clinical Commissioning Policy: Robotic-Assisted Surgical Procedures for Prostate Cancer. 2015
5. Cancer Research UK. Available at: https://www.cancerresearchuk.org/health-professional/cancer-statistics/statistics-by-cancer-type/prostate-cancer. Accessed November, 2020.
6. NICE Guidelines. Prostate Cancer Diagnosis and Management. 2019
7. Protopapa KL, Simpson JC, Smith NCE, et al. Development, and validation of the surgical outcome risk tool (SORT). Br J Surg 2014;101:1774e83.
8. Barnett S, Moonesinghe SR. Clinical risk scores to guide perioperative management. Postgrad Med J 2011;87:535e41.
9. Hollenbeck BK, Miller DC, Taub D, et al. Identifying risk factors for potentially avoidable complications following radical cystectomy. The J Urol 2005;174(4 Pt 1):1231e7.
10. West MA, Lythgoe D, Barben CP, et al. Cardiopulmonary exercise variables are associated with postoperative morbidity after major colonic surgery: a prospective blinded observational study. Br J Anaesth 2014;112:665e71 4.
11. Snowden CP, Prentis JM, Anderson HL, et al. Submaximal cardiopulmonary exercise testing predicts complications and hospital length of stay in patients undergoing major elective surgery. Ann Surg 2010;251:535e41.
12. Copeland GP, Jones D, Walters M. POSSUM: a scoring system for surgical audit. Br J Surg 1991;78(3):355–60.
13. Protopapa KL, Simpson JC, Smith NCE, et al. Development and validation of the Surgical Outcome Risk Tool (SORT). BJS 2014;101:1774–83.

14. Bilimoria KY, Liu Y, Paruch JL, et al. Development and evaluation of the universal ACS NSQIP surgical risk calculator: a decision aid and informed consent tool for patients and surgeons. J Am Coll Surg 2013;217(5):833–42. e423.

15. Schlonborn JL, Anderson H. Perioperative medicine: A changing model of care. BJA Education 2019;19(1):27e33.

16. Karl A, Rittler P, Buchner A, et al. Prospective assessment of malnutrition in urologic patients. Urology 2009;73(5):1072e6.

17. Gregg JR, Cookson MS, Phillips S, et al. Effect of preoperative nutritional deficiency on mortality after radical cystectomy for bladder cancer. The J Urol 2011;185(1):90e6.

18. Pang KH, Groves R, Venugopal S, et al. Prospective implementation of enhanced recovery after surgery protocols to radical cystectomy. Eur Urol 2017;73:363–71.

19. Wong J, Lam DP, Abrishami A, et al. Short term preoperative smoking cessation and postoperative complications: a systematic review and meta-analysis. Can J Anaesth 2012;59:268e79 15.

20. Tønnesen H, Nielsen PR, Lauritzen JB, et al. Smoking and alcohol intervention before surgery: evidence for best practice. Br J Anaesth 2009;102:297e306.

21. Jensen BT, Lauridsen SV, Jensen JB, et al. Prehabilitation for major abdominal urologic oncology surgery. Curr Opin Urol 2018;28(3):243–50.

22. Minnella E, Carli F, Kassouf W. Role of prehabilitation following major uro-oncologic surgery: a narrative review. World J Urol 2020. https://doi.org/10.1007/s00345-020-03505-4.

23. Jones C, Kelliher L. Enhanced recovery after surgery: past, present and future. Dig Med Res 2019;2:19.

24. Patel HR, Cerantola Y, Valerio M, et al. Enhanced recovery after surgery: are we ready, and can we afford not to implement these pathways for patients undergoing radical cystectomy? Eur Urol 2014;65:263–6.

25. Kehlet H. Multimodal approach to control postoperative pathophysiology and rehabilitation. Br J Anaesth 1997;78:606–17.

26. Varadhan KK, Neal KR, Dejong CH, et al. The enhanced Recovery after surgery (ERAS) pathway for patients undergoing major elective open colorectal surgery: a meta-analysis of randomised controlled surgery. Clin Nutr 2010;29:434–40.

27. Tikkinen KA, Agarwal A, Criagie S, et al. Systematic reviews of observational studies of risk of thrombosis and bleeding in urological surgery (ROTBUS): introduction and methodology. Syst Rev 2014;3:150.

28. Herling SF, Moller AM, Palle C, et al. Robotic-assisted laparoscopic hysterectomy for women with endometrial cancer. Dan Med J 2017;64:A5343, pii.

29. Parisi A, Reim D, Borghi F, et al. Minimally invasive surgery for gastric cancer: A comparison between robotic, laparoscopic and open surgery. World J Gastroenterol 2017;23:2376–84.

30. Knox ML, El-Galley R, Busby JE. Robotic versus open radical cystectomy: identification of patients who benefit from the robotic approach. J Endourol 2013; 27:40–4.

31. Backes FJ, El Naggar AC, Farrell MR, et al. Perioperative outcomes for laparotomy compared to robotic surgical staging of endometrial cancer in the elderly: a retrospective cohort. Int J Gynecol Cancer 2016;26:1717–21.

32. Shabsigh A, Korets R, Vora KC, et al. Defining early morbidity of radical cystectomy for patients with bladder cancer using a standardized reporting methodology. Eur Urol 2009 Jan;55(1):164e74.

33. The British Association of Urological Surgeons. BAUS Enhanced Recovery Pathway. 2015

34. Hu X, Xiong SC, Dou WC, et al. Minimally invasive vs open radical cystectomy in patients with bladder cancer: A systematic review and meta-analysis of randomized controlled trials. Eur J Surg Oncol 2020;46:44e52.
35. Nix J, Smith A, Kurpad R, et al. Prospective randomized controlled trial of robotic versus open radical cystectomy for bladder cancer: perioperative and pathologic results. Eur Urol 2010;57:196e201.
36. Lin T, Fan X, Zhang C, et al. A prospective randomised controlled trial of laparoscopic vs open radical cystectomy for bladder cancer: perioperative and oncologic outcomes with 5-year follow-upT Lin et al. Br J Canc 2014;110:842e9.
37. Parekh DJ, Reis IS, Castle EP, et al. Robot-assisted radical cystectomy versus open radical cystectomy in patients with bladder cancer (RAZOR): an open-label, randomised, phase 3, non-inferiority trial. Lancet 2018;391:2525–36.
38. Mottet N, Bellmunt J, Bolla M, et al. EAU-ESTROSIOG Guidelines on Prostate Cancer. Part 1: Screening, Diagnosis, and Local Treatment with Curative Intent. Eur Urol 2017;71:618–29.
39. Tewari A, Sooriakumaran P, Bloch DA, et al. Positive surgical margin and perioperative complication rates of primary surgical treatments for prostate cancer: a systematic review and meta-analysis comparing retropubic, laparoscopic, and robotic prostatectomy. Eur Urol 2012;62:1.
40. Lin C, Wan F, Lu Y, et al. Enhanced recovery after surgery protocol for prostate cancer patients undergoing laparoscopic radical prostatectomy. J Int Med Res 2019;47(1):114–21.
41. Abaza, et al. Same Day Discharge after Robotic Radical Prostatectomy. J Urol 2019;202(5):959–63.
42. Thomas L, Lacarriere E, Martinache G, et al. Experience of day case robotic prostatectomy. About thirty-two patients. Prog Urol 2019;29:12.
43. Ljungberg B, Bensalah K, Canfield S, et al. EAU guidelines on renal cell carcinoma: 2014 update. Eur Urol 2015;67:913–24. 19.
44. Minervini A, Siena G, Carini M. Robotic-assisted partial nephrectomy: the next gold standard for the treatment of intracapsular renal tumors. Expert Rev Anticancer Ther 2011;11(12):1779-1782.
45. Open versus robotic partial nephrectomy: Systematic review and meta-analysis of contemporary studies. Tsai et al. Int J Med Robotics Comput Assist Surg 2019;15:e1963.
46. Nygren J, Thorell A, Ljungqvist O. Preoperative oral carbohydrate nutrition: an update. Curr Opin Clin Nutr Metab Care 2001;4:255–9.
47. Smith I, Kranke P, Murat I, et al. Perioperative fasting in adults and children: guidelines from the European Society of Anaesthesiology. Eur J Anaesthesiol 2011;28:556e69.
48. McCracken GC, Montgomery J. Postoperative nausea and vomiting after unrestricted clear fluids before day surgery: A retrospective analysis. Eur J Anaesthesiol 2018;35(5):337–42.
49. Xu R, Zhao X, Zhong Z, et al. No advantage is gained by preoperative bowel preparation in radical cystectomy and ileal conduit: a randomized controlled trial of 86 patients. Int Urol Nephrol 2010;42:947–50.
50. Wigmore T, Jhanji S. Long-term Survival for Patients Undergoing Volatile versus IV Anesthesia for Cancer Surgery: A Retrospective Analysis. Anesthesiology 2016;124:69–79.
51. Soulié M, Straub M, Gamé X, et al. A Multicentre study of the morbidity of radical cystectomy in select elderly patients with bladder cancer. J Urol 2002;167:1325–8.

52. Klein A, et al. Association of Anaesthetists guidelines: cell salvage for peri-operative blood conservation 2018. Anaesthesia 2018;73:1141–50.
53. Gustafsson UO, Scott MJ, Schwenk W, et al. Guidelines for perioperative care in elective colonic surgery: Enhanced Recovery After Surgery (ERAS) Society recommendations. World J Surg 2013;37(2):259e84.
54. Maffezzini M, Campodonico F, Canepa G, et al. fast Track surgery and technical nuances to reduce complications after radical cystectomy and intestinal urinary diversion with the modified Indiana pouch. Surg Oncol 2012;21:191–5.
55. Hughes MJ, Ventham NT, McNally S, et al. Analgesia After Open Abdominal Surgery in the Setting of Enhanced Recovery Surgery A Systematic Review and Meta-analysis. JAMA Surg 2014;149(12):1224–30.
56. Forastiere E, Sofra M, Giannarelli D, et al. Effectiveness of continuous wound infusion of 0.5% ropivacaine by On-Q pain relief system for postoperative pain management after open nephrectomy. Br J Anaesth 2008;101:841–7.
57. NICE guideline 65 Hypothermia: prevention and management in adults having surgery
58. Giglio MT, Marucci M, Testini M, et al. Goal-directed haemodynamic therapy and gastrointestinal complications in major surgery: a meta-analysis of randomized controlled trials. Br J Anaesth 2009;103(5):637e46.
59. Cerantola Y, Valerio M, Persson B, et al. Guidelines for perioperative care after radical cystectomy for bladder cancer: Enhanced Recovery After Surgery (ERAS) society recommendations. Clin Nutr 2013;32:879–87.
60. Campaign N, Mcgrath J, Jackson L, et al. "Same day discharge" RALP – the ultimate form of enhanced recovery. Eur Urol 2014;13:15–6.
61. Fitzgerald JE, Ahmed I. Systematic review and metaanalysis of chewing-gum therapy in the reduction of postoperative paralytic ileus following gastrointestinal surgery. World J Surg 2009;33:2557–66.
62. Lassen K, Soop M, Nygren J, et al. Consensus review of optimal perioperative care in colorectal surgery: Enhanced Recovery After Surgery (ERAS) Group recommendations. Arch Surg 2009;144(10):961e9.
63. Novotny V, Hakenberg OW, Wiessner D, et al. Perioperative complications of radical cystectomy in a contemporary series. Eur Urol 2007;51(2):397e401.
64. Chandler JG, Corson SL, Way LW. Three spectra of laparoscopic entry access injuries. J Am Coll Surg 2001;192:478e90.
65. De Oliveira GS, Castro-Alves LJ, Nader A, et al. Transversus abdominis plane block to ameliorate postoperative pain outcomes after laparoscopic surgery: a meta-analysis of randomized controlled trials. Anesth Analg 2014;118:454e63.
66. Older P. Anaerobic Threshold, is it a magic number to determine fitness for surgery? Peri-operative Medicine 2013;2:2–13. Submitted for publication.

Emergency Laparotomy

Geeta Aggarwal, MBBS, MRCP, FRCA[a],*,
Michael Scott, MBChB, FRCP, FRCA, FFICM[b,c,d],
Carol J. Peden, MBChB, MD, FRCA, FFICM, MPH[e,f,g]

KEYWORDS

- Emergency laparotomy • Emergency general surgery • Enhanced recovery
- Surgical outcomes • Geriatric management

KEY POINTS

- Emergency laparotomy is a high-risk surgical procedure with a high mortality.
- Patients frequently present with deranged physiology and sepsis.
- Outcomes have improved with measurement and targeted enhanced recovery type approaches, as described in this article.
- Many patients presenting for emergency laparotomy are elderly and frail, and geriatric conditions should be managed proactively.

INTRODUCTION AND DEFINITION

Emergency laparotomy is an overarching term used for the exploration of the abdomen for many diverse underlying intraabdominal pathologies. The term, as used in this article, will be applied only to nontrauma, nonvascular emergency general surgery procedures. The commonest conditions requiring emergency laparotomy are hernias with obstruction or gangrene, bowel ischemia, bowel obstruction, peritonitis, and gastrointestinal ulcers.[1]

The publication of the international Enhanced Recovery After Surgery (ERAS) guidelines on emergency laparotomy in 2021 generated worldwide interest and are freely available through Open Access.[2] In addition, the AHRQ Safety program for Improving Surgical Care and Recovery (ISCR) published a technical evidence review in 2020 for emergency major abdominal surgery including emergency laparotomy.[3] Recent guidelines for anesthesia for colorectal surgery from ISCR[4] and updated elective ERAS colorectal guidelines overlap with key components of care for emergency

[a] Royal Surrey Hospital NHS Foundation Trust, Egerton Road, Guildford, Surrey, GU2 7XX, UK;
[b] Hospital of the University of Pennsylvania, 3400 Spruce Street, Philadelphia, PA 19104, USA;
[c] Leonard Davis Institute of Health Economics, University of Pennsylvania, Philadelphia, PA, USA; [d] Surgical Outcomes Research Centre, University College London, London, UK; [e] Keck School of Medicine, University of Southern California, 1975 Zonal Avenue, Los Angeles, CA 90033, USA; [f] Perelman School of Medicine, University of Pennsylvania, Philadelphia, PA 19104, USA; [g] Clinical Quality the Blue Cross Blue Shield Association, Chicago, IL 60601, USA
* Corresponding author.
E-mail address: geetaaggarwal@nhs.net

Anesthesiology Clin 40 (2022) 199–211
https://doi.org/10.1016/j.anclin.2021.11.010
anesthesiology.theclinics.com
1932-2275/22/© 2021 Elsevier Inc. All rights reserved.

laparotomy particularly in the intraoperative and postoperative phases.[5] This article does not duplicate the evidence in those guidelines but highlights specific considerations and components of care in the enhanced recovery emergency laparotomy pathway. The ERAS emergency laparotomy guidelines include consensus-based components, some of which are traditional ERAS steps such as early mobilization after surgery, and some aspects of care (particularly in Part One: Preoperative: Diagnosis, Rapid Assessment and Optimization) that are new to ERAS pathways, such as comprehensive geriatric management and delirium and postoperative neurocognitive disorder prevention.[2]

HISTORY

In the United States (US) the burden of nontrauma emergency general surgery (EGS) is significant, with data showing that EGS accounts for 11% of total surgical cases but 47% of surgical deaths.[6,7] Emergency laparotomy is one of the highest mortality conditions contributing to this burden, with data published in 2012 from the National Surgical Quality Improvement (NSQIP) database showing mortality for emergency laparotomy of 14% at 30 days.[8] There has been a worldwide focus on emergency laparotomy in the past few years with programs such as the National Emergency Laparotomy Audit (NELA),[9] the Australian and New Zealand Emergency Laparotomy Audit (ANZELA), and the emergency surgery component of the American College of Surgeons Improving Surgical Care and Recovery (ISCR) project. With this dramatically increasing clinical focus and research interest, outcomes are improving for this previously overlooked group of patients. The Emergency Laparotomy Network, which preceded NELA in the United Kingdom, found mortality in 2012 of 14.9% at 30 days,[10] very similar to that reported on the NSQIP data.[8] The first 30-day mortality reported by NELA on more than 20,000 patients in 2015 was 11.8%; the mortality reported in 2021 on 2020 data had reduced further to 8.7%. The use of clinical pathways and an enhanced recovery approach has likely contributed to the improvements seen in the UK data. Another driver of improvement in the UK has been the setting of standards for emergency surgery and emergency laparotomy by national bodies. A call has been made for a similar approach to be taken in the US coupled with standardized EGS patient care using evidence-based guidelines and clinical care bundles.

Background to an Enhanced Recovery Approach to Emergency Laparotomy

Enhanced Recovery After Surgery (ERAS) approaches have usually been applied to elective surgical pathways, but there is mounting evidence that ERAS principles apply to high-risk emergency patients and help reduce morbidity and mortality. The preoperative phase of an enhanced recovery pathway is focused on getting the patient in the best possible condition for surgery. In the emergency setting, this still applies, but the time frame available must be truncated from days and weeks to just a few hours. The intraoperative and postoperative enhanced recovery approach of best possible management during surgery and optimal postoperative rehabilitation are equally applicable to emergency patients.

One of the first studies to demonstrate improved outcomes using an ERAS approach was the "ELPQuIC" or emergency laparotomy quality improvement care pathway study.[11] This relatively small quality improvement study focused on 5 evidence-based components within a care bundle thought to be essential to improving outcomes as part of an enhanced recovery type pathway. The 5 components were as follows:

- Early assessment and resuscitation

- Early antibiotics if signs of sepsis present
- Prompt diagnosis and early surgery
- Goal-directed fluid therapy for all patients
- Postoperative intensive care for all

As with any care bundle approach, part of the improvement was likely to be due to enhanced measurement and teamwork, as clinicians developed approaches to delivering the care components reliably to all patients. None of the 4 centers involved in ELP-QuIC reached high reliability (that is more than 95% delivery) of any component. However, improvement did occur in the delivery of all care components with an associated significant reduction in risk-adjusted mortality. When this approach was scaled up and delivered across 28 major acute hospitals in the South of England in the Emergency Laparotomy Collaborative (ELC), a reduction in mortality and length of stay was seen when compared with baseline data.[12] For ELC the care bundle was modified and made more specific, with a 6-point bundle that included prompt measurement of blood lactate levels, early review and treatment of sepsis, transfer to the operating room (OR) within defined time goals after the decision to operate, use of goal-directed fluid therapy, postoperative admission to an intensive care unit (ICU), and multidisciplinary involvement of senior clinicians in the decision and delivery of perioperative care. Change management and leadership coaching were also provided to ELC leadership teams. At the end of the 2-year study, 30-day mortality had reduced to 8.7% following the intervention, from a baseline of 9.6%. Associated improvements in key process delivery such as lactate measurement and faster time to the OR were also seen.

Another major UK study called EPOCH—"Evidence-based Perioperative Care for the High-risk surgical patient"—focused on the delivery of a much more extensive pathway of care with 37 components (a similar number to most enhanced recovery pathways).[13] This study took the form of a stepped-wedge randomized controlled trial, and with that design, many of the 90 hospitals that participated had a very short period of time to engage in implementing the pathway. Although 279 of the potential 800 pathway components measured in the 90 hospitals improved,[14] that was not enough to reduce mortality at 90 days between the active pathway implementation and the control phase of the study. Lessons learnt from this study and ELC applicable to improving enhanced recovery pathways for high-risk patients include allowing adequate time for improvement, understanding the social aspects of change, and if time and resources are limited focusing on a small number of high impact changes.[15]

In the US, the final phase of the American College of Surgeons ISCR program is on EGS with emergency laparotomy as one of the key conditions.[16] This program also takes an enhanced recovery approach with a focus on preoperative detection and management of sepsis, multimodal pain management, care of the older patient, and patient and family education and shared decision-making. Results are not yet available.

The Need for a Proactive Enhanced Recovery Approach for Older Patients Undergoing Emergency Laparotomy

Although the mortality for emergency laparotomy is very high and much higher than for a similar procedure performed electively, the deaths do not end in the hospital. Mortality for emergency laparotomy patients has always been much greater for older and frail patients A fifth of older adults undergoing emergency laparotomy are frail, which is associated with greater mortality and morbidity. In 2015 Cooper and colleagues using Medicare data recorded mortality of 49% at 180 days for patients aged 85 years and older, 29.4% for those aged 75 to 84 years, and 20.8% for those aged 65 years and older.[17] Using an ERAS approach has been shown to improve outcomes to a greater extent for older patients than for younger,[11] and the need for rapid proactive management of acute physiologic derangement emphasized in the ERAS emergency laparotomy guidelines[2] is likely to have a significant impact in older, frail patients with less physiologic resilience. A recent paper on US surgical trends has shown that outcomes are improving for older patients undergoing emergency colorectal procedures, encompassed by emergency laparotomy, but although a growing number survive, an increasing percentage are discharged to skilled nursing facilities.[18] Based on these poor outcomes the international ERAS guidelines include guidance on cognitive and frailty assessment preoperatively, as well as delirium screening and a reminder on the avoidance of Beers' criteria drugs such as benzodiazepines in older patients.[2,19] The rationale for inclusion preoperatively, even though it is acknowledged that multiple assessments may not be feasible in the preoperative period when correction of physiologic derangement is most pressing, is the need to alert perioperative care teams that these patients are very high risk and that geriatric conditions must be considered and managed as soon as possible.

An Enhanced Recovery Approach to Emergency Laparotomy, Preoperative Considerations

All surgeries attract the surgical stress response, but with emergency abdominal surgery the response can be extreme and prolonged before presentation in the OR.[20,21] ERAS aims to attenuate the surgical stress response and minimize the physiologic insults that occur.[22] This approach works well in elective surgery, but the situation is very different in emergency abdominal surgery where the physiologic insult and potentially systemic inflammation response has already been triggered.[20] To overcome this, patients require a rapid pathway to diagnose and manage the underlying problem, with ERAS components modified to account for the ongoing physiologic stress.[2] Organization of care delivery before emergency abdominal surgery is very important. Patients undergo several tests, imaging, and assessments before they enter the emergency OR, which should be carried out with urgency. In addition to this, best practice should include open and clear communication with the patient and their advocates about the next steps and escalation.[23]

Key preoperative components

- *Use Early Warning Scores to screen for physiologic derangement and deterioration*

In emergency abdominal surgery, the physiologic insult starts before the patient arrives in hospital.[20,21] The use of a physiologic track and trigger or Early Warning Score ensures timely and appropriate management of deteriorating patients by assigning a numeric value to several physiologic parameters, giving a composite score to identify a patient at risk of deterioration and facilitate communication among perioperative team members about patient risk and management.

- *Use a sepsis screening tool*

There is a high incidence of sepsis in patients presenting for emergency laparotomy, and this needs to be detected and managed proactively.[2] Patients should be screened for signs of sepsis using an appropriate scoring system and local management algorithms.

- *Measure and manage physiologic derangement*

Measure blood lactate that might be high due to anaerobic metabolism. There may be acute electrolyte disturbance, and fluid shifts may occur due to sepsis, an inflammatory reaction, or bowel obstruction. The patients may be hypovolemic and may have vasoplegia.[1,21] Evidence suggests that surgery should not be delayed for optimization, rather that skilled clinicians should be resuscitating and optimizing the patient during the initial diagnostic phase and ongoing during surgery.[11,24,25]

- *Urgent diagnostic imaging*

Hospitals with a higher number of facilities for diagnostic imaging have improved outcomes for emergency laparotomy.[1,26] Early computed tomography scans facilitate surgical planning but should not cause undue delay to surgery.

- *Formal risk assessment*

Risk assessment helps with optimization of perioperative pathways and organization of services as well as adding to informed decision-making for emergency laparotomy care.[2] Use of a validated score is recommended, and several scores are available; however, the NELA risk score developed using several emergency laparotomy patient data in the National Emergency laparotomy database has been shown to be the best performing predictive model when compared with other scores.[27]

- *The need for a nasogastric tube* should be assessed on an individual patient basis, as patients may require gastric decompression[2]; this is different to elective colorectal surgery where it is discouraged to use nasogastric tubes for risk of respiratory infection as well as delay to feeding[28]
- *Reversal of anticoagulants and management of antiplatelet drugs*

Bleeding is the most common complication from EGS and the one that causes the most morbidity and mortality.[29] However, increasing numbers of patients are now on anticoagulants and antiplatelet drugs, some of which have no direct drug to reverse them. A balanced, patient-specific assessment should be carried out to reverse the antithrombotic medication based on the risk of bleeding, the risk of thromboembolism, and the urgency of the surgery.[2]

- *Venous thromboembolism prophylaxis*

Patients undergoing emergency intraabdominal surgery have an increased risk of venous thromboembolism and should be assessed preoperatively. If pharmacologic prophylaxis is not appropriate before surgery, mechanical prophylaxis should be initiated promptly.[30]

- *Age-related evaluation of frailty and cognitive assessment* should ideally be performed preoperatively; the ERAS guidelines[2] acknowledge this may not always be possible, but the perioperative care team should be aware of the impact of frailty and abnormal cognitive function on outcomes and take steps as early as possible to mitigate these issues. Baseline delirium screening should be performed and Beers criteria drugs such as benzodiazepines and anticholinergics avoided whenever possible in patients older than 65 years.
- *Patient and family education and shared decision-making*

This is one of the most important aspects of the surgical pathway and one that is the most difficult. There are multiple factors involved, with a high level of complexity with a short amount of time.[31] The discussions should include the risk of death and more detail on the morbidity that the patient could face, including quality of life, independent living, and other factors that affect a patient's life such as stoma formation.[32] Ceilings of care and advanced care directives should also be discussed. Guidance has been written on how best to have these difficult conversations, such as using the "best case/worst case" scenario[33] or using the "Serious Illness Conversation Guide" from Ariadne Labs.[34,35] Using multiple facets of communication including written information and decision aids and ensuring detailed documentation of discussions is very important.

Key intraoperative components

- *Antibiotic prophylaxis*

Usually, a single dose of antibiotic is delivered before the start of surgery to prevent surgical site infection, and a second dose is delivered if procedures last for more than 4 hours. However, in an emergency laparotomy, the patient may already be septic, antibiotics may have already been given, and appropriate further management may require consultation with a microbiologist. Compliance with on-time antibiotic administration in emergency patients is poor, with only 50% of patients receiving timely administration as compared with elective colectomy.[36]

- *Rapid sequence induction* is carried out to decrease the risk of gastric contents being aspirated during tracheal intubation. It consists of a short-acting induction agent (traditionally thiopentone) with a short-acting muscle relaxant (suxamethonium) and the application of cricoid pressure. However, there are no clear recommendations on whether a rapid sequence induction should be carried out in every emergency abdominal surgery. The technique of a rapid sequence intubation (RSI) has been modified with the use of propofol and rocuronium being used (the latter being reversed easily with sugammadex). In addition, there may be a nasogastric tube in situ that will prevent effective cricoid pressure. The principles of an RSI remain valid, to secure a safe airway with the least possible risks, but an individual assessment should be carried out to establish how to carry this out safely.[37]
- *Minimally invasive surgery*

In some centers, minimally invasive abdominal surgery may be undertaken depending on the pathology of the patient and the skill of the surgeon; this can improve postoperative recovery with lower pain scores, decreased blood loss, and early mobilization and when appropriate results in improved outcomes including shorter length of stay and decreased morbidity and mortality.[3] However, emergency laparotomy is usually an open procedure, traditionally with a large surgical incision, sometimes from xiphisternum to pubic symphysis, needed for access and ability to examine all the bowel in detail and to wash the abdomen out.

- *Prevention of intraoperative hypothermia*

Hypothermia is associated with poor wound healing, increased blood loss, and a high surgical stress response.[38] Warmed intravenous fluids, forced air warmer blankets, and invasive temperature monitoring can help with warming the patient. However, caution must be taken to the patient who is septic and has a high temperature. Usually, an open abdomen will cool the patient significantly.

- *Monitoring*

In addition to standard monitoring, invasive monitoring should be used on an individualized patient basis; this includes the use of arterial lines, central venous catheters and minimally invasive cardiac output monitoring. Arterial lines offer continuous blood pressure monitoring and arterial blood gas analysis, providing acid-base and electrolyte dysfunction. Cardiac output monitoring has been used extensively in emergency surgery, and some quality improvement studies included it as part of the care bundle.[11]

- *Perioperative fluid management*

Goal-directed hemodynamic therapy is a term used to describe the optimization of intravascular volume, cardiac output, oxygen delivery, and maintenance of mean arterial pressure with vasopressors if needed. Minimally invasive cardiac output monitors can help ensure that stroke volume is optimized before vasopressors are used. Intravenous fluid administration should be a balanced solution such as PlasmaLyte, rather than 0.9% sodium chloride, to avoid hyperchloremic acidosis and increased risk of acute kidney injury.[39]

- *Analgesia*

Optimal analgesia reduces stress and aids restoration of function and mobility. No one technique is proved to be better than another in patients undergoing emergency laparotomy, but a multimodal opioid-sparing approach should be used. These patients may not be suitable for a neuraxial technique due to anticoagulation or deranged clotting studies due to sepsis. A rectus sheath catheter, continuous wound infusion catheter, or a transverse abdominal plane block may be appropriate.[3]

- *Choice of anesthesia*

Mode of anesthesia for emergency abdominal surgery is not widely studied despite the high workload in hospitals. General anesthesia is normal practice. Short-acting inhalational agents should be used. Bispectral Index monitoring to titrate anesthesia delivery to the lowest levels may be of advantage in the elderly to reduce the risk of delirium.[40]

- *Reversal of neuromuscular block*

With an increase in older patients undergoing emergency surgery, it is important to be mindful of age-related changes in physiology and drug distribution and clearance. Appropriate neuromuscular monitoring should be used to guide the administration of neuromuscular blockers, and neuromuscular blocking agent reversal drugs should be given[5]; this can be with anticholinesterase drugs such as neostigmine or with newer agents such as sugammadex for aminosteroidal agents such as rocuronium. Residual neuromuscular blockade is higher in elderly patients, leading to hypoxic events and increased postoperative pulmonary complications and airway obstruction[41] and increased adverse events in all patient groups.[42]

Postperative Considerations in an Enhanced Recovery Approach to Emergency Laparotomy

Patients who have undergone emergency laparotomy are likely to have ongoing requirements for monitoring and management of physiologic derangement, acidosis, hypothermia and fluid shifts, and vasopressors. These patients are at significant risk of reintubation in the early postoperative period and of postoperative pulmonary complications (PPC) and failure to rescue for several days following surgery. Therefore, a careful assessment and evaluation should be made before extubation, and plans should be made for management in a high care area or ICU postoperatively. Some published standards suggest repeating a risk score before the end of surgery to provide an objective score of patient risk and guide discussion among the surgical, anesthesia, and ICU team if appropriate, about postoperative management.

Other components of postoperative care are similar to those for elective colorectal enhanced recovery pathways with a focus on early oral feeding, removal of drains and catheters, and mobilization as soon as possible. The large numbers of older patients undergoing emergency laparotomy demand a proactive comprehensive geriatric approach to ensure an increased likelihood of returning home, rather than deconditioning and discharge to a skilled nursing facility. Investment in such an approach has been shown to improve outcomes for older patients and to be cost-effective.[43,44]

Key postoperative components

- #### ICU/ high dependency unit (HDU)

Evidence has shown that when emergency laparotomy patients go to a monitored high care area with a high patient to nurse ratio such as an ICU or surgical high dependency unit (HDU) postoperatively as part of a care bundle, there is a decrease in mortality.[11,12] The National Emergency Laparotomy Audit in the United Kingdom recommends patients who have a mortality risk of greater or equal to 5% to go to an ICU or HDU.[9] Local bed availability and policies will dictate resources, but teams should develop protocols for managing these patients proactively, in appropriate care areas following surgery.

- #### Failure to rescue

Patients who have undergone emergency laparotomy are particularly at risk of "failure to rescue."[45] An initial complication, if not detected and managed early, develops into a cascade of events that can lead to a poor outcome. Complications continue for several days after surgery, requiring close monitoring and protocols for escalation.

- #### Postoperative multimodal analgesia

Multimodal analgesia based on opioid-sparing regimens has been a component of enhanced recovery for many years; this is to decrease the side effects of ileus and respiratory depression as well as removing the addiction potential.[3,46] Regular acetaminophen (paracetamol) is used combined with other opioid-sparing drugs and local anesthetic nerve blocks. The use of epidural analgesia has also been found to be associated with a decreased risk of mortality in emergency abdominal surgery but can be difficult to manage effectively due to hypotension and the need for vasopressors[47] as well as the increased risk of epidural hematoma and infection due to systemic sepsis and coagulopathy. Regional techniques such as rectus sheath catheters, transversus abdominal plane blocks, and wound catheters can be efficacious and reduce opioid requirements.

- #### Removal of urinary catheter

Although there is little evidence in emergency laparotomy patients, extrapolation from elective pathways[5] suggests that early removal, unless needed for monitoring, is appropriate.

- #### Early mobilization

Early mobilization decreases skeletal muscle loss and improves respiratory and gastrointestinal function; this will be facilitated by an adequate analgesic regimen and physiotherapists to help mobilize patients. Again, there is little direct supporting evidence for emergency laparotomy; recommendations are taken from the elective colorectal and ICU literature.[5]

- #### Comprehensive geriatric management and discharge evaluation

Several recent major studies have shown the importance of involving geriatric physicians in the management of emergency laparotomy patients at the earliest opportunity. They can also take over the care of the patient once surgical and critical care is no longer required.[43,44]

Discussion

There has been a great deal of progress in the management of the emergency laparotomy patient in the last few years, with the publication of the international ERAS Society guidelines on emergency laparotomy and technical evidence reviews from the AHRQ ISCR program. In addition, large quality improvement studies have added to the knowledge around what changes can affect outcomes for these high-risk patients and how change can be achieved.

The adaptation of the UK national emergency laparotomy audit in Australia and New Zealand and the final phase of the American College of Surgeons ISCR program focused on EGS have raised awareness about the high mortality and complication rate for this group of patients.

Anesthesiologists have an important role to play in improving outcomes for emergency laparotomy patients. In the preoperative phase, this should include assessment and management of deranged physiology and sepsis before transferring to the OR and continuing management and resuscitation in the OR. In the OR these patients require optimal management of fluids and electrolytes and close monitoring of hemodynamics and perfusion. The patients' physiologic status at the end of surgery and the findings at surgery must be considered before extubation, and the high risk of reintubation and postoperative pulmonary complications should inform where the patient is managed in the immediate postoperative phase. Optimal intraoperative and postoperative analgesia is likely to facilitate pulmonary function and early mobilization.

NONBENEFICIAL SURGERY AND END-OF-LIFE CARE

Despite recent progress, challenges remain in the management of patients undergoing emergency laparotomy. With an aging population, inevitably, there are large numbers of older patients undergoing emergency abdominal surgery. There needs to be a balance between the urgent nature of the surgery, versus ensuring that the surgery is the best treatment option, avoiding surgery that is ultimately nonbeneficial. Emergency surgery can increase the risk of nonbeneficial surgery. There is no formal definition for nonbeneficial surgery but usually, it is death within 48 to 72 hours after an emergency operation.[48] Most risk scoring tools predict 30-day mortality and very few give predictions for early death.[12] Patients can develop complications related to the underlying condition before admission to the hospital, adding to their premorbid state and their increased risk of death. Conversations between patients and doctors can be hasty in a bid to get the patient into the OR, with more junior members of the team often carrying out the discussion without using information such as risk prediction, including detailed morbidity and frailty measurement. Such difficult conversations might be avoided altogether.[49]

UK guidelines have advocated for an ad-hoc multidisciplinary meeting when predicted mortality for a patient is 25% or greater, with intensivists, surgeons, anesthesiologists and care of the elderly physicians all involved as required; however, of course there are major challenges of organizing such a meeting within a limited time frame.

It has been reported that almost two-thirds of the US population already had baseline palliative care needs before their emergency laparotomy.[50,51] Patients who are eligible for an emergency laparotomy but do not undergo it are not as widely understood as those who undergo surgery. Those that undergo the nonoperative path should have palliative care specialists involved early.[52] There are still very few studies recording outcomes of all patients referred for surgery and comparing those who are operated on with those who are not. More work is required in this area.

QUALITY OF LIFE

Health-related quality of life measurements are just as important to measure as binary outcomes such as mortality. Patient's self report their quality of life with tools such as EQ-5D, which has an extensive evidence base for use in elective surgery and is increasingly being used in emergency surgery (http://www.euroqol.org). Some work has been carried out looking into the quality of life after emergency surgery using EQ-5D tool.[53] Investigating quality of life after emergency abdominal surgery will help plan care postoperatively but also help shape the discussions that are needed before the surgery and lead to a decrease in nonbeneficial surgery.

SUMMARY

There has been a rapid synthesis of a lot of studies in the last 10 years on emergency laparotomy patients. Evidence-based pathway-driven care for patients has been demonstrated to improve outcomes. Compliance with ERAS pathways is important for optimal outcomes, and the outcomes of emergency laparotomy patients seems also to depend on addressing, optimizing, and treating many different physiologic issues. The age and comorbidity of the patient are also key factors affecting outcomes.

CLINICS CARE POINTS

- The morbidity and mortality for emergency laparotomy is high although data show that outcomes are improving.
- An enhanced recovery pathway approach seems beneficial to these very high-risk patients, and studies using ERAS have shown reductions in morbidity and mortality.
- An initial approach with rapid identification, correction of acute physiologic derangement and management of sepsis, and minimal delays to surgical intervention is essential for optimal outcomes.
- Consideration and management of the impact of age-related conditions such as frailty and cognitive dysfunction should begin as early as possible in the ERAS pathway.

DISCLOSURE

C.J. Peden has received consultancy fees from the Institute for Healthcare Improvement and the American College of Surgeons. She is a shareholder and advisory board member of Somnus Scientific. M. Scott has received consultancy fees, Honoraria, and travel expenses from Edwards, Deltex, Baxter, Trevena, and Merck and Grant funding for Studies from NIHR, United Kingdom, Merck, Untied States, Merck, Fresenius, Lidco, and Deltex Medical.

REFERENCES

1. Symons NRA, Moorthy K, Almoudaris AM, et al. Mortality in high-risk emergency general surgical admissions. Br J Surg 2013;100(10):1318–25.
2. Peden CJ, Aggarwal G, Aitken RJ, Anderson ID. Guidelines for perioperative care for emergency laparotomy enhanced recovery after surgery (ERAS) Society Recommendations: Part 1—Preoperative. World J Surg 2021;45(5):1272–90.

Available at: https://link.springer.com/article/10.1007/s00268-021-05994-9?wt_mc=Internal.Event.1.SEM.ArticleAuthorOnlineFirst&utm_source=ArticleAuthorOnlineFirst&utm_medium=email&utm_content=AA_en_06082018&ArticleAuthorOnlineFirst_20210307&error=cookies_not_supported&code=ac0943a4-c1c8-4928-bd6a-4bc6f766b7b4.

3. Hu QL, Grant MC, Hornor MA, et al. Technical evidence review for emergency major abdominal operation conducted for the AHRQ safety program for improving surgical care and recovery. J Am Coll Surg 2020;231(6):743–64.e5.

4. Ban KA, Gibbons MM, Ko CY, et al. Evidence Review Conducted for the Agency for Healthcare Research and Quality Safety Program for Improving Surgical Care and Recovery: Focus on Anesthesiology for Colorectal Surgery. Anesth Analg 2019;128(5):879–89.

5. Gustafsson UO, Scott MJ, Hubner M, et al. Guidelines for perioperative care in elective colorectal surgery: enhanced recovery after surgery (ERAS®) Society Recommendations: 2018. World J Surg 2019;43(3):659–95. Available at: https://link.springer.com/article/10.1007/s00268-018-4844-y.

6. Gale SC, Shafi S, Dombrovskiy VY, et al. The public health burden of emergency general surgery in the United States: A 10-year analysis of the Nationwide Inpatient Sample–2001 to 2010. J Trauma Acute Care Surg 2014;77(2):202–8.

7. Ogola GO, Gale SC, Haider A, et al. The financial burden of emergency general surgery: National estimates 2010 to 2060. J Trauma Acute Care Surg 2015;79(3):444–8.

8. Al-Temimi MH, Griffee M, Enniss TM, et al. When is death inevitable after emergency laparotomy? Analysis of the American College of Surgeons National Surgical Quality Improvement Program database. J Am Coll Surg 2012;215(4):503–11.

9. National Emergency Laparotomy Audit. Available at: https://www.nela.org.uk. Accessed February 20, 2021.

10. Saunders DI, Murray D, Pichel AC, et al. UK Emergency Laparotomy Network. Variations in mortality after emergency laparotomy: the first report of the UK Emergency Laparotomy Network. Br J Anaesth 2012;109(3):368–75.

11. Huddart S, Peden CJ, Swart M, et al. Use of a pathway quality improvement care bundle to reduce mortality after emergency laparotomy. Br J Surg 2015;102(1):57–66.

12. Aggarwal G, Peden CJ, Mohammed MA, et al. Evaluation of the Collaborative Use of an Evidence-Based Care Bundle in Emergency Laparotomy. JAMA Surg 2019;154(5):e190145.

13. Peden CJ, Stephens T, Martin G, et al. Effectiveness of a national quality improvement programme to improve survival after emergency abdominal surgery (EPOCH): a stepped-wedge cluster-randomised trial. Lancet 2019;393(10187):2213–21.

14. Stephens TJ, Peden CJ, Haines R, et al. Hospital-level evaluation of the effect of a national quality improvement programme: time-series analysis of registry data. BMJ Qual Saf 2020;29(8):623–35.

15. Stephens TJ, Peden CJ, Pearse RM, et al. Improving care at scale: process evaluation of a multi-component quality improvement intervention to reduce mortality after emergency abdominal surgery (EPOCH trial). Implement Sci 2018;13(1):148.

16. Wick E, Fischer C, McSwine S. AHRQ Safety Program for ISCR expands scope to include emergency general surgery in 2020. 2020. Available at: https://bulletin.facs.org/2020/01/ahrq-safety-program-for-iscr-expands-scope-to-include-emergency-general-surgery-in-2020/. Accessed July 28, 2021.

17. Cooper Z, Mitchell SL, Gorges RJ, et al. Predictors of mortality up to 1 year after emergency major abdominal surgery in older adults. J Am Geriatr Soc 2015; 63(12):2572–9.
18. Rubin DS, Huisingh-Scheetz M, Ferguson MK, et al. U.S. trends in elective and emergent major abdominal surgical procedures from 2002 to 2014 in older adults. J Am Geriatr Soc 2021. https://doi.org/10.1111/jgs.17189. jgs.17189.
19. Panel BT. 2019 AGSBCUE, By the 2019 American Geriatrics Society Beers Criteria® Update Expert Panel. American Geriatrics Society 2019 Updated AGS Beers Criteria® for Potentially Inappropriate Medication Use in Older Adults. J Am Geriatr Soc 2019;67(4):674–94.
20. Desborough J. The stress response to trauma and injury. BJA 2000;85(1):115–9.
21. Peden C, Scott MJ. Anesthesia for emergency abdominal surgery. Anesthesiol Clin 2015;33(1):209–21.
22. Ljungqvist O, Scott M, Fearon KC. Enhanced recovery after surgery: a review. JAMA Surg 2017;152(3):292–8.
23. Barry MJ, Edgman-Levitan S. Shared decision making–pinnacle of patient-centered care. N Engl J Med 2012;366(9):780–1.
24. Tengberg LT, Bay-Nielsen M, Bisgaard T, et al. Multidisciplinary perioperative protocol in patients undergoing acute high-risk abdominal surgery. Br J Surg 2017; 104(4):463–71.
25. Møller MH, Adamsen S, Thomsen RW, et al. Peptic Ulcer Perforation (PULP) trial group. Multicentre trial of a perioperative protocol to reduce mortality in patients with peptic ulcer perforation. Br J Surg 2011;98(6):802–10.
26. Chana P, Joy M, Casey N, et al. Cohort analysis of outcomes in 69 490 emergency general surgical admissions across an international benchmarking collaborative. BMJ Open 2017;7(3):e014484.
27. Hunter Emergency Laparotomy Collaborator Group, Hunter Emergency Laparotomy Collaborator Group. High-Risk Emergency Laparotomy in Australia: comparing NELA, P-POSSUM, and ACS-NSQIP Calculators. J Surg Res 2020; 246:300–4.
28. Nelson R, Edwards S, Tse B. Prophylactic nasogastric decompression after abdominal surgery. Cochrane Database Syst Rev 2007;(3):CD004929.
29. Scarborough JE, Schumacher J, Pappas TN, et al. Which complications matter most? Prioritizing quality improvement in emergency general surgery. J Am Coll Surg 2016;222(4):515–24.
30. Murphy PB, Vogt KN, Lau BD, et al. Venous thromboembolism prevention in emergency general surgery: a review. JAMA Surg 2018;153(5):479–86.
31. Morris RS, Ruck JM, Conca-Cheng AM, et al. Shared decision-making in acute surgical illness: the surgeon's perspective. J Am Coll Surg 2018;226(5):784–95.
32. Berian JR, Mohanty S, Ko CY, et al. Association of loss of independence with readmission and death after discharge in older patients after surgical procedures. JAMA Surg 2016;151(9):e161689.
33. Kruser JM, Taylor LJ, Campbell TC, et al. "Best case/worst case": training surgeons to use a novel communication tool for high-risk acute surgical problems. J Pain Symptom Manage 2017;53(4):711–9.e5.
34. Bernacki RE, Block SD. American College of Physicians High Value Care Task Force. Communication about serious illness care goals: a review and synthesis of best practices. JAMA Intern Med 2014;174(12):1994–2003.
35. Cooper Z, Koritsanszky LA, Cauley CE, et al. Recommendations for best communication practices to facilitate goal-concordant care for seriously ill older patients with emergency surgical conditions. Ann Surg 2016;263(1):1–6.

36. Eton RE, Highet A, Englesbe MJ. Every emergency general surgery patient deserves pathway-driven care. J Am Coll Surg 2020;231(6):764–5.
37. Avery P, Morton S, Raitt J, et al. Rapid sequence induction: where did the consensus go? Scand J Trauma Resusc Emerg Med 2021;29(1):64.
38. Wong PF, Kumar S, Bohra A, et al. Randomized clinical trial of perioperative systemic warming in major elective abdominal surgery. Br J Surg 2007;94(4):421–6.
39. Semler MW, Self WH, Wanderer JP, et al. Balanced crystalloids versus saline in critically ill adults. N Engl J Med 2018;378(9):829–39.
40. Shan W, Chen B, Huang L, et al. The effects of bispectral index-guided anesthesia on postoperative delirium in elderly patients: a systematic review and meta-analysis. World Neurosurg 2021;147:e57–62.
41. Murphy GS, Szokol JW, Avram MJ, et al. Residual neuromuscular block in the elderly: incidence and clinical implications. Anesthesiology 2015;123(6):1322–36.
42. Murphy GS, Brull SJ. Residual neuromuscular block: lessons unlearned. Part I: definitions, incidence, and adverse physiologic effects of residual neuromuscular block. Anesth Analg 2010;111(1):120–8.
43. Khadaroo RG, Warkentin LM, Wagg AS, et al. Clinical effectiveness of the elder-friendly approaches to the surgical environment initiative in emergency general surgery. JAMA Surg 2020;155(4):e196021.
44. Aitken RM, Partridge JSL, Oliver CM, et al. Older patients undergoing emergency laparotomy: observations from the National Emergency Laparotomy Audit (NELA) years 1–4. Age Ageing 2020;49(4):656–63.
45. Sheetz KH, Waits SA, Krell RW, et al. Improving mortality following emergent surgery in older patients requires focus on complication rescue. Ann Surg 2013;258(4):614–7 [discussion: 617–618].
46. Echeverria-Villalobos M, Stoicea N, Todeschini AB, et al. Enhanced recovery after surgery (ERAS): A perspective review of postoperative pain management under ERAS pathways and its role on opioid crisis in the United States. Clin J Pain 2020;36(3):219.
47. Vester-Andersen M, Lundstrøm LH, Møller MH, Danish Anaesthesia Database. The association between epidural analgesia and mortality in emergency abdominal surgery: A population-based cohort study. Acta Anaesthesiol Scand 2020;64(1):104–11.
48. Aggarwal G, Broughton KJ, Williams LJ, et al. Early postoperative death in patients undergoing emergency high-risk surgery: towards a better understanding of patients for whom surgery may not be beneficial. J Clin Med Res 2020;9(5):1288.
49. Cooper Z, Courtwright A, Karlage A, et al. Pitfalls in communication that lead to nonbeneficial emergency surgery in elderly patients with serious illness: description of the problem and elements of a solution. Ann Surg 2014;260(6):949–57.
50. Cooper Z, Lilley EJ, Bollens-Lund E, et al. High burden of palliative care needs of older adults during emergency major abdominal surgery. J Am Geriatr Soc 2018;66(11):2072–8.
51. Lilley EJ, Cooper Z. The high burden of palliative care needs among older emergency general surgery patients. J Palliat Med 2016;19(4):352–3.
52. Cauley CE, Panizales MT, Reznor G, et al. Outcomes after emergency abdominal surgery in patients with advanced cancer: Opportunities to reduce complications and improve palliative care. J Trauma Acute Care Surg 2015;79(3):399–406.
53. Gazala S, Tul Y, Wagg A, et al, Acute Care and Emergency Surgery (ACES) Group. Quality of life and long-term outcomes of octo- and nonagenarians following acute care surgery: a cross sectional study. World J Emerg Surg 2013;8(1):23.

Moving?

Make sure your subscription moves with you!

To notify us of your new address, find your **Clinics Account Number** (located on your mailing label above your name), and contact customer service at:

Email: journalscustomerservice-usa@elsevier.com

800-654-2452 (subscribers in the U.S. & Canada)
314-447-8871 (subscribers outside of the U.S. & Canada)

Fax number: 314-447-8029

Elsevier Health Sciences Division
Subscription Customer Service
3251 Riverport Lane
Maryland Heights, MO 63043

Printed and bound by CPI Group (UK) Ltd, Croydon, CR0 4YY

08/05/2025

01864694-0003